The

Irritable Heart

Also by Jeff Wheelwright

Degrees of Disaster (1994)

The

Irritable

Heart

The Medical Mystery of the Gulf War

Jeff Wheelwright

 W. W. Norton & Company New York London

Copyright © 2001 by Jeff Wheelwright

Excerpt from "The Second Coming" reprinted with the permission of Scribner, a
division of Simon & Schuster, and A. P. Watt on behalf of Michael B. Yeats from *The
Collected Poems of W. B. Yeats, Revised Second Edition*, edited by Richard J. Finneran.
Copyright © 1924 by MacMillan Publishing Company, renewed 1952 by Bertha
Georgie Yeats.

For information about permission to reproduce selections from this book, write to
Permissions, W. W. Norton & Company, Inc., 500 Fifth Avenue, New York, NY
10110

The text of this book is composed in Adobe Garamond
with the display set in Perpetual Bold
Composition by Gina Webster
Manufacturing by The Haddon Craftsmen, Inc.

Library of Congress Cataloging-in-Publication Data
Wheelwright, Jeff.
The irritable heart : the medical mystery of the Gulf War / Jeff Wheelwright.
p.   cm.
Includes bibliographical references and index.
ISBN 0-393-01956-X
1. Persian Gulf syndrome—Case studies. I. Title.
RB152.7.W48 2001
616'.047—dc21   00-058410

W. W. Norton & Company, Inc., 500 Fifth Avenue, New York, N.Y. 10110
www.wwnorton.com

W. W. Norton & Company Ltd., 10 Coptic Street, London WC1A 1PU

1 2 3 4 5 6 7 8 9 0

In memory of my father

Contents

To have great pain is to have certainty; to hear that another person has pain is to have doubt.
—Elaine Scarry, *The Body in Pain*

The presence of disease in the body, with its tensions and its burnings, the silent world of the entrails, the whole dark underside of the body lined with endless unseeing dreams, are challenged as to their objectivity by the reductive discourse of the doctor. . . .
—Michel Foucault, *The Birth of the Clinic*

The

Irritable Heart

Introduction

Basically there are two approaches to writing about a public health mystery: the personal and the scientific. Both start by gathering the stories of people who are sick. The personal approach cultivates the narrative, bringing forward the breath and blood of the individual. The scientific approach prunes the individual from the story and replaces him or her with medical analysis of the group.

This book will attempt to reconcile the two approaches.

The personal approach to a health mystery can't help but romanticize the individual, who is caught in a struggle that is wrenchingly recognizable even when the nature of the illness is unknown. You try to look *up* to such a person, for to look down would be to tempt a similar fate upon yourself. But the scientific approach can't help but diminish the individual. Science proceeds from the case to the pattern, from the particular to the general, from the inductive collection of information to the deductive tests of a solution, and in the meantime the ailing person, the patient, continues to bleed.

I shall try to steer between the two pitfalls.

Take the story of Bill Williams, the first patient I met after starting this work. Bear in mind that Bill is not typical of the characters in the book. In the first place, he wasn't angry. In the second place, he wasn't bleeding very much. I am fond of Bill because he broke the ice for me. When you have spent months studying the statistics of a strange malady and only then are introduced to an individual patient (the word means "sufferer" in Latin), you are liable to be a little apprehensive.

In March 1997, Bill came for an examination at a Veterans Affairs hospital in Los Angeles. He was a man who liked motorcycles and looked the part. He wore a black beard, long black hair pulled back, a black T-shirt, snug jeans with a clot of keys hanging off, and work boots. He had a wiry body and a lean face on which all the miles showed—forty-six, but Bill appeared older. When he coughed, his chest sounded soupy, the sign of a smoker, but I doubted he was here for that. He filled out a questionnaire about his symptoms, took a physical, and now he waited, affably, for a specialist to see him.

Bill used to belong to the National Guard. In January 1991, he and his unit of military policemen were summoned to the Persian Gulf War. Initially he was based in Dhahran, the large Saudi city on the coast. When the ground battle started, in late February, he was north of King Khalid Military City, near the Kuwait border. He heard the firing and spent an anxious night in the tent, his gun cradled on his chest. In three days it was over. Following the conflict, Bill was assigned to guard Iraqi prisoners at a desolate camp southeast of KKMC. This was a tedious interlude of several months that he remembers for its insects, "like ladybugs, but they bit," and for its black rain, emanating from the huge oil fires in Kuwait and smudging the tents and equipment.

"Did you ever see that movie about the oil fires? Man!" said Bill, shaking his head. Indeed I had, but what I saw was no movie.

Bill had been exposed to other nasty substances during the war, including diesel oil. The military's practice of spreading diesel on the desert roads to control the dust was "idiotic," in his opinion. Bill hurt his knee driving a truck that "lost its brakes" on a slick road. He was thinking of applying for compensation for the knee pain, but again, that wasn't why he was here. He was worried more about the accident waiting to happen. Sleeping poorly at night, he had found himself nodding off in the truck at work, as well as when driving his car or motorcycle. Moreover, his memory was shot with inexplicable holes, things like forgetting the exit to get off at or how to put the parts of his handgun together. Often he felt his heart flip-flop and speed up, and "some other weird stuff that goes on, like itches I cannot find.

"It started after the war," he said. "It was all that stuff we were breathing."

At this point the doctor summoned us—I'd attached myself to Bill—into the exam room. With the patient's preliminary results in hand but no explanation for his symptoms, the doctor recommended additional tests. "I'm concerned about the sensations you report in your chest," said the doctor. "So I want you to go to Cardiology. Sometimes it's normal that the heart can beat very rapidly, but we have to be sure."

Here is where Bill's story bifurcates. The medical information being drawn from him would go into a computer according to categories and scales. As the story of Bill was cleansed of its quirks by the antiseptic of numbers, Bill the individual was starting to disappear. Before my eyes he was becoming a case or, to be exact, an anecdote. To medical researchers an anecdote is a case that does not fit any previously established models of disease.

At the same time Bill became an increment in the grossest statistic of all, a staple in the news media, a source of national concern: that up to one hundred thousand veterans, one in seven who were deployed, suffered from a mysterious condition known as gulf war syndrome. The researchers planned to compare Bill's health story with others they had distilled and then come back to the group with answers derived from the pool of knowledge. Except the answers never came back. Why they didn't is a question I will take up in this book. Part of my task is to illuminate a medical inquiry that was imperfect and incomplete.

Bill Williams did not so much recover his health as put his health problems behind him. When we spoke a year later, his case had slipped through the cracks. None of the VA's specialized tests found anything concrete, at least not that he was told. "Forget it," he said, "if they don't want to give me an answer. I still fall asleep at work sometimes, but I'm letting it pass. I'm dealing with it. I go to my private doctor now for any complaints." Overall, he said, his health was a bit better.

Gulf war syndrome was and is real, don't misunderstand me. Ten years after it originated, it has not been solved and has not gone away. Although I suspect there are many like Bill, people dwelling in the borderland between health and disease, his story, as noted, isn't where I'm going in this book. The patients I will show you were sicker from the start, did not improve, and would not let it pass.

Whose fault is it when people lose their health for reasons that doctors can't explain? The bitter puzzle used to be laid to fate or God's will, but as often today an uncaring government or a selfish corporation is held responsible. The news media, advocacy groups, and political leaders put more faith in the patients' accounts of their health than in the cautious overview of the scientists and health professionals, most of whom are bureaucratically slow of foot even when they are not truly in the dark. The longer such illnesses fester unresolved, the more they become politicized, lending to the patients both a sense of strength and a sense of being wronged, but if they become victims, they do not get well by it. In this rendition of the health mystery, any one case stands for the plight of the group.

Gulf war syndrome is the newest member in a family of hard-to-figure millennial conditions. Quietly epidemic, long-running though not life-threatening, these ailments include chronic fatigue syndrome, fibromyalgia, and multiple chemical sensitivity. The illnesses are unique because patients are diagnosed without conventional measures of disease in their bodies. Objective findings are either lacking or inconclusive. Doctors can determine that the patients are sick all right, but they more or less have to take the patients' word on the nature and degree of the suffering.

Of course it is not a bad thing for doctors to have to listen to their patients. But sometimes the doctor, if he is a dim or busy doctor, will suggest that the symptoms are all in the person's head. Nothing gets my subjects angrier than to hear that. Be that as it may, the most ambitious goal of this book will be to dissolve the dichotomy between the suffering mind and suffering body, from which I hope a clear-eyed sympathy will flow.

A note about names: All the veterans I write about are real people. All provided me with medical and other information about themselves without any conditions on my using it. None of the major subjects of the book prohibited me from identifying him or her. In the end, however, I decided that patients' privacy would be served if I changed their names. Thus John Cabrillo, Carol Best, Pete Timmons, and Darren Moreau, the lead characters of Chapters One, Three, Five, and Six, respectively, are pseudonymous, as are Bill Williams, above, and the veterans described in Chapter Eight.

This policy extends to the relatives and companions of the subjects, as well as to their doctors. In the case of the veterans' doctors, a fictitious name is indicated by as a surname only (e.g. Dr. Smith, Dr. White). I mean to distinguish these people, included because of their connections to single patients, from the physicians of national significance to the gulf war health issue. The latter I have identified accurately and fully (e.g. Ronald Hamm, William Baumzweiger, Charles Engel). Likewise, real names apply to all scientists and researchers, military and government figures, and veterans who became nationally known.

1

John during Lent

The West Los Angeles Veterans Affairs Medical Center, as big as its name, consists of scores of buildings and 430 acres alongside the 405 freeway near Santa Monica. It is the largest medical complex within the largest health care delivery system in the United States.

The centerpiece of the complex is a six-story hospital. Built in the 1970s, it replaced a seismically shaky structure known as Wadsworth Hospital, which had been erected in the twenties on the site of an old soldiers' home, which in turn had been established for disabled veterans of the Civil War. Thus a thread of pain connected John Cabrillo, the disabled veteran occupying room 4011, to men whose lives were ruptured more than a century before.

John was sent to Wadsworth—still its informal name—from a VA facility in a southwestern state. If you telephoned his home hospital and were put on hold, a recorded voice would come on and announce: "If you are one of those veterans who either served us well during the Persian Gulf War, or who claims exposure to Agent Orange or atomic radiation, did you know that a free, comprehensive medical exam is available to you?" John had responded to the offer and to everything it implied. He was a victim of environmental history. He came to Los Angeles to pursue both a diagnosis and a disability pension for an illness he blamed on toxic exposures during the 1991 Persian Gulf War.

John's disability cut more ways than he knew. When the first Wadsworth was founded, in 1888, medical care and pensions for veterans of the Civil War absorbed nearly 20 percent of the federal budget. The editor of the *Nation* wrote that "the ex-Union soldier is coming to stand in the public mind for a helpless and greedy sort of person, who says he is not able to support himself, and whines that other people ought to do it for him."

Among the amputees, morphine addicts, and war-torn "insane" were pensioners who had been weakened by "irritable heart."

Veterans with this diagnosis had a rapid pulse and complained of palpitations, shortness of breath, chest pains upon exertion, fatigue, headache, dizziness, and disturbed sleep. First seen during the combat period and often leading to medical discharge, irritable heart was a vague sort of disease, even by the standards of the time. The structure of the heart did not appear to have anything wrong, nor was disease evident in other parts of the patient's body. To military doctors, irritable heart was a mysterious condition of diversely physical origin, since diarrhea, fever, or a hard march could bring it on. The same debilitating symptoms, the same mélange of causes, and the same mystery accrued to "gulf war syndrome" in the 1990s.

Wadsworth was a medical backwater until after World War II. Then, thanks to an infusion of newly wounded patients and the money to take care of them, the hospital was able to attract high-caliber staff. UCLA Medical School, founded in 1947, placed some of its faculty at Wadsworth. Conversely, the VA had some of its physicians appointed to the medical school. It was a good quid pro quo. The stature of the university boosted the status of the agency in medical circles, and in return UCLA got stipends for its doctors, laboratory space, and patients.

There was a third party to the arrangement, rather a silent partner, the Atomic Energy Commission. As the postwar guardian of U.S. nuclear materials, the AEC urgently needed to understand the biological effects of ionizing radiation. Starting in the late forties, the agency extended a series of research contracts to the medical school, some of which were channeled through the Veterans Administration. The AEC provided radioisotopes, the newborn elements of the atomic age, for experimental use, and select VA hospitals, including Wadsworth, provided the medical subjects.

The picture looks ominous, I know. The history to which John subscribed begins here. Abuses in the government's human radiation experiments were revealed years later; most of the problems centered on the failure to obtain the subjects' consent. In several instances radioactive substances were injected into unknowing patients just to see how their bodies would respond.

Upon review by a presidential panel, the VA escaped censure, as did the procedures performed at Wadsworth Hospital. The doctors used the radioisotopes as tracers—that is, testing their potential to illuminate and diagnose disease—and as therapeutic agents for otherwise untreatable conditions. Indeed what is known today as nuclear medicine began with the VA research. John, evaluated in 1997, had a PET scan of his brain, a test derived from the early tracers. He didn't mind the PET scan, but he did protest that other tests amounted to experiments upon him.

The VA solicited publicity in the late forties for its magical radioisotopes. Kept under wraps was the need for biomedical information about nuclear radiation in case of veterans' disability claims. With atomic testing under way and atomic warfare a possibility in the future, the agency wished to be prepared for the special illnesses that might result and the compensation that might be due. In the 1950s the military deliberately placed troops near detonations in Nevada, testing its men while it tested the bombs. As the "atomic veterans" got older, some contracted cancer. Eventually the government offered them compensation, acting on the assumption that exposures to radiation had harmed their health. There is some scientific basis for this assumption, for a few more leukemias have occurred among the atomic veterans than would be expected in men of their age.

The Agent Orange episode was similar. Soldiers were exposed to a chemical herbicide during the Vietnam War. Many years passed before the government awarded compensation for diseases and deformities occurring among the veterans and their offspring. Again there is some scientific evidence that Agent Orange was responsible, but it is slim. John, however, was convinced of the precedent. Of the cause of his own illness, he said, "It's important that it not take twenty years [to establish] like it did for the Agent Orange vets."

You see that before properly introducing him, I have put this man John in a context in which sickness and disability have long-standing political ramifications. Politicizing John's illness may make you angry on his behalf and spur you to seek redress for him and others like him, but the risk is that you will lose sight of John the patient, John who is suffering.

John too was removed from the sight of his suffering. The figure implanted in his mind was the soldier betrayed by his government—betrayed not as some exceptional necessity of service but insidiously and repeatedly, by means of slow-acting poisons. Even when the government poisoned its soldiers accidentally, as with Agent Orange, it didn't admit the truth behind the calamity. That's what John believed anyway, John clinging to his bed in room 4011, and many other Americans believed likewise.

The West Los Angeles VAMC had a special role in the care of Persian Gulf veterans. It was a referral center for special patients like John, who were just a trickle statistically, yet they were driving the political controversy. Their unresolved cases, like a hydraulic force being applied through the mass of concerned veterans, kept the pressure on Washington when the issue should have exhausted itself for lack of answers.

They were not walk-in patients. Any veteran of the gulf war who was no longer on active military duty could go to his or her local VA facility and register as an outpatient for special care. The VA called this step of the process Phase I. Bill Williams, the first gulf war vet I met, came to West L.A. for his Phase I evaluation. Most vets provided this single statistical snapshot of their health and then dropped from view. John by contrast, had been transferred to Wadsworth in order to undergo the more elaborate testing known as Phase II. His was a chronic case, well documented, and much thornier than Bill's.

The VA had set up referral centers at three facilities in addition to the one at West Los Angeles: Houston, Texas; Washington, D.C.; and Birmingham, Alabama. According to the promotional literature distributed to gulf war vets, "These centers provide assessment by specialists in such areas as pulmonary and infectious disease, immunology, neuropsychology, and additional expertise as indicated in such areas as toxicology and multiple chemical sensitivity."

This was considerably overblown. Separate investigations—by the American Legion, the Presidential Advisory Committee on Gulf War Veterans' Illnesses, the General Accounting Office of Congress (GAO), and even the VA's own inspector general (IG)—all were critical of the program.

"Misleading hyperbole," said the IG's report of the program's description. "Knowledgeable VA clinicians repeatedly told us that the referral centers do not have any more sophistication or expertise in treating Persian Gulf War veterans than many other major VA facilities."

"Delays of three months or more are not uncommon," said the Presidential Advisory Committee about the backlog of patients waiting to be referred. By the end of 1997 fewer than five hundred veterans had been evaluated of the fifteen thousand–plus who might qualify for the program because they had undiagnosed illnesses.

Especially harsh was a report to Congress from the American Legion, the nation's largest veterans' service organization. "During site visits several VA physicians admitted that they refer 'problem' patients to NRCs [national referral centers], those patients who 'make a lot of noise' concerning their care at VA. These physicians refer the patients in order to convince the patients that VA is doing all it can to diagnose their illnesses, not because of any particular merit in the NRC system."

Most unfortunate of all, some veterans who went through the testing were said to have become even more frustrated because they realized they could have got the same exam at home and in some cases already had. This particular criticism I can vouch for, on the basis of a sample of four patients. All having been referred to the West L.A. center, all complained that the program fell far short of what they had been led to expect. In fact two of the four stalked out before their tests were complete.

Again I am providing the context of his illness ahead of giving John his due. I am getting into the hospital elevator to go up and see him, to hear him talk and witness his suffering, but there is still context to dispense with: more of the political and journalistic constructions of "gulf war syndrome," those domineering abstractions that for a long time prevented me from seeing the patients whole.

Ironically, the political course of the illnesses was much easier to track than the state of the veterans. The controversy was like a pesky fever in Washington, flaring and subsiding repeatedly. The major flare-ups had to do with whether the American troops were exposed to low levels of poison gas during the war and whether the Department of Defense subsequently covered it up. In 1997, for instance, no less than eight federal entities, including the Presidential Advisory Committee and special task forces within the Pentagon, Central Intelligence Agency, and Congress, examined the possible exposure of U.S. troops to chemical warfare agents, this in spite of the conclusion by several scientific panels, including the presidential panel itself, that the health problems of the veterans were probably *not* due to warfare agents or to chemicals in general.

Why were millions of dollars spent on redundant and marginal investigations? For the truth? For the exercise, I finally decided, because an investigation promised to produce culprits—that is, high-ranking figures who might have obstructed information that might possibly pertain to the poor health of Persian Gulf veterans. Meanwhile the health mystery itself slipped off the stage, being far beyond the political investigators to solve. The errors of the VA referral program or the misfortunes of the referral patients were hardly noted in Washington. If an individual was called for, he or she was put forward as a generic sufferer, from the falsely coherent cohort of one hundred thousand, all wronged in equal measure, all of them John.

THE ELEVATOR DOOR opened, and I stepped out at the fourth floor. Dr. Ronald Hamm, who directed the referral program at West L.A., went ahead of me down the hall. Hamm, fifty, not your typical government doctor, had a walrus mustache and an auburn ponytail. He bade me wait at the nurses' station while he asked the veteran if he wished to meet with me. Hamm expected John to consent readily. "Some of his complaints are going to be valid," he said, putting the best face on what was to come.

About the patient's medical status I knew only that he had some kind of movement disorder that the neurologists were trying to fathom. John's case was unusual even by the standards of the referral patients. The most common symptoms experienced by Persian Gulf veterans were headaches, rashes, penetrating muscle and joint pain, diarrhea, memory deficits, shortness of breath, insomnia, and exhaustion. John attested to several of these, as I was to learn, but the florid expression of his movement disorder overwhelmed the more common elements.

The doctor fetched me, saying the patient was agreeable. John and I met only twice, on that day and again a year later, and both times he presented himself with panache. A handsome and strongly built man in his late thirties, Hispanic, with dark hair and fair skin, he was standing outside his room, talking to one or another of the attendants to his case. He used a crutch, the kind with a hand grip and a brace for the upper arm, but his body addressed the crutch condescendingly, leaning away from it rather than onto it. His posture, a straight line from hip to crown, was tipped slightly back from plumb, and the crutch was held more like a scepter. Or maybe it was just the assurance of his gaze, regally taking me in without deviating from the person in front of him.

Often gulf war patients don't look as though they are unwell. Not so John. He was trembling, I saw, and behind the posture of control he seemed to be fending off pain. His mouth writhed when he spoke. There was a pronounced quaver in his larynx.

According to his chart, a page of which John gave me later, his disorder consisted of "pendular movements of neck, speech impediment, breathing tic, & periodic titubation of trunk." Titubation means "stumbling" or "stuttering." To a neurologist titubation is a gross tremor of the head and body that occurs when the patient holds himself upright and that disappears when he is lying down. It is characteristic of a cerebellar disorder, in the part of the brain that coordinates the muscles and maintains equilibrium. But titubation is not a diagnosis. Something yet unnamed was causing John to titubate.

Dr. Hamm introduced me and then had a brief word with his patient. He said that in light of John's pending release, two final tests had to be scheduled. One was a lengthy psychological survey called the MMPI test, "to rule out psychological sources of your problem," and the other a speech pathology test. "We are looking for a tie-in between your speech disorder and your walking," explained Hamm.

Hamm was not a neurologist, but having seen a lot of gulf war vets, he had developed his own ideas about their health problems, most of which he kept to himself. Now he remarked to John that some of the undiagnosed cases might be chronic fatigue syndrome or fibromyalgia (a pain syndrome of multiple tender points), two conditions that, like the gulf war ills, are hard to delineate.

"My knowledge is that chronic fatigue and fibromyalgia were ruled out in my case," said John tartly.

He turned to me. "Do you have a card?"

I didn't.

"Do you work for the federal government?"

No, I said.

We withdrew to his room and sat down, he on the bed, I in a chair.

"Automatically it's assumed that it's a psychosis—out there in the world," said John, unhappy about having to meet with the psychologists again. "I told them I'm a straight shooter and I don't need this." More than that, he was unhappy about being discharged. Evidently a battle of wills was going on. He told me that the week before, the hospital had tried to discharge him prematurely. When he resisted, the mistake was admitted, but the move was on to get rid of him again.

"It's not a martyr thing," he stated. "It's my duty to stay. My president says he'll leave no stone unturned and I'll hold him to it. I want them not only to look under the stone but get rid of it. I'm doing this for thousands of sick vets. . . ."

Then: "What is the goal of your book? Does it lean more toward the veterans' side of the house? Or the other side?"

I stammered something—I was bemused—not only by the rush of his quivery words but also by the body language, a cacophony in itself. Periodically his head would roll on his neck, making him wince. Or his diaphragm would lock, and he would reach inside himself and forcefully grab a breath, like a diver working at great depth. He wore sandals, revealing that his second toe was crossed over and clasping his big toe, as if he were keeping a grip upon himself. Sitting straight in his chair, he gazed, from proud dark eyes, down a hawklike nose that had perfectly round nostrils.

John talked almost nonstop for four hours. We began in his room and then went outside, where an unseasonably hot afternoon was winding down. We sat in a gazebo next to the hospital and had mentholated cigarettes (his). We returned to his room and continued over an ordered-in pizza (mine). As I took down his story, I noticed something that the specialists had observed, that his tics and tremors were not regular or constant. Every now and then they would abate, and his body would grow still— except for a metronomic twitching of his left ear, maintaining the beat of John's illness in the interlude between the spasms.

He said little about what it was like to be sick, as if his disability could speak for itself. He wouldn't tell me anything of his personal life, other than that he was married and had children, because he said it wasn't relevant. His agenda, a fair word, I think, had three overlapping items, which he covered more or less in sequence: toxic exposures in the Gulf, his evidence being a document that "will open your eyes up"; the shortcomings of the diagnostic and disability assessment procedures of the VA medical system, which he sought to rectify out of obligation to his fellow veterans as much as for himself; and a narrative of his illness, spanning the period from its onset to his present struggle with the administrators of the hospital. Permeating the entire peroration was a powerful sense of duty to his family. Indeed, "duty" was the word I heard most.

He rarely allowed interruptions, turning aside my questions with "Let me get back on track" or "Hey, I'm only working on six cylinders here," a reference to the cognitive lapses of which Persian Gulf vets complain. When he got rolling, he stopped calling me sir and prefaced the increasingly diabolical turns in his account, amazing to him even now, with "Check this out" or "Now watch this, Jeff." At such moments of engrossment his body would nearly leave him alone.

"I got so many stories in my stomach—pocket, I mean," he began. The first topic, quickly covered because he thought it indisputable, was the issue of toxic substances on the battlefield. John had served with the air force in a noncombat role close to the front. He spoke of chemical weapons having been detected, but biological weapons were his main concern since he connected them to his symptoms.

"The bottom line is that I can help you with the knowledge that these chemical and biological agents existed. Weapons were sold to Iraq and used against us. They were weapons developed not only to have short-term effects but delayed effects too. Some of the symptoms lie dormant in your brain and organs and don't manifest themselves until later in life."

Intrigued, I asked to see John's documentation, but he waved me off. First he wanted me to understand the general argument about his health care. It was a rather sophisticated argument. Chronic illness had made John a savvy patient, an experienced consumer of medical services. Whatever information his document contained, he was using it to challenge the approach of the West L.A. staff.

"The missing link is, they place emphasis on the diagnosis and on treating the symptoms, but they don't address what causes it. If you don't know what it is, how can you treat it? Why are so much emphasis and tax dollars being spent on routine approaches that don't use the real knowledge?

"It's standard medicine on the one hand, but on the other hand"—he turned up his palms, one after the other—"the U.S. government has information on known exposures, proved on the Senate floor."

Now I really wanted to see what he had, but I would have to wait.

By "standard medicine" John meant the process of differential diagnosis. He defined it, accurately, as "the ruling out of known causes of symptoms using a standard process of elimination used on the general civilian populace."

If a diagnosis is a label for what ails a patient, differential diagnosis is the range of possible labels that the doctor considers in getting to the rightful label. John was concerned that his rightful diagnosis, "gulf war syndrome," had been prejudicially ruled out.

Having once been a mechanic, he likened differential diagnosis to the

mechanic's "troubleshooting chart for eliminating the causes of the problem. If I were in charge"—he chuckled—"a crazy world it would be, but I
would set up the elimination chart this way. I'd turn it around and look at
the probable causes. I'd start with the symptoms caused by the directly
applicable viruses and chemicals, all that jazz, and I'd rule those out first. I
know it'll work, that approach. They have ways to do it."

"Why aren't they doing it?" I interjected, not sure what his approach
would entail.

"Because it doesn't fit the political and financial status quo."

Indeed, the government had taken the standard approach. Confronted
with a novel set of symptoms, the medical researchers first tried to define
the symptoms, by tracking them to their sources within the veterans' bodies, and only then would they consider the possible causes. However,
because the scientists were still stuck on the definition of the problem, the
causes were still up for grabs.

"But what if," I asked him, "they did diagnose you with fibromyalgia,
say? That would mean they would have 'ruled out' Persian Gulf syndrome,
but it would be a step forward, wouldn't it? Because at least you would have
a finding."

"It wouldn't be the truth. Fibromyalgia could be something that wasn't
caused by the war. OK, I need to get back on track."

In John's opinion not only were the referral center doctors looking in the
wrong direction, but also their tests were invasive and heartless. "Data collection efforts," he called them. "It's at the expense of people. The guinea
pig theory. More emphasis should be placed on treatment." Again he circled through his reasoning, since correct treatment depended on correct
apprehension of the toxic exposures.

John paused. He gasped and he gaped. If his long-running movement disorder had been successfully identified and treated (or if not
diagnosed, at least treated), he couldn't be waging this argument. Like
many Americans who become dissatisfied with conventional doctoring, John was demanding an alternative medicine. But the Wadsworth
physicians weren't backing down. John sensed they meant to determine a label for his condition yet. Either that or throw him out of the
hospital.

He sprang a question on me: "Say you had a car, and you wanted to sell
it, and you fixed it only enough so it would go down the road. Or you real-

ize you have *concern* for the car, and you're doing everything you can for it. Do you have that certain level of compassion?"

I could honestly say I did. The politics on his agenda put us at cross purposes as writer and subject, not because I disagreed with him but because I knew I could learn the politics without his help. That was the easiest part of the story. I was more interested to hear of his personal suffering and, secondarily, to find out how much he knew of the epidemiology of the gulf war ailments—the scientific investigation bumping along beneath the headlines. Those two were my book's subjects. We didn't make headway with either topic, in the first place because though he spoke in favor of compassion, he did not court it for himself, and in the second place because to him the epidemiology was open-and-shut. "I've been to the Gulf and I've been blowing gaskets ever since," he said.

JOHN ENLISTED IN the air force when he was twenty-five. He spent five years as a mechanic on the flight line and then "cross-trained" to civil engineering, specializing in water supply and wastewater treatment. When his unit arrived in Saudi Arabia, in December 1990, "the mission was to develop base facilities twenty klicks [kilometers] from the border—water treatment, runway repair, bivouac preparation, all that jazz. We were the backbone of the success of the flying units that came later. We exercised our respective disciplines right in the middle of the most intense air operations."

His health problems started about two years after the war. "I was having problems articulating—cognitive problems, memory loss. Then my body was feeling creaky, and my joints started to inflame. As time went on, the fatigue came, but I fought it." He went to a series of doctors, including osteopaths and rheumatologists. Because of pain flaring in his right hip, he developed a limp, which was pointed out to him by another serviceman. He hadn't noticed the limp, but thereafter it got worse.

He enrolled in the health registry established by the Defense Department for active duty veterans of the war. (The VA registry and health exams are a separate program for nonactive duty and retired personnel. Some gulf war vets enrolled in both.) "The military ruled that I had degenerative joint disease and osteoarthritis," he said. "Also, I was forced to address mental health. They found cognitive deficits. There's a lot of emphasis placed on the psychosis of the person. It's a misconception that it's stress. As I've told 'em here, it's not stress."

Its budget declining, the Defense Department was in the process of reducing its forces. In many cases it offered bonuses to active duty personnel who would agree to resign. "For my family I decided to take a buyout," said John. "I separated from the service on June thirtieth, 1995.

"I was still working, you see. From July '95 until August '96 I worked in the mines. I had three kids. I had a family and I was doing my duty as always." A sarcastic thrust to "as always."

"OK, now watch this. The VA started sending me medical bills because they said I had income as a miner. But what I'm doing is buying time, so I can continue to support my family until my ship comes in. Before I got out, I had filed a compensation claim for disability with the VA. I knew I was sick. I did it right."

I noted earlier that John was pursuing a disability pension as well as a diagnosis. By all appearances he was disabled, but still he had to meet the criteria for his pension. The Department of Veterans Affairs would pay compensation for disabling illnesses or injuries if they were incurred in the line of duty. Following a medical examination, such conditions were rated as "service-connected," and the amount of the veteran's monthly payment was geared to the degree of his or her disability.

The trouble was, the gulf war illnesses, emerging many months after the fighting, did not neatly fit the criteria for service connection. The headaches, rashes, pain, exhaustion, etc., however severe or disabling, did not immediately suggest a consequence of war. They weren't bullet wounds or other traumatic injuries; they weren't battlefield infections or diseases endemic to the Gulf; nor, to reach further, did they accord with the textbook effects of chemical or biological weapons or with the health consequences of chemicals in general. In a word, the illnesses were new. The Veterans Benefits Administration therefore took a hard line on service connection, especially in cases that eluded diagnosis. As for the Veterans Health Administration, the other wing of the agency, many of its clinicians began to suspect psychological causes for the illnesses and told their patients so.

Congress passed a law in 1994 enabling the VA to pay disability compensation for undiagnosed illness among Persian Gulf vets. Such cases were presumed to have resulted from a service-connected environmental exposure, much as the Vietnam vets with cancer were presumed to have been exposed to Agent Orange, and the atomic veterans were presumed to have been exposed to health-damaging radiation during bomb tests. However, the VA stipulated that the undiagnosed illness had to have manifested itself during the war or within two years after the veteran had departed the Gulf.

John's symptoms met the qualification of the time period. He had filed for a 100 percent disability rating. The agency would pay about two thousand dollars per month to single veterans who were judged completely disabled and more to those with dependents. Yet John's application for compensation had been under review for eighteen months. What was the holdup? "Hey, how about breaking down and letting my ship come in?" he demanded. Wasn't he entitled to at least a temporary determination, on the basis of his three-week hospitalization in L.A.? He clung to his bed, sick and trembling, his condition getting worse. "I'm rolling with the punches," he vowed, "and I am going to take it for as long as I can."

"SOME DAYS—I'm glad you caught me tonight—I'm all messed up," John was saying. He was almost apologetic. While we sat talking outside, his tremors had eased, but now that we were back in the hospital room, with another night approaching and John a long way from home, his head rolled about on his shoulders and he didn't look so hot.

When his movement disorder started, in the summer of 1996, John succumbed to his disability. On the advice of a doctor, he said, he quit his mining job and went on unemployment. Looking for different work, he sought to invoke the Americans with Disabilities Act, but "they still didn't have to hire me." He sent the job rejection letters to the local office of his U.S. senator, in the hope that they demonstrated that he qualified for compensation under the Social Security disability insurance program.

Social Security decided John's claim relatively quickly. Just days ago he had been notified that he was approved for full disability benefits. "I get a cut that most people who work all their lives don't get," he admitted. He was still eligible for his VA disability pension, but if it came through, the SSD payments would probably be reduced.

"SSD is an entitlement, not a charity," he wanted me to understand. "It's hard-earned. It only covers my mortgage. . . . I have a family! If I could dump this thing now, I would. It's called living."

Then he told how he learned of the national referral program for gulf war vets. Characteristically he dug out the information himself from the small print on a leaflet in a VA office, after which the leaflets mysteriously disappeared from the rack. When he got himself on the list to come to Wadsworth, no small chore, he waited on the list for months. Twice he was told he was next up and was admitted to local VA hospitals in preparation for transfer, but both times he cooled his heels for weeks.

"Clinton's thinking everything's in place for gulf vets? I think not," he said disgustedly. "I'm a veteran trying to get help and I gotta fix all *their* problems. I'm tired of fixing the system."

So he turned once more to his senator's office. "They made the call, and boom, I'm in. Though I find out from Dr. Hamm that fourteen vets were ahead of me. Where are they? Do they exist?"

John was supposed to be met at the Los Angeles airport by a driver dispatched by the medical center. No one showed up. He telephoned the hospital, humped his bags back and forth across the terminal to two missed meeting points, and telephoned some more. The logistical shambles, later confirmed by Hamm, might have been told humorously by another person now that it was over. "It was a nightmare," John said. "They fired the cab company after that."

John, like many involved, did not find incompetence a sufficient explanation for the performance of the government in regard to the gulf war illnesses. He suspected dark purposes across the board. At any rate he was admitted to the West Los Angeles VA Medical Center on February 25, 1997.

"I was referred here because my home VA center couldn't diagnose me. I'm not an idealist-type person trying to change the world, but I am one, who with others, is going through this protocol process to establish"—he flinched and caught his breath—"what is the ultimate truth. I want to make changes for the common good of veterans and their children who are deformed."

What a mix of motivations, I thought. It was about time for me to go. Just then the phone next to his bed rang. John picked it up and spoke to the caller in Spanish.

"My family's kept out of this, right?" he said to me, after hanging up. Counting the period prior to his transfer, John had been apart from his family for over a month, since the beginning of Lent. A pious husband and father, he did not want to spend Easter in the hospital too.

When I got to my feet, John pleaded, "I need the pension to look after my family!" He looked as though he were going to cry. His eyes widened in uncertainty, his brow seemed to widen, new lines appeared on his extravagantly expressive face. From his seat on the bed he tried to stand. An arm shot out, flailed, and knocked over the crutch leaning on the wall. I bent over and retrieved it. Wow, I thought.

Since I had asked to see the evidence guiding his quest, his smoking gun on toxic exposures, John at last pulled it out. It was a copy from the *Congressional Record* of a speech by Senator Donald Riegle in February 1994. Riegle, a Michigan Democrat who has since retired, titled the speech "Arming Iraq: The Export of Biological Materials and the Health of Our Gulf War Veterans." On the cover page of the speech was a photocopy of a business card. It read: "James J. Tuite, Professional Staff, Committee on Banking, Housing and Urban Affairs."

John didn't know who Tuite was, but Jim Tuite happened to be the most important person in the political history of the gulf war illnesses. In 1993 and 1994, from his staff position on the Senate Banking Committee, which was chaired by Riegle, Tuite authored a series of powerful reports. The stalled response of the government health researchers was a green light to his independent analysis. Rejecting the official line that troops in the theater of operations were not exposed to chemical and biological weapons, Tuite interviewed dozens of veterans, studied news and weather reports about the war, and combed for clues in the medical literature and in unclassified documents.

The Banking Committee had reason to get involved because it oversees the U.S. Commerce Department. The Commerce Department had approved the sale and export of biological materials to Iraq in the late eighties, and Iraq had diverted the materials to military use. As Tuite discovered, a U.S. company provided bacterial stocks for anthrax disease and botulinum toxin, which became mainstays of the Iraqi germ warfare program. Although Iraq imported biologicals from Europe as well, the revelation of an American connection made a big splash in Congress, in the press, and in the veterans' community, rippling to John's bedside three years later.

Three years later, however, the revelation was moot. Tuite and others had shifted their focus to chemical agents because no evidence had emerged that the Iraqis used their biological weaponry during the war, let alone that such materials could have made the veterans chronically ill. No evidence didn't mean it was impossible to have happened, but it was very unlikely.

Try telling that to John, who seemed to find a kind of relief from his pain in the very inequities that he believed had contributed to his pain. His grievances (political, remunerative) distracted him from his body, but his body inevitably caught up with him. With one hand he fought off his advancing symptoms, and with the other he grappled with the medical authorities, whom he saw standing between him and his goal. So far he was tough enough to give both opponents a run for their money.

WE TALKED ON the phone several times before his discharge from the hospital. After that I didn't see or hear from John for a year. When we did meet again, he gave me further details of his ordeal in Los Angeles. The medical inquiry had ended badly. Some of what follows he told me himself, some is from his doctors, but most is taken from his written account, forty-eight pages, including attachments. John prepared his chronicle shortly after getting home and passed it to his senator's office for action. He prefaced it:

> It took me a great deal of effort to compile this information for you. I ask you to closely review this report as it is my hope to clarify the process in which Persian Gulf Veterans from [his home state] will be subjected to in the event they are referred to the West Los Angeles VA Medical Center. I ask for a full Federal investigation. . . .
>
> Senator, in no way are my accounts a result of a distorted analysis or some concocted dream. I am by no means paranoid or suffer from any delusions. The medical staff at West Los Angeles instilled a high level of distrust in me, and clearly minimized Persian Gulf War Veterans' concerns. I feel that the West Los Angeles VA Medical Center will do anything in their power to discredit me as manifested during my stay there.

After being admitted, John was turned over to the neurologists. According to the Phase II protocol for gulf war cases, he would be examined by other specialists too, and Dr. Hamm, head of the referral program, would remain his primary physician; but the Neurology Service took the lead because of his perplexing movement disorder.

John underwent the basic neurology examination. This takes several hours to complete because the nervous system has many overlapping parts. One set of neurons collects sensory information and sends it to the brain, another transmits motor impulses to the muscles and organs, and a third enables the brain to make sense of the incoming and outgoing signals. The neurologist has a lot of wiring to test.

Thus John had his heels pricked, pupils stimulated, knees tapped. He walked on a line, rotated his tongue, identified smells, pushed against resistance, touched the neurologist's fingertip with his own fingertip, grasped his own extended thumb while keeping his eyes closed. He named presidents and recollected words from a sequence that was read to him. The wobbles in his speech and limbs affected his performance, but the examiner was trained to look past them to what John was able to accomplish. In some brain diseases, like chorea, the tremors have a pattern specific to the disorder, but John's movements were too general to abet the diagnosis.

On the basis of the exam the doctors ruled out the great majority of neurological disorders. From John's blood work they determined he didn't have diabetes, cancer, vascular disease, or any other of the conditions that might cloak themselves in neurological symptoms.

John's neurologists at home had come to the same pass. Test results that are normal are helpful because they tell what a condition isn't (differential diagnosis), but they are no substitute for abnormal findings that may point to what the condition is. The hope was that Wadsworth's experts might uncover the abnormalities. Yet fresh images taken of his brain and spine—by CT scan, MRI scan, PET scan—offered no clues. Nor did the nerve conduction test, in which electrodes pressed to his skin measured the speed through the nerve of small shocks to his arms and legs.

A test of his muscle function, called electromyography (EMG), had to be called off. The procedure involves the insertion of tiny needles into the muscle. When John's leg was probed, he flopped about like a fish (his own description), and readings were impossible. The doctors tried the EMG again a few days later, prompting the same spasmodic reaction.

He was given a strong tranquilizer, Haldol (haloperidol), to see if it might suppress his symptoms. When I visited him, the treatment had been stopped, but he was still complaining about it, saying he hadn't been properly informed. Subsequently John read the fine print about Haldol on the manufacturer's advisory and concluded that he'd been abused.

Haldol has a range of applications. Depending on the dose, it may be used to calm hyperactive children, self-destructive Alzheimer's patients, or violent psychotics. It is also a treatment for chorea. Any condition of spasms and tics, including John's, ought to yield to Haldol, again depending on the dose, which may range from half a milligram to one hundred milligrams daily.

John was started on an amount that one neurologist recalled as "very low, almost at the placebo level, because the patient was very labile, fragile, reactive." It seems he did tell John something of the properties of the drug, for John was concerned about its "psychotic nature" and possible side effects and maintained that he didn't need it because his "thinking was clear." The doctor insisted.

Immediately John was alarmed by the effects. He complained of "paralytic feelings . . . limitations in my arms, legs, and hands . . . very slow motion feelings in my entire body." He felt "lethargic, dizzy, and very weak." All this might be expected from Haldol, but then John might also be extremely sensitive to it.

The trial of the medication coincided with, and in his view conspired with, the failed electromyographs. "After the second [EMG] test I experienced cramps and severe pain in both legs and was very shaky. Now I cannot raise my arms up higher than my shoulders. I cannot lift my legs straight up. I did not have these limitations before I was hospitalized at West Los Angeles VA Medical Center. I believe these to be caused by a combination of the Haldol use coupled with EMG tests."

Later in his account John took note of "VA Patient's Rights No. 11 which states, 'You have the right to be informed of any human experimentation or other research/educational projects affecting your care and treatment.'" In addition, on the manufacturer's sheet for Haldol he starred two ominous side effects: tardive dyskinesia and tardive dystonia, movement disorders themselves, which can sometimes afflict long-term users of antipsychotic medications. These syndromes have "the potential of becoming irreversible," John underlined.

The VA neurologist had no qualms about the episode, calling Haldol the standard treatment for symptoms that John presented. "He claims that ten days of Haldol made him more disabled?" said the doctor. "Maybe he's the first patient in the world to have that reaction after ten days.

"He went off the drug because there was no drug that would help this patient. Haldol wasn't the only one we tried. He is truly disabled, and I have full sympathy for him, but he wouldn't stay on any one medication for any length of time. He complained and made us change them."

What was going on here? John may have been frightened by Haldol's power, even at the low dose. He told me that he didn't like taking Valium, a weaker relaxant prescribed for him. He really didn't like pills of any kind. I think what scared him about the tranquilizer was not that it dampened his limbs but that it dulled his edge to fight. The medication was meant to manage him rather than diagnose him. If another patient might have appreciated the relief from the tremors—not caring what he had so long as he was better—John was one for whom getting better was not as important as obtaining a proper diagnosis and winning his disability claim.

On March 13 the Haldol was withdrawn, and the next day the hospital attempted to discharge John for the first time. He had been a patient for more than two weeks. "I felt this to be an irrational and suspiciously urgent decision," John recalled, "due to the events following the use of Haldol and EMG tests and subsequent upper and lower extremity limitations." He insisted to the medical staff that he had further testing to undergo. Unfortunately Dr. Hamm, his primary physician, was out of town that day.

A case manager appeared in his room. She asked if he was upset. John said he wasn't. She asked what was the matter. He said there was no problem. "She insisted on me leaving today. She requested my airplane ticket [an open ticket needing a reservation]. I refused to give it to her. I told her I needed to talk to Dr. Hamm when he gets back. Case worker left frustrated."

Somewhat later the psychiatrist assigned to his case told him it was all right to stay. The Neurology Service having finished with him, he was transferred intramurally to the department at the hospital that normally handles Persian Gulf cases. Put it down to a failure of communication between departments.

Over the weekend John was visited by two neurologists. One was the man who had been treating him, and the other man I'll call Dr. Gray. He was the head of the Neurology Service at West L.A. VAMC and would have the final say on John's diagnosis. Dr. Gray was frosty, blunt, and sixty-three years old. His temperament I know from my very brief dealings with him (he refused to deal with me), and his age was supplied by John, who researched Dr. Gray's medical biography in the VAMC library.

The two doctors repeated that they had found no known cause for his condition. John gave the doctors a copy of Riegle's speech, with an appendix by the senator's aide, Tuite, listing the biological materials exported to Iraq.

"I asked Dr. Gray, 'Do you know about our exposures?'" John said. "He made a copy of my protocol, but he blew me off. He said that stuff was already in the newspapers. This is the guy who had tried to boot me out of there. He insulted my intelligence, like I was an ignorant bean picker or something. This guy didn't realize who he was dealing with."

Ordinarily John's Latino accent was faint, but as he elaborated on this incident, the accent welled up indignantly. "A smart-ass," he said of Dr. Gray. Granted there are as many sides to a story as there are participants. But if you talk to any gulf war veteran who is or was sick, invariably you will hear of an encounter with a physician who sounds a lot like John's Gray. Multiply this by tens of thousands: What a grand disconnect between patients and doctors.

John suspected that his body was infected, and some of his suspicions were reasonable. Two months prior, for example, he had tested positive for exposure to the tuberculosis bacillus. He did not have an active case, but the skin test, by eliciting antibodies to TB, suggested that the germ might lurk within his system. If so, it might flare into active disease in the future. His VA doctors at home had put him on a prophylactic antibiotic therapy, to knock out the bacillus if it was there. But what if, he wondered, they were treating the wrong agent?

A second concern was leishmaniasis. Several dozen veterans of the war had come home with a serious form of this condition, caused by a protozoan parasite endemic to the Gulf. The symptoms were abdominal pain, fatigue, and fever; in the worst cases the spleen and liver were found to be enlarged. The Defense Department therefore banned blood donations by all active duty personnel who had served in the war. The ban was revoked in late 1992, when additional cases did not crop up, but John still worried whether his blood was safe to donate. Giving blood, he said more than once, was his civic duty, interrupted since his illness.

His third concern was the germs that might have been weaponized by the Iraqis. John brought the Riegle "protocol" to Dr. Hamm, highlighting the symptoms of the biological pathogens on the list. Anthrax, John noted, caused difficulty breathing, botulinum toxin caused paralysis of the muscles involving swallowing, and brucellosis caused chronic fatigue and joint pain. Didn't it fit? He demanded to be tested for exposure to these and two other agents.

The Infectious Diseases department at Wadsworth had already run some basic screens of John's blood and stool, which were negative. Hamm saw no point in investigating further. It was not that the biological agents on his list had definitely been ruled out. Indeed no tests exist to show whether or not John might have been exposed in the past to these pathogens. Rather it was that there was no sign in his body of a rampant infection. Brucellosis, for one, is accompanied by a fever. The effects John noted for anthrax and botulinum poisoning advance quickly to death, yet this patient was most certainly alive. Moreover the conditions had not turned up in other chronically ill veterans.

However these facts were put to him, John did not get satisfaction. "I feel that I was set up," he wrote, "and I am being used as a pawn to further deny the truth regarding Persian Gulf Veterans and their symptoms and illnesses." Unhappy with the doctors' performance, coming on top of the move to discharge him ("this hurried fiasco"), John marched his complaints over to the office of the West L.A. VAMC medical director. He didn't get to see him, but the director's assistant went to John's room later and heard him out.

How unusual a patient he was. In a hospital population noticeable for its grizzled amputees and crestfallen, limping wraiths, John Cabrillo stood out: a young veteran on a mission, chin high, shoulders square, a pack of Kools in his breast pocket, trembling proudly. Technically he wasn't a patient like the others. The VA could have housed him at one of its domiciliary facilities while he was being evaluated, but as an inpatient he could be kept handy to the specialists. He didn't hang around his room, though. Hamm, who liked to pop in at the end of the day, often found him out.

AMONG HIS MANY consultations, John was examined by experts in rheumatology. Joint pain was a long-standing concern, more bothersome to him than his movement disorder and as difficult to diagnose. His write-up of the rheumatology consult is vintage John. It demonstrates his exasperating and insightful behavior, the bull in the china shop, except that the VA medical organization wasn't fine china and the bull never lost his head:

During the week following originally planned departure date of 14 March, 97, I asked medical staff for X-rays to be taken to further provide a thorough, comprehensive approach to determine why, for a long period of time, I have been experiencing pain and stiffness in my joints. These X-rays were not offered to me. It was not until I asked for them that I received a consult to the X-ray Department. Shortly thereafter, the Rheumatology Chief said I did not have rheumatoid arthritis. He said he looked over the full body X-rays which I requested. I asked him about my concerns with having multiple degenerative joint disease and osteoarthritis. The Chief said according to my X-rays there were no signs of multiple degenerative joint disease in my body, and only a trace amount of osteoarthritis in my neck area. I asked him how this was so. I told him that when I was in the military, I had extensive work done by military doctors from several disciplines and many tests taken to determine if I had these ailments. The military ruled that I had both multiple degenerative joint disease and osteoarthritis. Subsequently, I told the Chief that my [home] VA Medical Center records indicate that I have both of these conditions. I've been receiving treatment for these since I started with the VA system in [hometown] during the Summer of 1995. The Rheumatology Chief said this was not a "progressive" problem. How is this so, given the fact that these conditions have progressively gotten worse since my service in the Persian Gulf? This does not make very much sense to me. The Rheumatology's staff make-up on this matter is redundant with respect to a thorough approach already taken by both the Department of Defense and the [home] VA Medical Center. It is a repeat of work already accomplished comprehensively. In fact, the majority of testing done on me at the West Los Angeles VA Medical Center was already accomplished in regards to my medical condition. This includes testing from several medical disciplines. It was my experience, after 37 days spent at the West Los Angeles VA Medical Center to undergo testing through the Persian Gulf Referral process, that there is a high level of redundancy which I feel needs addressing. Each respective medical discipline which is tasked to diagnose the patient is not briefed appropriately regarding patient's past medical history. As a result, the patient is subject to extensive questioning concerning the history and medical problems unique to himself. This is duplication of services at its finest. It is very tasking to continually answer the same questions over and over and over again. It is almost ridiculous. This is highly non-conducive to efficient Government-provided, taxpayer-funded medical service. On several occasions during my stay, I had to wait hours and sometimes days for each medical discipline to provide their services. I have always made every attempt to inform nursing staff of my whereabouts. If I stepped out for five to fifteen minutes—after waiting extensively for respective medical discipline to show up—on several occasions they would show up while I was out. Then the medical people would peg me as unavailable or hard to find. All they would have had to do was ask a nurse at the station where I was. I highly resent these implications. I was very cooperative during my stay at the West Los Angeles VA Medical Center. And to hear otherwise would be a blatant lie.

After nearly four weeks at Wadsworth John had only one test remaining on his schedule, a probe of his speech disorder. The overriding conundrum was the source of the tremors resonating in his speech and limbs. The problem did not lie in his peripheral muscles or nerves, most probably, because they were not wasted or impaired. As John himself might have put it, when the wiring and moving parts check out, it is time to look under the hood. The doctors came to agreement that his tremors must originate in his brain, but that hardly concluded the issue. An injury, or a degenerative disease, or an obscure immunological reaction to an environmental toxin might be centered in his brain without being recognized. All would qualify as "organic" conditions. By this line of thinking, John manifested a kind of dystonia, a neurological debility characterized by involuntary muscular contractions. His dystonia would have to be of an unusual pattern, however, encompassing his vocal cords.

Or he might have a somatoform disorder. Somatoform is the updated medical term for psychosomatic, and is assigned when an explanation is needed for a farrago of symptoms for which all other labels have been ruled out. Thus John's unexplained tremors, unexplained joint pain, unexplained fatigue, and unexplained respiratory and vocal quirks would be the disparate elements of a single disorder. To be more specific, his would be a subtype of the somatoform condition called conversion disorder. It meant that John had converted his mental distress into neurological symptoms: pseudoneurological, actually.

John would never accept that his mind could be so powerful as to cause tremors and pain throughout his body. To him, as to most people, physical symptoms driven by the mind indicated a failure of character, a defective personality, rather than a genuine illness. But manufacture is not the only mechanism of somatoform disorder. The other is that the mind becomes engaged with the body's troubles secondarily, by magnifying an existing pain or embellishing existing symptoms. In effect, the mind won't let the body recover.

On the eve of the speech test the neurologists were leaning toward conversion disorder for their diagnosis. Ronald Hamm was a holdout for an organic explanation. "Did you notice his left ear?" Hamm asked me, referring to John's most idiomatic motion. "How could Mr. Cabrillo be wiggling just one ear? He does have a kind of dystonia. The question is, how it is mediated?"

Hamm endorsed John's disability claim whatever the nature of the illness. "He is not feigning, even if it's psychogenic," the doctor said. "Faking would require too much energy. Anybody who'd go to these lengths if it *were* conscious has got real problems. With a repertoire like that he has got a real disorder, and it ought to be compensable."

Hamm was suggesting that the diagnosis was irrelevant. It would be much better for John to finesse it somehow, avoiding labels, and to focus the patient's attention on managing his chronic condition and his life. That way no longer was possible. If the differential diagnosis of the gulf war illnesses can be compared with a chess match, under play in the national arena for years, then on this board the two sides had reached the endgame. The medical profession insisted it could decide the case in its own uncompromising language, and the veteran insisted he could prove a disability in his.

A SPEECH PATHOLOGY test, like the basic neurology exam, requires many exercises of the subject. Most are formal, such as the drill to elicit a stutter, but some consist of observation, as when the patient and examiner make conversation and the examiner takes mental notes. The speech pathologist who worked with John spent seven hours with him over the course of four sessions. "There was an intermittent quality to his communication problems," she recalled, "and a considerable variability in his performance. He was aware when he was being evaluated." She made note of his vocal tics and tremors and his occasionally disrupted breathing but also recorded that he would speak normally "when he forgot why I was there. He expressed himself as fluently as you and I do. Neurological disorders can be exacerbated by fatigue, but they are not usually an on and off sort of thing."

Part of the examination was by videostroboscope. A tiny camera, placed at the back of John's throat, peered down his windpipe at the larynx and the vocal cords inside it. Unable to talk, he was instructed to make a series of sounds, such as the letter *E*. Because the vocal cords vibrate too fast for the eye to follow, a strobe light, flashing on and off rapidly, captured frames of the action while a videotape recorded the results.

Screening the tape, the pathologist studied the membranous cords and the muscles controlling them. She looked for what she called neurological indications. If the nerves or muscles were damaged in some way, the vibrations of the cords would reveal it, their "symmetry" and "amplitude" departing from normal. Maybe she would find that John had a mild form of spasmodic dysphonia, a disorder that can strangulate speech, or that one of his cords was partially paralyzed. But the instrument illuminated nothing organic, no pathology, that would cause John's voice to tremble.

Perhaps the pathologist was missing something that was slowly progressing, something too subtle to be seen. As she pondered this "extremely rare and difficult case," she invited professional colleagues to observe the patient. Their impression of John was the same: The ebb and flow of his vocal symptoms pointed away from an organic condition. Although she did not use the term somatoform in her written report, her findings settled the matter for Dr. Gray. Checkmate.

Somatoform it was, but John would not accede to the diagnosis. Moreover, although nothing now stood between him and his release, he absolutely refused to go. Maintaining that he was in worse shape than ever, he tried again to see the hospital medical director. He demanded that his 100 percent disability check be "in the mail" before he would consent to leave.

The next day, Thursday, March 26, a hospital social worker beseeched John to relent. "I'm sorry I can't accommodate you," was his reply.

Friday, Good Friday, was the day they put the screws to him. When I phoned John in the morning, he was gasping for breath. He said that Hamm was headed for his room bearing a plane ticket and that the medical director was expected soon afterward. "I'll have to make a decision what to do after the meetings," he said shakily. "You know, my senator's looking at me; my VA at home is looking at me. It's an *entitlement* that they're holding out on. I'm not going to die not having got what I deserve."

John waited. The director never showed, and Hamm did not arrive until the end of the day. According to John's rendition of the meeting, Hamm told him "it was imperative that I leave tomorrow. He said I was complete with the Persian Gulf referral process. He gave me my instructions. I told him I was still not satisfied with what had happened during my stay."

The doctor handed over the final pages of John's medical chart, containing the diagnosis. Although the neurologists had already informed him of it, John asked Hamm to explain "somatoform." "He said it entails my body manufacturing these symptoms. I understood this to be my condition was not valid and that I was causing my own symptoms."

The veteran had found, in a wastebasket in the hospital, a leaflet describing the VA regulations for the transfer or discharge of patients. He was to be transferred to his home facility since that was where he had originated. Now he pointed out to Hamm the line that read: "NO transfers on weekend or holidays." He couldn't travel tomorrow, for it was a matter of safety. Hamm said John had a point but must go on Saturday nonetheless.

"I felt very uneasy about the situation. Dr. Hamm then shook my hand and also gave me a hug, wishing me well, and then proceeded to leave. As he was walking away, I told him that I really felt unsure about this. He said, with a smile, 'I'll see you on Monday, Mr. Cabrillo.'"

Over the weekend John waved the transfer leaflet at the two or three staffers who attempted to dislodge him. They backed off. On the telephone he was pugnacious. "What, are these guys on drugs? Weekend travel isn't safe. I'm sticking to my guns, doing what I feel is right.

"It's disappointing to my family that I can't be with them for Easter, but my ship hasn't come in. What do they expect me to live on—my good looks? Am I going to bend over and take it? I have come too far to look the other way."

John also said he was dissatisfied with his diagnosis, but when I inquired what it was, disingenuously, I confess, he was vague. "They don't know what's wrong with me," he said. In a strong sense he was right. John had mounted no counterarguments to "somatoform," having only an old document from Senator Riegle and James Tuite to refer to. These two advocates, had they materialized at his bedside, would have attacked the diagnosis. They would have claimed that John was suffering from a bona fide neurotoxic injury and that if the VA physicians could not discover its source, theirs was the failing, not his. Shortfalls in neuroscience, where much remained unknown, should not lead the doctor to conclude that the illness was all in the patient's head.

MONDAY PASSED WITHOUT incident. On Tuesday the assistant to the medical director took the well-trod path to room 4011. He proposed to involve John's senator's office, but John would not give the man the telephone number.

Desperate for allies, John placed a call to the patient representative at his home VA. She wasn't in. Next he telephoned the secretary for veterans affairs, Jesse Brown, at VA headquarters in Washington, D.C. He was not put through, but a receptionist agreed to take down a message. It was verses from Proverbs, dictated from the Gideon Bible:

> Do not withhold good from those to whom it is due, when it is in the power of your hand to do so.
> Do not say to your neighbor, "Go and come back, and tomorrow I will give it," when you have it with you.
> Do not devise evil against your neighbor, for he dwells by you for safety's sake.
> Do not strive with a man without cause, if he has done you no harm.

Brown didn't respond. (When the VA chief resigned a few months later, John took satisfaction and even part of the credit.)

On Wednesday, April 2, John left Los Angeles at last. He folded after Ron Hamm and two nurses, arriving in the morning, presented him with an ultimatum. If he didn't go voluntarily in the afternoon, he would be forcibly turned out to the street and billed for his medical care since Saturday.

"I'm tired, I don't feel too good," he told me. "Even a bear knows when its stomach is full." But before leaving John had the doctor type up two communications. One was a note of commendation from John to the nursing staff ("With rare exceptions, they treated me courteously and were compassionate and supportive of my needs"), and the other was a memo to the medical director of the hospital, whom John chastised for not facing him "man to man."

In the letter to his senator John complained that "Dr. Hamm seems to have minimized my concerns and belittled the validity of my issues." However, as he was packing to go—on this day I was on the phone to John several times—he said about Hamm, "As a veteran I have respect for the man. He made every effort." He also observed, sourly, that "Hamm is a hugger."

The taxi was ordered for 3:00 P.M. Hamm insisted on gathering the necessary paper work for John while John fetched his bags and medications. After spending, by his own estimate, fifteen to twenty hours with this patient, the doctor had mixed feelings. He was glad to be rid of John, but he considered him the most interesting case he had ever seen among gulf war veterans.

The taxi was outside. Handed his discharge form to sign, John noticed several errors in it. The form indicated he was being discharged to his home rather than transferred to another VA hospital—a minor mistake perhaps. Also, it listed, under the heading of "Final Diagnosis": "Gulf War Syndrome, Movement Disorder and PPD+." Astounding, on two counts. First, these were the conditions that John had been *admitted* with and no one bothered to revise them at the end. "PPD+" referred to his positive result on the TB antibody test, and "movement disorder" was self-explanatory. But how could Wadsworth admit a person with "gulf war syndrome," a label that the VA eschewed? The mistake was terrible, Hamm conceded later, a double goof. He told me he had meant to cross it out. Yet by not doing so, he probably assisted John's cause.

Seizing on the discharge/transfer error, John asked Hamm to issue a corrected form. When Hamm would not, John refused to sign. Hamm entered his own signature on the form as the patient's representative.

"Dr. Hamm then helped me haul my luggage to awaiting taxicab. I asked Dr. Hamm if I would have a VA escort to accompany me to Airport. He said no. Then he insisted on driving me to the Airport himself. I told him I felt this was not appropriate. Upon my initial arrival to Los Angeles and the West L.A. VA Medical Center, I experienced many problems. It was a serious logistical problem. I felt hesitant to take a taxicab to the Airport, but decided to leave as it was apparent that Dr. Hamm could not wait to see me go. We shook hands and then Dr. Hamm proceeded to give me a hug. The taxi driver told me he waited a total of 45 minutes to pick me up."

THE PATIENT RETURNED to his home—physically worse off, by his own assessment, and set back as well on his disability claim. The diagnosis of somatoform disorder was an unforeseen blow. Not only did it offend him, but the labeling of his condition also undercut his claim of undiagnosed illness. A somatoform disorder that kept him from working might be compensable, but only if it was service-connected under normal VA rules— i.e., that he was able to show he had acquired the illness while on active duty. This he could not, would not do.

John therefore fought to overturn the diagnosis. First he wrote about his dissatisfactory evaluation at West L.A. and forwarded the account to his senator's office. Next he dug into news reports and commentary having to do with the gulf war illnesses. More than four years into the controversy, a lot of material was available for his soon burgeoning binder.

Using an Internet connection at his local library, John downloaded articles from a veterans' Website. "On the Misdiagnosis of Somatization Disorder" was one. Its author, a proponent of multiple chemical sensitivity, argued that the veterans' symptoms typified an organic reaction to chemicals, not a psychosomatic problem.

Another find was titled "Persian Gulf Illness: Is It All Just 'In Their Heads'? New Report Shows Evidence of Brainstem Encephalitis." John recognized the name of William Baumzweiger, formerly of the VA. While treating veterans in Los Angeles, Dr. Baumzweiger had developed a complicated theory of the genesis of the illnesses, starting with an inflammation of the brainstem. The inflammation probably was triggered by an exposure to neurotoxic chemicals as revealed by the investigator James Tuite.

John also learned of the debate over pyridostigmine bromide, PB for short, a drug given to the troops as protection against Iraqi nerve gas. John recalled taking his "Ptabs" in the field. Certain scientists and members of Congress speculated that PB's effect on the nervous system, supposedly temporary, was pernicious in the long term, especially in concert with the other chemicals that the troops had encountered.

All of it rang true. His neurological disorder, John decided, was probably due to chemicals rather than to biological toxins. Flush with information, he seems to have convinced his local VA doctors and his senatorial contact to disregard the diagnosis of the specialists at Wadsworth. John's supporters sent letters to the regional benefits office of the VA, pressing his claim for a disabling, undiagnosed illness. The West L.A. discharge form, referring to his "gulf war syndrome," must have helped.

Meanwhile he kept his distance from the inquiring writer. On leaving the hospital, John had given me his mailing address (a post office box), but not his telephone number, and he'd been vague about keeping in touch. He didn't answer a couple of my letters, nor messages passed through his senator's office. When I eventually read his L.A. narrative, I saw that I had become one of the players in his unhappy drama.

I had appeared at his bedside out of the blue. "At the time," he wrote, "it was appropriate to converse with him and maintain his interest until I could come to terms with why he was referred to me by Dr. Hamm." I doubt John was that calculating, considering how torridly he talked, but he did seem to recognize the value of a reporter, for he spoke about "going public" if he got "the short end of the stick."

Wariness won out, however. "In light of other concerns which I had with regard to my hospitalization here at West Los Angeles VAMC, I started feeling suspicious and uneasy as to why I was maintaining contact with Mr. Wheelwright." He concluded: "I am not sure why Dr. Hamm referred Mr. Wheelwright to me, and what connection they have with the Persian Gulf Referral process. What does Dr. Hamm stand to gain from this connection and why was I included in this ordeal? I feel this situation not to be appropriate."

Well, John is owed an explanation, and so are the three referral patients whom I met later by leave of Ronald Hamm. There was nothing more to the arrangement than a doctor doing a favor for a writer, on a matter that the doctor and writer agreed was important. No quid pro quo was discussed. Moreover, the patients understood they could refuse to talk with me, and the VA public affairs office was informed. I won't deny being grateful to my subjects for the entrée. Still, like all journalists, I am quite capable of biting the hand that feeds me. I think John for one realized the risks and withheld large portions of his story in order to protect himself.

In July 1997 John's ship finally came in. The VA approved his claim of a complete service-connected disability from a "neurological disorder of unknown origin," and his monthly compensation was put through. Yet to his great annoyance he did not get all that he requested. John wanted his disability to be declared of a "total and permanent nature." The designation would mean that he wouldn't have to be periodically reexamined and, more important, that his wife and children would qualify for health and education benefits in their own right.

He sent the paper work to the claims office all over again. More letters were rounded up from doctors, family members, a VA social worker and the senator's aide. That summer his physical condition got no better. If anything, it was a little worse.

In August he was examined by a team of private neurologists on consultation to the VA. Stumped by what they saw, the specialists asked to videotape his tremors and spasms for further scrutiny. John refused, calling the taping "inappropriate." This familiar judgment of his was not rendered casually, for you must appreciate that propriety mattered greatly to him. Here was no freak, no specimen for medical analysis, but a veteran in need of redress. Why couldn't they see that?

If he expected their report to buttress his latest appeal, once more he was disappointed. Though finding "dystonialike symptoms" and doubting that John would improve, the consultants cautioned, "It is difficult . . . to state that Mr. Cabrillo has a permanent medical condition since we are not fully aware of the Gulf War syndrome and there is debate as to the extent of chemical warfare used during the Gulf War."

John tried repeatedly to reach the lead doctor of the group by telephone. He wound up writing a long letter of complaint, urging the neurologist to put down on paper what he had told John orally— namely, that he and his colleagues disagreed with the West L.A. diagnosis of somatoform disorder. John also pressed the doctor to amend the prognosis of his condition to "total and permanent in nature." Not being employed by the VA, the doctor needn't worry about reprisals, John assured him. "Your considerations may help enable me to provide my family with much needed health insurance coverage and other benefits."

You have the picture of him now, don't you? It's not very flattering, the portrait that John and I have fashioned: the grasping for compensation, the badgering of the medical system, the insistence on forcing the round peg of his symptoms into the square hole of his convictions. I wish it were a more complete portrait. John provided me only part of himself, and the part that I relay to you glances over the generosity of his suffering. I can't convey the sense I felt of his physical sacrifice.

EARLY MARCH 1998, the time of Lent again. Unannounced, I drove up to his house. I had passed word through the VA that I was in the area and wished to see him, but I didn't hang around waiting for a reply. The town was small enough that I easily got directions.

The one-story white stucco house was neatly presented. It sat back from the road on a pretty rise with a view of the desert mountains. Off a beam near the back door hung a heavy bag, the kind that boxers use, and parked beside it was a motorized wheelchair, which a clever mechanic had outfitted with three wheels, no doubt to handle the rough terrain around the house. The wheelchair and the heavy bag were the yin and yang of John.

He was out, as it happened. I left a message with a family member that I could be found at Marie's Café downtown.

I had brought along a health professional who was interested in the case. About an hour later we were finishing our lunch, disappointedly, when the door to the café swung open. Not saloon doors, but there should have been, because he stood there in the backlight, legs apart, like some western hero.

He came forward on two crutches and sat down at the table. We were flustered and excited. He was collected and courteous, and gently made it known that it was improper for me to have gone to his home.

Point taken. We began to discuss the ground rules for an interview, which I proposed to set for the next morning. Again I found it hard to pay attention both to what he was saying and what he was doing. He was physically different from a year ago, not displaying the same tremors of the extremities but rather a contracted posture. Yet his trunk, neck, and face were even more active than before. An undulating movement, the head rolling as if it wanted to float free of his body, and the everted lips, like a grouper's, called to mind a marine creature.

My colleague, who was quite charmed by John but who was after all a clinician, had the identical impression. She supplied this description: "He'd twist his shoulders, lean in slowly, tilt his head down and to the side, then swivel a bit. His lower lip would fold under, and his eyes would go lateral. His forehead would furrow, and always there was a movement, a tense flow in his face and trunk, bizarre and captivating. A fish dance with eyes popping to the sides of his head and moving independently from one another, an internal war manifesting in his face.

"His hands would freeze up with fingers stiff and arched like a swan's neck. All of these changes and movements happening at once while talking and then suddenly: a stillness, softening. The muscles in his face would relax, and he would appear normal, but only for a second. Then, as if taken over by a force beyond his control, a firing of synapses would return him to a tormented flow of energy, from a particle to a wave."

Both flattered and affronted, John took his time committing to a meeting. He asked himself, as he confided later, "Why am I talking to Jeff? Is anyone really helping me medically? Are they knocking on my door, trying to offer me something? What have I got to lose?"

I disarmed John by saying that I was just a guy trying to make a living like everybody else. Looking me in the eye, he said he knew what it was like to have to support a family. So we made the appointment for nine the next morning, same place. Before we parted, I said (this time with no calculation) that I was truly sorry to see him worse.

John's preferred table at Marie's was in the far corner. The waitresses seemed to know and appreciate him, the minor celebrity who had been mysteriously wounded in the Persian Gulf. Today he wore a pressed blue and white striped shirt, pleasant cologne, and a watch in a leather case on his belt. He set his crutches against the wall and unzipped a backpack full of papers and documents.

He appeared to have lost weight in battling his illness; he looked smaller and more sallow than I remembered. He mentioned that he was trying to eat better and to quit smoking. Over a light breakfast and decaffeinated coffee, he went into familiar topics: the failure of the West L.A. doctors to "face the plate" regarding his medical concerns, their administration of Haldol ("I still can't raise my arm"), their conflicting advice on whether it was safe to give blood.

"We waited months to receive the comprehensive report," John said, "and then the speech pathology report was not even included."

"What did it find?" I asked.

"It said 'unknown etiology.' But the records of the tests were never sent. I had to hammer on the local VA to get them. It's the veteran who has to initiate everything. . . ."

But the bravado was missing from the declamation. Better informed, John no longer suggested that his own illness qualified him to answer for all cases. He was taking a craftier approach. Instead of bulling toward his goals under a banner of idealism, he was bobbing and weaving—literally.

"A lot of possibilities could account for my progressive deterioration," he said. "I'm leaving it up to the experts. But I think it was probably some of the toxic stuff in the Gulf."

He told me that his disability award from the VA had been incomplete. "The regional office was saying that there's a chance I'll get better. But they misread my claim. It wasn't special benefits for *me* that I wanted. Hey, I need the insurance for my family. My condition is permanent—don't look the other away," he implored, as if I represented the VA.

Did I represent the VA? In his view anyway? A not unreasonable question.

He allowed that in the past year he'd had so much pain he could barely walk. "I feel the sockets grind; my leg feels like it's going to pop out of the socket. But the X rays don't show any inflammation in my hip, so they can't do anything about it." Also, he occasionally suffered "spasms" that sounded to me like seizures. But since strong medication didn't agree with him, he had stopped taking Valium in favor of Tylenol and salsalate, a mild anti-inflammatory similar to aspirin.

"You're supposed to go from diagnosis to treatment," he observed. "But I never did reach the diagnosis or the treatment phase. At the VA they say that since they can't tell me what it is, they have to go to case management, just managing symptoms, including physical therapy and speech therapy."

Like his movement disorder, his speech pathology had drifted or modulated from tremors toward contractures. He was hard to understand at times. There was so much tension around the purse of his mouth that he pronounced "recommend" as "wecommend." He demonstrated the problem, frighteningly, grasping the front of his face with both hands. "My face was cramping up. It kind of scared me."

I had long been curious about his life before he went into the air force—his upbringing, his siblings. His parents, I had discovered, lived in the same little town; there was a John senior in the phone book. I tiptoed into these waters as innocently as I could: "What did you want to be when you graduated from high school?"

No way. "A writer can't always get everything he wants," he said with a small smile. He would go no farther back in time than his decision to enlist. Ironically, the reasoning then—"to get health care" for his wife and first child—was the same that was driving him now.

"I don't regret my career," John said. "I got a lot of schooling in the service." Like many aggrieved veterans I met, he had only positive things to say about his time in the military, as opposed to his experience afterward. For these men and women it was more than the difference between being well and being sick: They had enjoyed serving their country. John became animated, a natural animation.

"Did you have any excitement during the war?" I asked.

My voice brought him back to himself. "Excuse me," he said, his head and face twisting. His lower lip turned out and over, almost a simian gesture, so that I could see his gums.

"We had lots of alarms [chemical weapons alerts] but they always said they were false. Once we experienced a Scud [missile] attack right on the flight line. Kaboom! Kaboom! That was the sound of the Patriot [antiaircraft] batteries going off on either side of the runway. I guess they intercepted it. We took cover, laying down. We just had time to put our masks on. The ground shook, and there were these dramatic colors in the sky. *Then* the alarms went off."

He remarked that alarms were recorded on Pentagon logs that now were missing, an issue much in the news. . . . How easy it was, for both of us, to draw away from the unspeakable loneliness of individual suffering into the language of the political debate. But even he seemed to find the terms shopworn and hollow.

"Since I saw you, there has been a slew of manifestations relating to veterans' concerns," he said, taking out his binder. "The report of this congressional committee. . . ."

"I have read it cover to cover," I said. An interview is like a fox-trot, where one partner has to lead, and today was my turn. John did not resist when I steered him back to his case.

"I've been struggling, juggling this for a long time. Jeff, this is very draining for me [he made another grimace, a sharp askance look]—I'm going to keep going, but my biggest fear is that with my neurological condition my body is going to stop. Probably there's a better way to state that [writing furiously, I shook my head], and who's going to take care of them?"

I put down my pen and I put my hands to my face. He paused, obliquely acknowledging the emotion.

"When I found out what my diagnosis from L.A. meant, my whole world fell apart."

"What was the diagnosis, John?"

His voice dropped to a whisper. "It's called somatoform disorder. . . .

Jeff, it means that the mind manufactures the symptoms. In other words, they think I'm crazy.

"I felt let down. But then I found out I wasn't alone among veterans who are misdiagnosed. And the three main doctors on my team do not concur with the diagnosis."

"What do they call it?"

"They have categorized it 'chorealike symptoms.'"

He continued, "Somatoform disorder is not ratable." He became indignant. "These people who were tasked to help me, how dare they put a label on me that will affect me for the rest of my life? And not only me, a lot of vets."

At last I understood his obsession with diagnosis. In his long struggle with the medical system John had pitted his symptoms against every test thrown before him, his object not to achieve a label but to defeat one—to defeat them all. What he wanted to be told (so as to be able to reiterate it on his claim) was that his illness, an incontestable illness, could not be explained.

John's hands were hooked at the wrists, his thumbs interposed between long fingers in a kind of fist. He eyed my notebook. "From an outside perspective this sounds like a story. But this is *real* to me."

He described the consultants' exam of the previous summer and showed me his letter of complaint about their report. I thought it only fair to tell him how I'd make use of his letter if he would give me a copy. I'd call up the neurologists and try to obtain a sense of their side of the story. Journalists call this triangulation, I explained.

He understood me. "Jeff, you're taking a third-party approach. Well, now I'm having doubts." He put the letter away. His face contorted. "One of the issues in this story is the veterans' credibility. But on my level it's not an open question. It's my *direct* experience. You do not have me in a corner because I have nothing to hide."

Insisting that he pay for our breakfast, he wrote out a check in a small, neat hand. His face was relaxed except for the bulging eyes.

"Your dilemma," he said acutely, as we got up from the table, "is that you're dealing with the *human* element." For the second time he seemed to commingle my identity with the VA, the system, the doubters, the diagnosticians—all one looming force. His mouth labored and emitted the most pathetic plea, reminding me of how he had spilled his crutch at the end of our first meeting. "Yoou help mee get bettew!" he said.

But outside, leaning forward on his crutches in the strong light, he was the gruff, kind, independent, and faintly ironic fellow whom I knew better. We said good-bye—I restrained myself from hugging him—and he climbed into his truck. Walking away, I thought I heard him say, "God bless you."

NONE OF WHICH deterred me from ringing up his latest doctors. When John discussed his case with them, he must have exercised a selective hearing, but were the doctors as clear as they might be? Was an uncertainty about his condition permitting him to hear only what he wanted to hear?

A neurologist with the consulting group that examined John told me that equivocating in such cases is not only proper—the lack of organic findings doesn't prove a psychological disorder—but also safer. "If I say it's somatoform," observed the specialist, "the patient may break up the office. If I put down on the form that it's *not* a somatoform, maybe the VA will sue me. But where I have a doubt, I always give it to the patient.

"Unfortunately the compensation issue muddies it. Almost everything on the basic neurological exam can be faked except for certain tests of reflexes. Handwriting is a good key. You say his handwriting is good? That's a red flag. Someone with a neurological condition shouldn't have control to that degree. Some patients can control it, but then you do see the tremor break through—in a pattern, with a certain change in the lettering.

"Still, if he's got a conversion disorder, conversion means that he actually has had a change of spirit. The patient comes to believe in what he has."

John's neurologist at his local VA voiced a similar opinion, but with different emphasis: "It's a pretty strange case. He tests consistently negative on the diagnostic studies. We doctors don't do well with that. We like to find something positive, and we get insecure when we can't make a diagnosis.

"There is factitious stuff with John, but he does have some kind of a movement disorder. Some of the underlying things are real—and that's the part he hears—but there's a lot of somatization too.

"I just can't believe he's faking. He's not a malingerer, but it is a conversion disorder of some kind. I'd like to see him get his benefits. He has deteriorated. I just sent another letter supporting his claim for his [total and permanent] disability.

"The other thing about John is that he's confrontational. He can piss people off. But I don't think his condition involves his Persian Gulf experience. There are family issues at work, perhaps, and cultural aspects. He has a lot of Hispanic pride."

I asked the neurologist, "Do you think if he were finally able to get all the benefits he's seeking that he would be open to dealing with the somatization?"

The doctor was not sanguine. "You'd think that would be the rational course to take, but then these things aren't rational. It would be a sign of weakness for John to talk about psychological stuff."

After I got home from our second meeting, I sent John a card of thanks, ending with the thought that he was in Lent now but that Easter was coming. By return mail, the last contact I have had to this day, he sent me the account of his stay in Los Angeles, a few news clippings, his letter to the neurological consultants, and the quotation from Proverbs that he passed to VA Secretary Brown.

The cover note was executed in small, neat printing: "When an individual becomes involved with the media, it sometimes compels government agencies to react, but also we might not like the answers given. Therefore, I will not have unrealistic expectations.

"I share this info with you Jeff, for I know what it is like to make a living and provide for a family. . . . You have been privileged in life Jeff. Remember that God Knows your heart and your ways."

2

On the Coast of Arabia

After the start of the bombing campaign, on January 16, 1991, the authorities closed the Dhahran airport to nonmilitary traffic. Dhahran is a Saudi city on the Persian Gulf, some two hundred miles southeast of Kuwait. You flew as far as Riyadh, in the center of the kingdom, and then made your way by road to the staging ground of the war.

Joined by an Indian businessman, I bargained a price with a taxi driver. I had a meeting to make in Dhahran in the afternoon. Would we get there in time? "*Insha'allah*," said the driver, shrugging. "God willing." The gold in his front tooth gleamed at the challenge. He averaged 105 mph over a smooth, straight highway for two and a half hours.

The winter air was cool, the desert sun hot. The roadside was conspicuously littered and fenced off with wire, beyond which camels foraged like shorebirds on the sloping sand. The wastes rippled; the rock outcrops flashed by with hardly a shred of vegetation. Now and then the barren landscape would be broken by the juicy green of an agricultural plot, irrigated by a center-pivot system.

A convoy of American trucks, minus their trailers, were slouching toward Dhahran. High and truncated, they must be part of the auxiliary force going to support the imminent invasion of Kuwait. The names painted on the back read: "Maine Exchange," "Coop da Vill," "Janie's Mom." The gibe at Janie's mother escaped me completely, because my heart was pounding.

Or maybe it wasn't. When you pick through the past in search of something you did not anticipate or recognize at the time, you might try to infer too much. If I was anxious en route to Dhahran, it was in anticipation of people being killed, not of people getting mysteriously sick after not being killed.

Launched just one day before, already I had experienced unusual excitement. The war's whirlpool had sucked in all comers. On the flight to Saudi Arabia, for example, were several contractors from Texas, who hoped to work on the cleanup of the oil spill caused by Iraq, the world's biggest; a Boeing employee, ex-army Special Forces, now advising the Saudi air force; a Sudanese with an airy smile and a bouffant turban; an Egyptian named Hassan, late of Red Bank, New Jersey, who carried boxes of gas masks that he intended to sell in Dhahran. The Iraqi leader, Saddam Hussein, had been rattling his chemical weapons, and past conflicts in the region had proved he would use them. The entrepreneurial Egyptian didn't know how his gas masks were supposed to fit, until the Boeing man showed him.

I sat next to a Westernized Saudi in his late twenties—Michael, his name was—who I later learned was being expelled from the United States. A few hours before the plane landed in Jidda, where I was to connect to Riyadh, Michael went into a drug withdrawal and began to groan and rip his shirt and crush the airline's plastic cups. I clutched his hand while a nurse on board took down his pants and shot him in the thigh with Valium. Drooling and drowsy, he smiled and mouthed, "Thank you," as we taxied to the terminal. In a marbled foyer off the main concourse, where scores of Arabs were praying on the floor, a phalanx of bare heels faced directly away from Mecca.

My hotel was the Algosaibi in the Khobar district. The management had printed an advisory on what to do in case of poison gas. When the air-raid sirens sounded, guests were to proceed to a conference room in the lobby (named the Pearl of the Gulf), which had been made airtight and stocked with provisions. No Scuds had struck the city of late. At sunrise on the first morning I peeled the tape from the windows and flung them open to the Gulf, a half mile distant.

I wish to establish, from my very first hours, the chemical threat and the psychological threat, bridging the external and internal environments, touching everyone there in some manner. It was both unsettling and stimulating. The sensations were a kind of stress, for me more positive than negative, like the jolts of arousal from the Turkish coffee, Saudi Arabia's only legal drug. Indeed I rarely felt the stress of the war except when I administered it to myself in small doses.

If I sometimes felt disoriented, I had come by the condition willingly, unlike the army reservists, who with little notice had been dispatched from their homes in the States to cramped tents in the desert, where they awaited, so far as they knew, the chemical wrath of the Iraqis. Whenever I had enough of the devilish stimulation of crisis, I retreated to my hotel room, knowing I could leave for home the next day. The menace of the missiles was pushed to the back of my mind. One night the air-raid siren went off at 2:30 A.M. As I closed my window and returned to bed, I heard abrupt sliding noises from windows all over the hotel. The people exposed on the front were not so cavalier.

America and its allies won a smashing victory in the Persian Gulf War. The victory was dimmed by the emergence of the veterans' illnesses and the failure to resolve them. The political wrangle over the problem eventually petered out. A number of veterans have remained sick. There is no medical consensus on what happened to them. The scientific inquiry continues.

What were, what are the gulf war illnesses? Earlier, in telling you about an individual, I kept my general thoughts about the issue to a minimum. John Cabrillo I still believe to be sui generis, his medical case representing only the vessel for his own suffering. But since his was not the only case among those who had been to the Gulf, I was obliged to look at others, so as to make reliable generalizations if there were any to be made. The same exercise was conducted on a grand and formal scale by government investigators and by private teams as well, all of them in pursuit of the identity and cause of the illnesses. These paramount questions of identity and cause, or diagnosis and etiology, were like Siamese twins, because to capture one would surely reveal the other. However, for reasons to be explained later, the two key fugitives escaped.

When the initial pursuit began to flag, the researchers took up two subsidiary questions. What was special about the experience and the environment of the war, if anything, that might have led to the ill-defined conditions, and second, what was special about the veterans who became sick, if anything, that had made them more susceptible than the majority who kept their health? The latter question was ticklish, pointing as it did to personal characteristics and perhaps straying into judgments upon individuals. There wasn't much work undertaken on this subject. But the broad issue of environmental agents attracted a lot of attention. To study the forces affecting a military cohort of seven hundred thousand not only might yield significant generalizations about the group's health but also would relieve the individual veteran of any role, let alone fault, in his or her illness.

As I have suggested, the environmental factors themselves were split into camps. When the researchers went back to 1991 and reconstructed the wartime conditions, inevitably they were guided by preconceptions—hunches about what to look for. "We hear and apprehend only what we already half know," as Thoreau once put it. Opinion was divided between what might be called the toxic hypothesis and the stress hypothesis. One side argued that the illnesses must spring from hazardous substances that were rife in the theater of the war. The other position was that the illnesses were either caused by or greatly amplified by psychological stress.

They were dueling paradigms. In any of the investigative reports released about the gulf war illnesses you could anticipate the conclusion by reading the opening statement about the wartime environment. It was either a particularly toxic situation or a particularly stressful one. The better reports weighed both sets of circumstances, but I took exception to the dualism: It implied there were separate objects of exogenous attack, the mind affected by stress and the body affected by chemicals.

In my mind I have come back to Arabia to search for the origins of the rival schools of thought. This morning of February 10, 1991, finds me staring once again from a hotel window in Khobar at a big sun squatting upon a stripe of green sea. Illnesses are germinating upon this flat and battered coastline. It has been six years between my experience of this place and my starting this book. Of course I have followed the health mystery in the interim, but trained as a journalist, I was aware of receiving the journalists' version, a picture that was high in contrast and low in resolution.

During the war some eight hundred foreign correspondents were based in the kingdom, half in Riyadh and half in Dhahran. Most of the Dhahran contingent stayed at the Sheraton, which was the most secure hotel and the site of the media center. The military public affairs office ran small groups of journalists up to the front and back; their pool reports were produced daily. You could cover the entire war from the Sheraton by rewriting the handouts and taping the briefings. A number of my colleagues were content to do so, I suspect, though much was made afterward of the Pentagon's muzzling of the news media.

Some of the reporters who covered the war later covered the illnesses.

But I think I am the right one to gather the clues to the health mystery, particularly the environmental clues, for my original assignment, from a national magazine, was the unfolding environmental impact of the war, not the war per se. Because my subjects were the massive oil spill in the Gulf and subsequently the massive oil fires in Kuwait, I was attuned from the start to the notion that human beings would pay a personal cost for despoiling their environment.

Oil having instigated the war as a geopolitical matter, oil also caused part of the casualties. It was raw on the desert shoreline, from the spill created by Saddam Hussein, and thick in the desert air, from the ignition of hundreds of wells. Great concern was expressed, official and otherwise, about the health consequences of the oil pollution. The fires and spill set the terms not only for how the war was viewed but also for how the troops' illnesses were going to be viewed—in other words, for the conception of toxic exposures, which would apply to every environmental agent but stress.

The oil pollution even had a nickname in 1991. Occasionally, half jokingly (the joke cutting the fear), the oil that suffused the environment was referred to as Agent Oil, a play upon Agent Orange.

AFTER SEIZING KUWAIT in August 1990, Saddam Hussein had warned that if attacked, he would set Kuwait's oil ablaze or flush it into the sea. The threat was trumpeted for months by Jordan's King Hussein, who sympathized with Iraq, and by the more vehement of American and European environmental groups, which opposed going to war to preserve "an oil-based lifestyle."

What would happen if Iraq lit up the wells? Said Jordan's Hussein: "Lingering in the atmosphere for around 100 years, this massive carbon dioxide emission would promote the greenhouse effect and contribute to global warming, climatic changes, lower global food production, and human and animal health deterioration."

Carl Sagan, an independent U.S. scientist, stated on national television that an oil conflagration could trigger a "nuclear winter" in South Asia and beyond.

"Warfare in the Middle East," claimed the Friends of the Earth, "could result not only in the loss of many thousands of human lives but extend to a scorching of the Earth through the destruction of sprawling petrochemical complexes, mass bombings of communities and urban areas, chemical warfare, poisoned water supplies turning masses of civilians into refugees, and wholesale pollution of the Persian Gulf."

In late January, with the start of the air war, the destruction began as predicted. Opening the cocks of tankers and pipelines, the Iraqis loosed an oil spill at least twenty-five times the size of the *Exxon Valdez*. They aimed to disrupt the desalination plants of the Saudis and deter the invasion of Kuwait, if it were to come by sea. They succeeded in neither, but the oil slithered onto the Saudi shoreline in tumid, acrid bands.

Blackened and poisoned, cormorants and grebes began to die by the thousands. A wildlife rescue operation in the port of Jubail, heroically staffed by Saudis and Europeans, was able to accomplish little. On a peninsula named Abu Ali I watched a cormorant walking on the side of the road. It kept to the right of the yellow line like a dutiful pedestrian. Because of its dark plumage, I couldn't tell whether or not it had oil on it, but clearly something was wrong. The bird marched toward the gates of a pipeline pump station as if it had business inside. Later I heard of other seabirds sick from the spill that walked confusedly into the desert.

Sluggishly the slick spread. Abu Ali, shaped like a fishhook and sticking out into the Gulf, blocked the oil from reaching Jubail and Dhahran to the south. For several hundred miles north of Abu Ali, however, as far as Khafji on the Kuwait border, the beaches were fouled.

The Eastern Province, where oil is king, is not Saudi Arabia's prettiest. From Dhahran I sped north through salt flats, yards full of junked cars, unfinished construction projects, and gas vents flaring bright orange. I passed petrochemical plants and tank farms. Huge pylons shouldered high-voltage wires; pipelines snaked here and there. The prostrate geography of the coast offers little resistance to pollution, although at unspoiled junctures west of the highway the desert is piled up in prominent pinkish dunes. Blown in from the interior, the beautiful sand consists of quartz grains tinged with iron oxide. To the east, on the approach to the dead flat shore, the sand whitens from the calcareous contributions of marine life, the atomized shells and coral.

The littoral landscape consists of tawny shallows and lagoons, with occasional mudflats and a few patches of mangrove. The beach vegetation is halophyte, the indestructible saltbush, which even the camels can't stomach. The intertidal animals are snails and crabs. Life becomes more interesting in the broad subtidal zone. There are waving belts of sea grass, which serve as the spawning grounds for shrimp and fish and as shelter for the sea turtles and the dugongs, the mermaidlike sea mammals.

From a low bluff above the beach I could hear the altered lapping. More than the sight of black waves breaking gently, more than the sharp, alien smell, the sound of the spill was most terrible. It was a muffled plooping, a heavy lilt, a perversion of the restful sea sound. Inky fumaroles popped up behind the glimmering waves, releasing fumes. When a wave withdrew, only then was water revealed, a transparent film between the floating oil and the packed sand. I took a palm frond, dipped it into the black, and dripped Saddam's name onto the pale strand.

The extent of the slick and the deaths of the seabirds gave rise to alarm about the health of the entire Gulf. The week I arrived, *Time* magazine, under the headline DEAD SEA IN THE MAKING, reported: "This complex ecosystem, already pushed to the limits of survival by years of pollution, is now threatened with total collapse by the inexorable spread of the smothering, toxic oil."

As a student of the *Exxon Valdez* spill, which had taken place in Alaska two years earlier, I knew this to be an exaggeration. However terrifying the immediate losses, the environmental damage of marine oil spills rarely lasts, since the ocean purges itself readily. Though more embattled than most marine bodies, the Persian Gulf had come to grips with its years of pollution. At least one hundred large oil spills had occurred as a result of the Iran-Iraq war during the 1980s. I was actually standing upon a bench of asphalt, embedded in the sand, stemming from that war. The Gulf's operational spills, as they were euphemistically called, included dribblings and periodic blowouts from a thousand offshore platforms, pipeline leaks, tanker ballast discharge, and runoff and dumping from coastal facilities. Yet for all its inputs of petroleum, the Gulf had remained a tolerant marine habitat, supporting a commercial shrimp fishery. The latest spilled oil, except where it stranded onshore, would likely be diluted, degraded, and accommodated as the rest.

I was not the only observer who believed this. THE GULF ISN'T DEAD, was the headline of an op-ed piece in the *New York Times* in early February. Subsequently, in *USA Today*: WARTIME OIL SPILL NOT AS BIG OR BAD AS FEARED. Like the huge slick itself, which drifted offshore one day and smacked new areas of coastline the next, opinion about the Gulf's ecological future seesawed in the news media as a kind of sidebar to the war.

A *New York Times* reporter on the scene interviewed an oil company "ecologist" named Costello. Costello was very pessimistic about the Gulf. The reporter wrote: "Although some scientists who analyze the effects of oil at sea believe that the spill may not be the environmental catastrophe once predicted, Mr. Costello and others who have spent years studying the peculiar nature of the gulf believe that the slick will ravage the fish, the wildlife and the luxuriant coral reefs that have long existed here on the edge of extinction."

Note the reporter's tack. He has sampled the different opinions and, by his choice of expert, has decided to go with the dire point of view. This to me is an interesting document, because the *Times* reporter was Philip Shenon, who was to galvanize the political debate over the gulf war illnesses five years hence. As before, Shenon's stories would acknowledge the divided opinion about the cause of the illnesses and then favor the dire point of view. He promoted the importance of nerve gas exposures at a time when such exposures, allegedly covered up by the Pentagon, were the prime agent of the toxic hypothesis.

Well, I can report to you that the Persian Gulf did not die from the oil spill, nor was it ravaged. The fertile sea grass beds were undamaged. Dugongs, sea turtles, and fish were unharmed. An estimated thirty thousand birds perished, a disaster in itself, but seabird populations routinely suffer big losses and rebound. The shrimp fishery was hurt for a few years, but most likely it was because of overfishing in the relaxed climate after the war. Likewise, the coral reefs in the northern Gulf seemed to decline, but they were declining before the conflict. The only biological effect that could be laid exclusively to the oil spill was the smothering of intertidal life. Tar mats persist today on the northern Saudi shoreline, cracked and lifeless spaces, like the parking lots of old drive-ins, facing a still-vibrant tableau.

I TURNED NORTH again, toward Kuwait. Past the city of Jubail, jittery over Scud attacks, the six-lane highway narrowed to two. Military convoys dominated the traffic, and coveys of helicopters wheeled overhead. The ground war would happen any day. I stopped at the small airport at Tanajib on the coast. Next to the Chinooks and Blackhawks on the tarmac, young marines were doing bench presses, their arms as big around as tank treads. They looked good to go.

Yeats wrote:

. . . somewhere in sands of the desert
A shape with lion body and the head of a man,
A gaze blank and pitiless as the sun,
Is moving its slow thighs, while all about it
Reel shadows of the indignant desert birds.

John Cabrillo, what are you thinking at this moment, hunkered by the runway at KKMC? Paul Johnson, were you one of the marines I saw at Tanajib working out? And Pete Timmons, a less gung ho marine, what are you feeling now, at the rail of the ship, the landing zone in sight? Darren Moreau, in Oman, far from the front, I know you are preparing to receive the American corpses in a professional manner. And Carol Best, still in the States, wishing to participate, piqued by excitement, not yet called up.

Daily the sky became more palpable, as a tincture of slate was added to the blue. The Iraqis had begun to ignite the oil wells in earnest around February 20. The smoke went up fast to twelve thousand feet, whereupon like coral at the sea surface, it spread laterally. The pilots flew above it and dropped their bombs through the sooty ceiling.

The late-February winds were light and moved the smoke most often out into the Gulf, but occasionally the same easterly breeze that pinned the slick onto the beaches pushed the smoke over the mainland. Black rain fell on the troops. As much oil fell into the Gulf from the emissions of droplets and soot as was spilled from the pipelines and tankers.

At a coastal promontory named Ras as-Zawr, oil and water came together in a dark mist, a man-made sea smoke. The desert, powerfully lit from the west, issued its own yellow light. With the sky full and dark, and the sunset radiating from the sand, the optics normal to Earth were put upside down, and I felt I was walking on the desert Moon, black heaven above, in danger of falling off into space. The Gulf, the third element to the piece, hung nearby in brooding purple, like something out of Spiritus Mundi.

It grew windy and cold. A huge tanker passed in the distance. Empty and bound for loading, the ship floated on the horizon as high as a house.

Day and night the Saudi kingdom continued to dispense energy to a needy world. The oil production had increased, in fact, in support of the war machine.

When the invasion finally occurred, on February 24, the Iraqis crumbled. They did not use their chemical weapons. They fled, surrendered, or were cut down in retreat. After a six-month buildup the Persian Gulf War ended anticlimactically, if a spasm of noise and blood can be called anticlimactic. A cease-fire was declared on February 28, leaving Saddam Hussein in power.

Another reporter and I crossed into Kuwait the next day, hard on the heels of the liberators. At the border town of Khafji, empty for months, the acacia trees drooped for lack of water. Camels grazed above the oil-stained beach. It looked like a paradise for car thieves, there were so many abandoned and stripped vehicles.

The barriers were only partly cleared from the highway, causing traffic to slalom. As U.S. troops blew up land mines in the distance, the booms reached the road more as pulses of air than of sound. Overhead the sun's disk had no power, no capacity to throw shadows; you could look right at it through the sullen atmosphere.

We weaved our way north. Traveling in the hollow land of Kuwait was like waking from a trance and finding all about you strange clues from an experience you couldn't remember. What to make of the shell casings beside the gate of the equestrian club? Or the artillery piece mounted on the patio of the beach house? The big piles of shoes on the highway? The photo album of an Iraqi soldier's family, in a bunker full of stolen cosmetics?

The occupiers seemed to have trashed the nicest places especially. At Al-Fuhayhil on the coast, dismayed people came out of hiding to inspect their gutted residences. There were mountains of garbage in the courtyards. My companion and I stopped and ate a picnic lunch, our table a door placed atop a shopping cart, and afterward, curious to examine a shoreline fortification, I strolled down to the beach. I felt a pressure on my boot and looked down stupidly at a wire that was connected to a round object in the sand. The mine, resembling a plastic smoke alarm with spikes, didn't go off.

Kuwait City was totally blacked out. We circled the roundabouts in the dark, beneath a heavily smudged moon, until we were welcomed into an apartment building by a mixed bag of Arabs. They were a Syrian, a Jordanian, some Palestinians and Egyptians, who had banded together and resisted eviction by the Iraqis. They fed us like royalty. The next morning people were waving flags in the streets and joyously firing their automatic weapons. They had big smiles and free gasoline for the Americans.

Angling toward the source of heavy smoke in the southwest, we came upon the fires consuming Al-Ahmadi, the country's largest oil field.

I don't think I've ever witnessed a more appalling scene. Spread across an empty plain, jagged columns of fire jetted uncontrollably. The earth rumbled from the pressure of oil escaping at sixteen hundred pounds per square inch. Great heat filled my face, the sky was a swirling lid of black, yet the view to the horizon was unblemished because clean winds blew in low, pulled by the need of the flames.

The fires roared from sixty spouts, and each well that we passed was burning a little differently. One had flames rolling upward with lavalike consistency; another had straining tongues. The wind shifted and sent a barrier of fire across the road, instantly raising the temperature within the car. Venturing outside, I leaned against an Iraqi tank in awe. Raw crude flowed churlishly past my feet, on its way to the Gulf, a small tributary of the great marine spill. There were rivulets burning like lit fuses.

In my rubber boots I clomped about in this Styx a little too freely, for all at once the fumes—of benzene, toluene, etc., fresh out of the ground—hit me hard. I thought I would pass out. I was lucky that my friend got me back into the car and whisked me out of Al-Ahmadi. Had I been alone and collapsed in the oil . . . This was the second trip wire not to go off.

You see, bravado comes easily to the noncombatant. Having put myself in harm's way, I could hardly complain. Still, if I had become sick afterward, I might have looked back askance at the oil smoke and fumes, which are neurotoxic and carcinogenic, depending on the dose. And so with the hostilities over (148 slain on the American side, untold thousands on the Iraqi side), the health inventories commenced.

OF THE THREE environmental systems assaulted by the war—terrestrial, atmospheric, and marine—the land of Arabia was left in the worst shape because it could not disperse the pollution. The desert was pockmarked with glowering lakes of oil, land mines, dumps of military junk, and tons of half-burned human waste from the resident armies. Vehicle movements had pulverized the delicate soil, increasing erosion, and the goats and camels, forced into smaller areas, had aggravated the already bad state of overgrazing.

A March 2 story in the *Washington Post* was apocalyptic: "The Persian Gulf War has been an environmental catastrophe that has poisoned the air, land and sea and could threaten the health of millions of people, scientists and environmental specialists said yesterday."

According to the article, the major health threats stemmed from the oil slicks, oil fires, water pollution, and devastation of the desert ecosystem. "In addition, unknown amounts of poisonous chemicals from bombed Iraqi factories and weapons stockpiles, and of carcinogenic uranium slivers from armor-piercing allied shells, may have been released into the atmosphere." Here was an ominous reference to two agents that later were implicated in the gulf war illnesses.

The focus at first was on the oil fires. Nuclear winter didn't seem so far-fetched because the plumes were thick enough to be tracked by satellite. More than six hundred wells were burning, and four million barrels of oil were going up in smoke every day. Another hundred or so wells gushed their contents onto the ground. Putting out the fires and capping the wells was a massive undertaking, requiring ten thousand workers and two billion dollars, and took eight months.

The Pentagon moved quickly to evaluate the health risks of the smoke. According to a congressional agency that looked into the matter later, the Pentagon responded expeditiously, given that "Grave concerns had been raised by U.S. officials in Kuwait that the pollution from the fires could cause severe acute health effects, including death." The danger was not only to the troops, who were gradually being pulled out of the country, but also to the Saudis and Kuwaitis, including exiles wanting to know if it was safe to return.

Starting in early March, scientists from the United States and other countries measured the constituents and concentrations of the smoke. They took air samples both at ground level near the burning wells and from aircraft within the plumes. To their great surprise, they found the smoke acting in a way to minimize its impact on health and environment. "It went where you would want to put it," a U.S. Environmental Protection Agency official told me. The emissions melded in a superplume whose bottom stayed a half mile above the ground and whose top was about three miles. Most of the time the smoke was lifted out of breathing range, yet because it kept below the clouds and collected condensation, it washed out rapidly. Moreover, the fires were efficient in combusting the oil's most dangerous gases, such as benzene and hydrogen sulfide.

Local temperatures did drop temporarily (the cooler air may have affected the coral in the Gulf), but there were no regional changes in meteorology, no demonstrable effect on the Indian monsoon. The much-feared environmental nightmare (atmospheric version) did not come to pass. Gritty to start with, the air in Kuwait contained unhealthy particulates and compounds, but the concentrations were found to be typical for urban industrial areas of the world.

Summarizing the findings a year later, the World Meteorological Organization reported: "The fact that the plume rarely (if ever) touched the ground drastically reduced human health effects. The fact that it did not reach the stratosphere drastically reduced global effects."

The oil fires did not pose a health emergency; the researchers were sure about that. Nobody was thought to be at immediate risk in the spring of 1991 unless he or she had a preexisting condition like asthma. But the long-term prospects of disease were uncertain. After all, the troops would be absorbing some measure of particulates and toxic chemicals until the fires were contained. Atmospheric inversions in the summer and fall could increase their exposures. Who knew what chronic illness might develop down the line?

Among U.S. policy makers the weight of opinion was that the fires would have dangerous consequences. Part of the judgment was empirical. The TV pictures showed tremendous black billows sweeping the desert and engulfing troop formations. Military doctors were sending back reports of respiratory ailments, red eyes, coughing, and sore throats. Commanders recommended masks, goggles, and scarves for protection. Although few soldiers cared to suit up again, having repeatedly donned masks and other gear against the threat of poison gas, everyone recoiled from the ubiquitous smoke. In short, to the layman a phenomenon so impressive could not *not* be harmful.

The other part of the judgment was historical. Pentagon officials expected that some veterans would claim damage to their health whether or not their problems were related to the smoke. In April Thomas Baca, a deputy assistant secretary of defense, wrote a memo to superiors urging that scientific data on exposures be collected at once. "Congressional, scientific and public interest in this issue is growing," Baca warned. "We view the above actions necessary to help protect the health of our personnel and to limit any future liabilities and controversies."

Officials at the Department of Veterans Affairs had discussed the need for a postwar health registry even before the fighting started. Subsequently, Dr. James Holsinger, chief medical director of the VA, told Congress: "[W]e are in the process of working with DoD [Department of Defense] to develop a registry of individuals that served in the Persian Gulf so that we can prospectively track issues that might deal with the oil fires and other environmental agents, so that we will not be in a position of having to deal with this thirty years from now without knowledge as we have done with both the atomic veterans and the Agent Orange issue. . . . We are trying to get ahead of the game this time on issues of environmental hazards."

You really didn't have to see the smoke on TV or study the draft of the plumes. If you were a military health official during the Persian Gulf War, the painful lesson of Agent Orange came to mind immediately. It was a more important precedent, being recent, than the radiation exposures of post–World War II soldiers. Indeed a controversy that had started while the war in Vietnam was being waged was still being argued on the floor of the U.S. Congress at the time of Desert Storm.

"I didn't know precisely what would come out of this war," recalled VA Deputy Secretary Anthony Principi, "but I knew it would be something. We had made some terrible mistakes in the Vietnam War. I saw all that smoke, and I conjured up images of dioxin and Agent Orange. Those kids were breathing the stuff in. If and when they fell ill, they were going to be raising the issue. If they developed bronchial conditions, or lung cancer, they would feel that a substance had caused it, and there would be questions in the media and in Congress. . . .

"We shouldn't go through it again. I thought we needed to have a database, so we could try to establish a causal nature of the illnesses or at least a statistical association. I felt this very strongly. I said, 'If someone comes in even for an unrelated injury, a leg injury, let's determine if the person was exposed to smoke. Let's find it out *now*, and five years later, if they have a problem, then give *that* to the scientists, and see if they get the statistical associations.' "

It would take a separate book to do Agent Orange justice, if justice were even possible, so poisonous was the debate over the inconclusive facts. By inconclusive facts I mean the statistical associations that were produced, as Principi indicated, between exposure and disease.

Agent Orange got its name from being stored in orange barrels. Its active ingredients were the herbicides 2,4-D and 2,4,5-T, and it also contained dioxin, or TCDD, as an unwanted by-product of the manufacture of 2,4, 5-T. Roughly twenty million gallons of Agent Orange were sprayed over about 10 percent of the area of North and South Vietnam. The purpose was to deny the enemy the cover of vegetation and destroy his crops, but to opponents of the war it smacked of environmental terrorism (only equaled, perhaps, by the oil spill and oil fires in the Gulf). Not just Vietnamese were hit by Agent Orange. Over the years many American personnel were exposed as well, but how many, and with how much of the herbicide, were not recorded.

The Pentagon stopped using the defoliant before the war ended because research was beginning to show that dioxin and the other two compounds could cause birth defects in laboratory animals. During the 1970s the chemicals in Agent Orange acquired reputations as bad actors. Laboratory evidence against them was buttressed by epidemiological studies of civilian populations connecting the chemicals to cancerous diseases and reproductive problems.

The epidemiologists did not connect cause and effect, a relationship that in science requires a stringent standard of proof. Rather, an association was shown—"link" is the word used in the news media—between exposure and risk. For example, a much-publicized EPA study, known as the Alsea study, linked one of the herbicides to miscarriage. Pregnant women in Oregon were found to have had a greater risk of miscarriage if they lived in counties where forests were sprayed with 2,4,5-T than if they lived somewhere else.

Now, an increased health risk qualifies as a real phenomenon only if it passes a mathematical test of its "statistical significance," without which the link between the exposure and the adverse outcome may be dismissed as pure chance: another of the hard knocks of life. Statistical significance conveys a rudimentary meaning to the finding. Suspicions (the hypothesis) have been fortified, but the true significance of the result is supposed to be explored further, with additional studies of risk and laboratory experiments. Eventually researchers may demonstrate a cause and effect relationship.

In the Alsea study the link between the herbicide and the miscarriages was declared statistically significant. What was the meaning? There were environmental factors other than spraying that might have contributed to the miscarriages, but the study was not intended to address any other factors. As for the exposures, it could not be proved that living in a county with sprayed trees actually caused pregnant women to absorb the herbicide into their bodies. The assumption was a reasonable one, however, and without reasonable assumptions science can not go forward. At any rate the imprimatur, "statistical significance," was sufficient for the politicians and regulators charged with protecting the public health. In 1979, 2,4,5-T was suspended from use in the United States. It went pretty much the same way for 2,4-D, the other herbicide in Agent Orange.

I am aware of having digressed from the smoky Gulf. But here come the parallels to the illnesses of concern to me. By the end of the 1970s Vietnam veterans began to report not only chronic health problems among themselves but also birth defects among their children. The medical conditions were of all types, hard to narrow down. The VA established a registry of the cases. Toxic chemical exposure was alleged, and scientific investigations were launched. The circumstances were much simpler than in the Gulf because only one environmental agent was implicated.

Federal researchers were hindered by the fact that the conditions manifested by Vietnam veterans, which, as the years passed, cohered around certain cancers, were not uncommon in men entering middle age. The hypothesis that Agent Orange caused their cancers was plausible, according to the studies of its components. Nevertheless, before the VA would pay compensation for disabling diseases, the conditions had to be rated as service-connected, which demanded of claimants a demonstration not only of exposure but also of cause and effect. So the veterans looked to the epidemiologists. The challenge put to the epidemiologists was to show that troops that had been exposed to Agent Orange were sicker than troops that had not. Ideally the studies would also show that the greater the exposure, the greater the likelihood of disease.

Such a fraught and thorny question could cost the VA a lot of money. Would the research be done fairly? Prodded by the press and veterans' groups, Congress in 1983 took the Agent Orange research away from VA and gave it to another agency, the Centers for Disease Control (CDC). The CDC floundered because it could not figure out a way, so long after the fact, to prove that Vietnam vets had been exposed.

Biomedical testing didn't work. Since the two herbicides themselves would have been rapidly expelled by the body, the scientists tested people for dioxin, which is stored in blood and fat. Dioxin was more toxic to boot. But the great majority of Vietnam vets, including those who were ill, had no more dioxin in their systems than ordinary civilians. The small minority who had actually handled and sprayed the stuff, known as the Ranch Hand cohort, showed higher levels of dioxin, but these men had no unusual incidence of disease.

Another approach was to infer the exposures from available records. The CDC sought to match the troop locations over the years with the times and places of the aerial spraying. This mammoth puzzle had too many missing pieces. Claiming that the picture of exposure was unreliable, the CDC abandoned the task.

It devolved into a scientific mess, leaving the VA and the vets at loggerheads over the validity of the compensation claims. In 1989 a court broke the impasse by ruling that the agency's demands were too strict. In considering the adverse health effects of dioxin, said the court, the VA ought to recognize those diseases for which there was a "significant statistical association," instead of a cause and effect relationship.

What a change ensued in the 1990s. With Congress pointing the way, the VA amended its regulations. Any veteran who had been to Vietnam was presumed to be exposed. The number of diseases presumed to have resulted from the presumed exposures grew. Except for one condition, non-Hodgkin's lymphoma, it was not demonstrated that Vietnam vets suffered from higher rates of any cancer than veterans who hadn't served in Vietnam. Almost all the statistical associations between the diseases and the defoliant had to be taken from studies of chemical workers, farmers, and populations elsewhere. In 1996 lung cancer and prostate cancer were added to the list of compensable conditions. As if lung cancer and prostate cancer had never been in the cards before Agent Orange.

I WANT TO return to the Arabian coast, where illnesses don't exist yet, though a fertile anxiety does, and where science still thinks it can escape the reach of politics. As they contemplated the awesome fires, the military health officials knew that if diseases eventually developed, data about smoke exposures were going to be critical to a proper understanding. Lack of such information had doomed the work on Agent Orange.

In April 1991 it was decided to send a research team from the U.S. Army Environmental Hygiene Agency to the area. The team's assignment was to gather enough information about the smoke to produce a risk assessment— a calculation of the probability of disease developing among the troops according to the amount of hazardous pollution they were exposed to.

A risk assessment is a quasi-scientific technique. It seeks to model real conditions with the help of a computer. The calculation of the risk depends on the quality of the assumptions used in the model, and in this instance they involved the volume of air passing in and out of people's lungs and the potency of the airborne chemicals and particulates to cause disease. Actual data went into the model too. I am not going to look hard at the mechanics of the procedure because the risk turned out to be minor. The exercise is what matters. The assessment of the Kuwaiti oil fires was the first of many attempts to define the toxic hazards of the war, and it was the only one with a chance of succeeding because the exposures were ongoing. The substances of concern later—nerve gas and prophylactic pills and uranium dust—were never measured and left fewer traces than Agent Orange, so that reconstructing their effects on the human body was nearly impossible.

The army researchers arrived in early May. They set up monitoring equipment at eight sites in Kuwait and northern Saudi Arabia. Over the next seven months they collected four thousand samples of the air and soil. As was the pattern, the smoke lofted and dispersed broadly. Critics said afterward that the sampling had missed those late-winter occasions when the plumes grazed the ground, a valid point, but the extra exposures from such events would not have changed the estimate of the long-term risks, according to the leader of the team, a physiologist named Jack Heller.

Not all the air pollution sprang from the fires. "I think a lot of what we were measuring," Heller said, in a statement to the Presidential Advisory Committee on the gulf war illnesses, "was the industrial activity in Kuwait and . . . in Saudi Arabia; the natural sand; and the metals associated with the natural sand. If you look at our lead levels, our lead levels tended to go up as the fires went out in Kuwait, and that is because more and more vehicular traffic went in. They burn leaded gasoline. . . ."

The overall risk calculations, as I indicated, were reassuring. For cancer, the most serious of the long-term threats, the risk at the sites with the highest pollution was two chances in a million. In other words, if a million people had been exposed at the smokiest place around the clock for seven months, two of them would be expected to contract cancer in the future. This rate is officially permissible. Given such a risk at a toxic waste site in the States, environmental regulators would take no action.

"No site had a higher cancer risk level," Heller told me, "than Khobar Towers, Saudi Arabia, in the city of Dhahran. The risk was from the benzene and heavy metals in the city air. I might add the levels we detected are probably no worse than you would breathe in the average U.S. city."

Khobar Towers, far from the fires, pricked my attention for several reasons. One, I had been by the location, a housing complex turned over to the military by the Saudis. Two, though I didn't meet her then, Carol Best, the subject of the next chapter, lived at Khobar Towers after being called up by the army reserves.

I asked Heller about Carol's risk of cancer as a result of her posting.

"Remember it's an incremental risk," he said. "Her two in a million is added on to her normal thirty percent risk." The overall probability of her contracting cancer was 0.300002, the last digit representing the faint input of Khobar.

The researchers also figured the noncancer risk—i.e., the general threat to health—using an EPA standard called the hazard index. The benzene and the particulates in the air at Khobar Towers and other sites made for a hazard that would be of modest regulatory concern, Heller conceded. "But because of EPA's conservatism," he said, "the index is set for a sensitive individual, such as a child or a person with asthma. The hazard index is designed to protect those people. Your reservist wouldn't have been deployed if she were among the most sensitive." He did not know Carol.

These reckonings for Carol had nothing to do with Carol the person, for a risk assessment is based upon a group or population. The results may be extrapolated to the individual as a point of interest, but the individual does not exist outside the realm of the group. The health risk is an average, and scientists recognize that no one person is average. So you might say that Carol and her two extra chances in a million of cancer do not have any significance, statistically.

She, and other veterans of the war, would naturally object. The picture of reality construed by the individual—the anecdote made general, the personal wrought large—clashes with the scientist's mode, which is to collect as many individual accounts as possible, compare them with accounts from other circumstances and then reduce them all to a general rule. On the one hand, you have people who remember being gravely exposed to the oil smoke, and on the other hand, a computer model showing their exposures to be minimal and their health risks negligible. How are the views to be reconciled? Science may hold the intellectual upper hand, but outside that arena our democratic system tends to value the convictions of individuals over any process, even an academic process, that treats individuals as grist.

That is my explanation, in any event, for Public Law 102-90, the second piece of legislation dealing with the consequences of the Persian Gulf War.

Heller's team had not yet reported its results. In late 1991, prompted by the persistence of the fires and the specter of Agent Orange, Congress mandated the health registry and medical program that the VA and Defense Department had been talking about (but not implementing). Congress further required the Pentagon to determine the exposures of all members of the armed forces who had been subject to the "fumes from burning oil wells."

The law gave the individual the right to know his or her risk. Heller's initial study, by contrast, only averaged the risks by means of representative sampling. His air pumps and filters had not followed soldiers moving about the desert but monitored the conditions at eight fixed locations. Heller assumed that nobody could get a higher dose of smoke than a hypothetical individual at his Al-Ahmadi site, for instance. The equipment here was situated less than a mile from the fires I have described previously.

Now a much more difficult chore befell him: to match the paths of hundreds of thousands of persons with the daily flux of the smoke and its hazards. The weather and pollution data were more or less in hand, but to quote from a report of the General Accounting Office of Congress, "Accounting for all individuals and their daily whereabouts during the war would be a massive and perhaps impossible undertaking."

With the help of intelligence officers, an army task force crunched the logs of the troop movements. When a unit's location was resolved for a given day, the information was turned over to Heller and his staff. They in turn figured the exposures according to the wind patterns and the unit's distance from the nearest of the eight sampling sites. In this manner exposures were estimated for each unit for every day the fires burned, with everybody in the unit assumed to get an equal dose. The final step was to calculate each individual's risk according to the number of days he or she had spent with the unit.

The monumental map took seven years to assemble, during which time illnesses did break out as feared, although few doctors, if any, believed that the oil fires were the reason. The risks derived for individual servicemen and women contained no surprises, no departures from Heller's initial estimates. If there were people likely to become ill from their exposures, they were not soldiers but those who had labored in the belch of the flames putting out the conflagration. Yet a survey of one hundred firefighters turned up none of the health problems reported by veterans.

This was a foolish exercise demanded by Congress, it seems to me, because it presumed that science could provide for every veteran a useful answer, in hard numbers, to the vaporous questions of health and risk. Indeed the sense was that the individual was *owed* such information, in recognition of his or her service to the nation. What did it mean in the full context of a person's perilous life? I am thinking not just of the baseline probability of cancer, Carol's one chance in three going in. She might have been called up five years later. If Carol Best had been billeted at Khobar Towers on June 25, 1996, as part of the force keeping an eye on Iraq following the Persian Gulf War, her health risk would have been sky-high. That day a terrorist truck bomb was exploded outside the fence of the complex, killing nineteen and injuring hundreds.

PUTTING ASIDE THE toxic hypothesis, a conception of health that, as I've tried to establish, includes equal parts Agent Orange, Iraqi poison gas, and Kuwaiti oil smoke, I go to dinner in the Algosaibi Hotel.

It is the evening of February 25, 1991. Yesterday marked the start of the ground war, the long-awaited thrust into Kuwait. On CNN in the lobby, blurred reports of the action. Outside, suddenly, an air-raid siren.

Scud missiles, everyone said, could not be aimed accurately, and besides, they often broke up in descent. Dhahran was a sprawl with many vacant pockets, the highways sprinting through. If you were going to get hit by a Scud, your odds were about the same as being hit by space debris in Times Square, or so I figured.

This Scud's warhead hit a warehouse in an area called Sport City, about five miles from the hotel. What a terrible fluke! The warehouse, standing nearly alone, like a bull's-eye on the scrubby plain, had recently been converted to a barracks. The barracks sheltered sixty-nine members of the 14th Quartermasters, an Army Reserve unit, which had arrived from Greensburg, Pennsylvania, six days before.

After the blast a fire burned intensely for about twenty minutes. By the time I got over there, ambulances were pulling out and helicopters were landing. The building had lost its roof. The skin was peeled away, exposing red-painted girders, some of which were akimbo. Insulation splattered the barbed wire ringing the complex, and an interior fence had been bent back from the shock. As a truck trained its strong headlights on the building, the beams passing through made it look like a grinning jack o'lantern.

Nineteen people died, including thirteen members of the Pennsylvania unit. Thirty-seven others of the unit were wounded, many sustaining deep cuts from the shrapnel and ruptured eardrums from the blast. With a casualty rate of almost three-quarters, the 14th Quartermasters were essentially wiped out. For Americans it was the worst single stroke of the Persian Gulf War.

A VA medical report picks up the story:

The 37 WIA [wounded in action] were treated at five different medical facilities in Saudi Arabia. There was considerable confusion within the unit concerning identity of the killed and wounded, as well as the status of the survivors. Members reported feeling considerable stress from what they perceived as intrusive contacts and aggressive reporting by media representatives, as well as concern about family members in the U.S. receiving these reports. Several members of the unit report being "debriefed" as a group by two chaplains shortly after the missile attack; however, it was generally agreed that this meeting was inadequate and poorly received. There appeared to no further organized effort to provide additional treatment for ongoing stress reactions. . . . Individuals reported substantial difficulty due to sleep disturbance, hypervigilance, intrusive recollections of the attack and its aftermath, and fear of separation from other unit members. . . . Surviving members of the 14th, reportedly against psychiatric advice, were evacuated early to medical facilities in Europe and then on to the United States.

The author of the report, Stephen Perconte, was a psychologist at the VA medical center in Pittsburgh, and after the 14th Quartermasters was brought home in March, he and a team of mental health counselors went to treat the soldiers' emotional wounds. Perconte believed the army had done a poor job. "These people were pissed off when we got them," he said. A month after the attack, better late than never, Perconte and his colleagues worked to head off the effects of posttraumatic stress disorder (PTSD). According to self-assessment questionnaires, five of twenty-four veterans were suffering from symptoms of PTSD already. Ironically, if they had been based at the front, the reservists might have been better off psychologically because specialists on duty there were prepared to treat the stress reactions to combat.

You recognize that I have come to the other hypothesis—to the idea that the gulf war illnesses must be rooted somehow in psychological stress. Like an old sweater, stress is a term that has grown baggy from overuse. I define it as a psychophysiological response to threatening events and, rather than expound (more will come later), note simply that stress has both internal and external components. There is substantial variation in how people are affected by stressful events, not unlike the range in biological responses to alien chemicals. Without much stretching you can consider stress an environmental agent like gas or smoke.

But now is posttraumatic stress disorder truly the way into the problem of the gulf war illnesses? The afflicted veterans always bridled at the mention of PTSD, and their supporters ridiculed it as an explanation for the health mystery. PTSD was to become a whipping boy in the political debate. I don't hold it to be the explanation for what happened either. It did occur, but statistically it was a separate item, though sometimes overlapping the unexplained physical symptoms.

Remember that in my retrospective treatment there are no ailments yet, only rival frameworks for thinking about sickness. The Vietnam War had left a second legacy for the medical management of the gulf war soldiers. Just as the Pentagon and VA tried to collect information on toxic exposures lest the debacle of Agent Orange be repeated, so the military agencies, even before the fighting started, planned for posttraumatic stress disorders, which, erupting in ugly and truculent forms, had ambushed them in the decade following Vietnam. I start with PTSD because it relates to the stress hypothesis in the same way that oil pollution relates to the conception of toxic exposures: PTSD was an important red herring.

The disorder arises from an unusual horror or a near encounter with death and consists of three categories of symptoms. There are flashbacks and nightmares of the traumatic experience; an emotional remove from anything that might evoke the experience, sometimes called numbing; and a jumpy, hyperaroused state, prompting the startle response. This is very serious stuff, seemingly hard to miss in any individual. Yet PTSD did not attain a formal diagnostic entity and a place in the psychiatric manuals until 1980.

Why the delay? The condition must have appeared among warriors before Vietnam. It is not the same as battle fatigue or the earlier shell shock, well known terms for the acute reactions to stress, which are quickly apparent. Posttraumatic stress may develop weeks later, as after the Scud attack on the Quartermasters, yet the sufferers may not be noticed for months or years, as after Vietnam. The delay in recognizing PTSD was as much social as medical because society's disapproval of psychological ailments tended to keep veterans of the earlier wars under wraps. Ashamed, a man would not admit, even to himself, that he was not in full control of his nerves. Oprah and the modern forums of confession have eased things in that department.

At any rate, the prevalence of PTSD among Vietnam vets turned out to be extraordinarily high. According to surveys taken in the eighties, the phenomenon affected hundreds of thousands. Almost one-third of veterans reported having PTSD symptoms at some point in their lives. Reified by the Vietnam experience, posttraumatic stress then came to be regarded as a hallmark scar of rape, child abuse, earthquakes, airplane crashes, and disasters in general. Here is an excellent example of a diagnosis that becomes common once doctors have agreed upon an identity.

During Operation Desert Shield, the deployment and planning phase of the Persian Gulf War, military health officials made ready for as many as fifty thousand killed or wounded, including five thousand psychiatric casualties. The Defense Department planned to handle the first wave of the injured at its medical facilities at home and abroad, and the VA would take the spillover. To do its part, the VA staged a force of one thousand psychiatrists, psychologists, social workers, psychiatric nurses, and counselors at its hospitals and outreach centers around the country. Each VA medical center already had a PTSD clinical team, under the direction of the agency's National Center for PTSD, which had been established some years before.

There is nothing complicated about the clinical approach to traumatic stress. Talk therapy, which the military calls debriefing, would be offered to the returning veterans. In groups and private sessions, individuals would be encouraged to recognize their feelings and to respect the power of the events that caused them. Debriefing was also a tool in place for the front-line psychiatrists. The procedure was to counsel troops as soon as possible following grisly incidents or deaths, to reassure them that their feelings of shock were normal, and to return them to duty. Before the fighting a small number of soldiers broke down even without a trigger. The army was proud of its record of turning them around.

When the bombing began and Desert Shield became Desert Storm, the tension in the forward units increased. Anxiety reached its height on the eve of the invasion; the predictions were that twenty thousand Americans might be killed by chemical and biological weaponry. Mental health professionals from the Walter Reed Army Institute of Research queried several thousand of the troops before and after the action:

> Most soldiers interviewed described the beginning of the Ground War as the greatest stress reliever of the months of deployment. Confidence in training was extremely high. The major underlying fear during the initial assault appeared to be the threat of chemical and biological warfare. This was compounded for many by concerns about the effective life of MOPP [mission-oriented protective posture] gear and conflicting beliefs about anti-chemical and biological agents (drugs and vaccines). Some soldiers worried as much or more about the potential harmful effects of these protective measures as they did about the enemy's chemical and biological weapons. Clearly training in this aspect of combat preparations was inadequate.

Because the combat ended quickly, the contingency plans for massive psychological injuries were left on the shelf. Relieved, the commanders did not think about PTSD developing, and if they did, the thought was, How could there be PTSD from a four-day war? Debriefings took place in the field after the fighting, but the efforts were spotty. In hindsight military health officials are a bit embarrassed by the execution of their postwar mental health programs. "We didn't do them very well," Ronald Blanck, the army surgeon general, told me. "We were prepared but fell short."

As I have noted, a number of investigators have revisited the wartime conditions, interpolating psychological stresses and toxic hazards, depending on their points of view, but I think it's better to view the conditions metaphorically. Alternately tedious and tense, set in a land raked by smoke and strange chemicals, with alarms going off and officials telling you not to worry—the war was a nightmare version of postindustrial life that would tax anyone's health.

Safe in my hotel, I was too wrapped up in what I was going to see the war from another's perspective. But I met an officer at breakfast there one day who had endured an acute exposure. Several men in his unit had died in a friendly fire incident. He described the file of soldiers in the middle of nowhere, a plane appearing, a plane wheeling and attacking them, an American A-10. "We kept waving them off," he said, "but it turned and came back." The soldier searched my face entreatingly, holding me at the table, as if I had the power to shut off the plane's cannon. He needed to tell me some more, or perhaps to tell it again, because repeating it was the only way of deleting it. Sorry, man, I gotta go.

I went home and started to write about the environmental damage of the war. I had a deadline to meet, a kind of debriefing on paper. Six days after returning I was taken to the hospital with severe chest pains. I heard voices yelling, "Stat," just like on TV, as I collapsed at the admissions desk. My heart rate fell to twenty-eight beats per minute, prompting the emergency room attendants to inject me with atropine.

Atropine, how fitting. The vets in the Gulf had carried atropine injectors in order to save themselves, or try to, if they were being overcome by nerve gas. Atropine reduces the biochemical havoc at nerve junctions. In my case it blocked a particular nerve that was depressing my heartbeat.

Fortunately I had pericarditis, an inflammation of the membrane around the heart, and not an infarction. I was soon released from intensive care since the condition can be treated with aspirin and ibuprofen.

The cardiologist said that pericarditis is caused by a virus, often an unknown virus. He speculated that I had been exposed to something unusual in the Gulf. I considered it one of those things that happen and go by. I declined to undergo further tests to see if there might be anything wrong with my heart. In my study that spring, gobbling Bayer and Motrin simultaneously, I strained to complete my magazine article. I scribbled furiously and fought with my editor. In short, I was not in good shape, mentally or physically.

Some of the veterans were not feeling well either. On the one hand, the medical support for them had been excellent. The accident rate and disease rate were lower than in any previous American conflict. Having been segregated from a skittish Saudi society, the troops were better off for the lack of alcohol, drugs, and sexual contacts. On the other hand, large numbers of men and women had suffered from fatigue, diarrhea, colds, flu, back strains, and muscle injuries. People felt worse because of the heat, dust, smoke, overcrowding, and pressure.

Whereas after prior wars the troopships had made possible a period of decompression, a chance to digest the experience on the long trip home in the company of people who understood, the Persian Gulf vets were rapidly reintegrated with their families. Regular military personnel resumed life on the base, and the reservists and National Guard were dropped back into their civilian existences as abruptly as they had been snatched out of them. It was a good move on the surface, yet it left feelings of disorientation in it wake. Spouses and children had not stood still in the interim. Veterans had to adjust to newly independent wives, upset kids, and uncertain employment. Some reservists found they had lost their jobs. Meanwhile the Pentagon started again to cull its active duty ranks, a process interrupted by the war.

In April 1991, at the height of the pullback, Congress stipulated that the Defense Department and VA should "assess the need for rehabilitative services for member of the Armed Forces...who experienced PTSD." Six months before the legislation on the smoke exposures, this was the first congressional measure regarding the health of the gulf war veterans.

The Pentagon, as I indicated, minimized the need for this task. In fact the Pentagon never turned in the comprehensive report that was stipulated. The Department of Veterans Affairs, because it had PTSD programs in place, responded better. The point I wish to make is that in the latter half of 1991, the top health officials at both agencies were more concerned about the threat of the oil fires than about damage to the troops' mental health.

But you must also understand the difference in medical posture between the two agencies. It will be critical when the baffling illnesses break out. The Defense Department would take care of acute injuries to its forces, including nervous breakdowns on the battlefield, but it was not in the business of managing chronic conditions. It didn't want to know about them. A person with a chronic medical or psychological condition was by definition unfit for duty and had to leave the service, at which point he or she became the VA's responsibility. The VA was used to chronic conditions and would provide free care and even compensation for them, but only if they were ruled to be service-connected and disabling. Thus the regular soldier had an incentive to stay well or to suppress a health problem, while the retired soldier or reservist had to call attention to a health problem in order to receive government benefits.

Harry Becnel, Ph.D., a mental health counselor who was activated for the war by the army reserves, ran one of the better Defense Department programs. Becnel was posted to Fort Benning, Georgia, which processed five thousand returning soldiers. He got the army brass to agree to a pilot program of readjustment counseling. He and two colleagues debriefed about eleven hundred of the troops and one hundred spouses, concentrating on the combat units because he thought they would be the most vulnerable to PTSD. Some 80 percent of the Fort Benning cohort, in other words, was not seen by the counselors.

Gathering the men in groups, Becnel had them make lists of the wartime events that affected their mental outlooks. They discussed stressors (e.g., the waiting for combat, the sound that your armored vehicle made as it rolled over dead bodies at night, officers constantly changing their orders); stress defusers (mail from home, the support within a cohesive unit, the news that the war was over); and intrusive or upsetting memories (having to shoot at fleeing, ill-equipped teenage Iraqi soldiers). Becnel did not formally assess if men were suffering from PTSD symptoms; his judgment was that serious mental disorders were few. He noticed, however, that many complained of gastrointestinal problems.

By contrast, the VA's evaluation of PTSD was methodical. Ten VA facilities screened a total of forty-five hundred people, mainly reserve members and recently retired soldiers. Combining the results of the surveys, the VA reported that about 9 percent of the veterans met the criteria for PTSD. Additionally about a third of those sampled experienced "other forms of significant distress during the months after their return from the Middle East," such as depression. The vets who needed psychological treatment were offered it, though not all would accept it. The VA provided less structured debriefings and counseling at its hospitals and outreach centers around the country.

There was an unforeseen consequence to the VA focus on PTSD. All the mental health professionals who looked for the condition among gulf war veterans were successful in finding it, according to their surveys. But by the time the doctors published their results—the papers appeared in professional journals in 1992, 1993, and 1994—many gulf war vets were undergoing a different sort of travail, and to them the PTSD publications were just another way of telling them that their physical symptoms were all in their heads. That is when PTSD became the whipping boy of the controversy.

Though I am jumping ahead of my story, again I aver that PTSD and the gulf war illnesses were separate creatures. However, the former did contain a useful portent to the latter, for those who had been trained to recognize it.

Experts who had studied the fallout of traumatic events knew that in addition to jumpiness, nightmares, and avoidance, the subjects often had problems with their physical health. It was true of Vietnam veterans, as well as of flood victims, battered women, Israeli combat veterans, prisoners of war, prostitutes, refugees from Cambodia, and Pennsylvania residents who had fled the Three Mile Island nuclear accident, to name some of the various populations studied. All these people had in common an increase in health complaints, things going wrong with their bodies quite apart from the emotional effects of their frightening experiences.

At the height of Operation Desert Storm, in February 1991, an expert panel of civilian psychologists predicted there would be both physical and mental health repercussions to the gulf war experience. Under the leadership of Stevan Hobfoll, a psychologist at Kent State University in Ohio, the panel put together a list of the symptoms that the military should expect among returning veterans and their families. One half of the reactions were obviously within the purview of mental health: shame, uncontrolled crying, flashbacks, suicidal thoughts, substance abuse. But the other half, drawn from the understanding of "stress-related physical illness," matched the hallmarks of the illnesses to come. Mentioned were sleep problems, headaches, gastrointestinal disorders, musculoskeletal pain, difficulty in concentrating, weakness and lack of stamina. Only rashes and shortness of breath, of the most frequently reported gulf war symptoms, were not on the psychologists' list.

A report by Hobfoll and colleagues, titled "War-Related Stress," was published in a professional journal in August. It was both a warning and a plea to the government to plan for treatment. Apparently the article was not widely read; no doubt it seemed overblown in light of the easy victory in the Gulf. I searched for references to the report in the publications of VA researchers who had tracked PTSD following the demobilization. I found that Hobfoll's predictions were discussed only in the work of Patricia Sutker, a psychologist at the VA medical center in New Orleans.

Bear with me on this twisting paper trail, for it is about to lead to the first sight of the gulf war illnesses, the pure cases, I call them, glimpsed here by Pat Sutker during the triumphant summer of 1991, many months before the problem escalated to the notice of health officials, political leaders, and the press.

Sutker was no novice. She had worked for years with veterans who had been held in prisoner of war camps during World War II and the Korean War. The Korean POWs in particular made an impression her. On the threshold of old age these men spoke about their brutal experiences for the first time. Many still wrestled with feelings of posttraumatic stress and depression, and they also conveyed to her their numerous bodily complaints.

In a review paper published around the time of the Persian Gulf War, Sutker observed that "somatic distress and psychological disturbances seem to be inexplicably intertwined." For the former she listed "fatigue, headaches, gastrointestinal disturbance, problems with respiration, hearing and vision losses, and chronic pain." She did not argue that these ailments were psychosomatic because after all the POW camps had truly assaulted the men's health, by exposing them to malnutrition, frostbite, and infectious disease, and because the men were at an age when health naturally declines. Cause and effect were not addressed; Sutker discussed only the correlation between mental and physical states.

As the director of the VA's PTSD team in New Orleans, Sutker was asked to evaluate the local gulf war veterans. She and her colleagues, visiting armories on summer and fall weekends, handed out questionnaires to measure the reservists' moods. On the face of it these vets on weekend drill were nothing like her elderly ex-POWs. Nevertheless, if they were harboring PTSD, she would try to arrest it.

After hearing Sutker talk, some of the vets made appointments for individual therapy. She recalled that in the first session or two, as she conducted a formal psychological interview, "I kept hearing about how they were feeling today." As a few more came to see her, she paid more attention to the theme of general health. "I was struck, I was floored by what they reported. Not at age twenty should they be so tired, as they were saying. These were young men talking about their dizziness or their headaches. Women go to doctors more, and they endorse these kinds of symptoms, but men *never* say they have all this."

Now when she went out to the armories, Sutker distributed a health symptom checklist in addition to the questionnaires about anger, depression, and startle reactions. The same spectrum of health complaints showed up. "I thought, Is that what happened to them in the war?"

Sutker did not assume that the maladies being reported to her were the products of stress. She proceeded cautiously because, as in her previous work, she was handicapped by an inability to verify what she was being told. "Complaints are fine and dandy, but more needs to be done than just recording them. We would have needed a physician to really go after these symptoms—take their blood, et cetera."

"Also," she added dryly, "it would be nice to know who we sent off to war." She was referring to the lack of a baseline: good prewar medical information about reservists who developed health problems afterward.

Sutker and her team wrote up their assessment of 215 gulf war vets. They first divided the subjects according to the amount of stress they had experienced. Having been asked about austere living conditions, Scud missile attacks, perceptions of injury and death, and other sources of discomfort, the veterans were assigned to either a high-stress or a low-stress category, depending on how they had rated the items.

Then the researchers looked at the two groups' scores on the psychological batteries. "Based on the Hobfoll . . . model," they explained, "we hypothesized that as war-zone stress severity increased, the frequency and severity of psychological symptoms would be greater. . . ." This correlation was borne out, as the high-stress group scored higher on scales measuring anger, anxiety, depression, and PTSD symptoms.

But the difference between the two groups was most stark in terms of general health. The high-stress veterans "endorsed twice as many complaints about bodily discomfort and physical well-being than did their low war-zone stress severity counterparts, particularly feelings of nervousness and tension, general aches and pains, and disturbed concentration, a symptom picture unusual for young to midlife adults. . . ."

Unlike the psychologists at other VA centers, Sutker administered the same tests to reservists who had never been sent to the Gulf, so as to have an unaffected group for comparison. Her nondeployed group scored roughly the same as the low-stress veterans, suggesting that there was a level of stress that warriors could tolerate without aggravating their mental or physical health. For half the veterans in the study, this threshold had apparently been breached.

When she looked closer, Sutker found that the most troubled vets came from a reserve unit whose job had been to identify corpses and sort human remains. Their high rate of PTSD and somatic complaints skewed her entire sample. For this and other reasons I must not overstate Sutker's findings or extend them too far in the direction of the as yet unrecognized ailments. But because she recorded the health problems of scores of people who were not yet seeking medical treatment, her work is a valuable early snapshot. It indicates that the gulf war ills did not break out a year or more after the conflict, as they seemed to the public. The rough beast didn't come out of nowhere.

In July 1991 the Senate Committee on Veterans' Affairs held a hearing in Washington on the readjustment problems of Persian Gulf War veterans and their families. Most of the testimony centered on domestic and financial stresses. But a veteran named Steve Robertson, who worked as a lobbyist for the American Legion, warned the senators about "health problems that I believe are in the future."

Of his own problems, Robertson mentioned increased family strains, a cough and diarrhea that were not getting better, and startle reactions, triggered by the sirens in Washington. He was concerned about microorganisms in his body, for which, he said, he had never been tested on leaving the Gulf. He talked about the oil fires, the smoke drifting as far as Khobar, and about garbage being burned, adding fumes of plastic and rubber to the air. Robertson's health was indeed on the skids. Soon he became one of the most outspoken sufferers of the "syndrome."

Another witness before the Senate committee, Lieutenant Colonel Darlene Anderson, told of her young son's reaction to her when she came home on a break from the war: "He said that I was more distracted, that I didn't seem to listen as well and was more preoccupied. He was very concerned about chemicals and that I would either come back dead or that the chemicals would make me different, so he kept asking what was wrong with me."

A third witness, a psychologist named Dennis Embry, was the most prophetic. PTSD and the Vietnam experience were misleading us, he said. "If we keep looking in that direction over our left shoulder, which is where we got hit the last time, we will not notice the truck that might hit us from the right. . . . I don't think it is just a mental health issue here. Again, if we look back at the stress research which has been funded by NIMH and NIH [federal health agencies], we are also looking at issues of physical illness which will have unknown impacts."

Clearly something was gaining strength in the aftermath of Desert Storm, a minor chord beneath the fanfare, like a motif by Stravinsky drowned out by Sousa. I have tried to distinguish between constructs of illness, asking what did the health authorities know and when did they know it, but in real time, of course, it was coming together in a rush and a jumble.

In the late fall of the year two young doctors at Walter Reed Army Medical Center in Washington, Alan Magill and Robert Gasser, began to see patients who perplexed them. The two doctors were specialists in infectious diseases, and when they examined gulf war veterans, they were most on the lookout for viscerotropic leishmaniasis, a feverish condition caused by a desert organism. Leishmaniasis was the third red herring of the medical mystery, after the oil fires and PTSD.

I mentioned leishmaniasis in connection with John Cabrillo. The military had halted blood donations by active duty veterans of the war, such as John, largely because of the work done by Magill and Gasser in detecting this disease. Its characteristics included headache, fatigue, diarrhea, sweating, and sometimes a swollen liver and spleen, but it proved very difficult to diagnose. The bone marrow test for the organism wasn't foolproof. Magill and Gasser had identified eight cases for certain and were gearing up for a lot more, although as it turned out, they recorded only a dozen cases in total.

After the news about leishmaniasis had gone out, referrals to Walter Reed increased. The patients included active duty personnel and reservists from around the country. But though obviously unwell, these veterans of the war did not have infectious diseases. "There was something different about them," Gasser recalled. "We couldn't identify leishmaniasis in spite of aggressive workups. I am talking about an hourlong exam and then bringing them back in for more tests. We couldn't find it. Yet we were convinced that something had happened to them. Some of them had become nonfunctional."

The two doctors wondered if they were studying the wrong thing. "I became concerned about the tenor of these patients," said Magill. "They were angry. They were cooperative with us, yes, but they were ticked at what they had to do to be seen by us." He didn't think they had psychological problems. "Some were into what I call the sickness model, but most were real straight shooters. I didn't know *what* their problems were. I remember telling my superiors, 'Hey take this seriously. This might be the next Agent Orange.' "

Almost here, so the poet warned, "its hour come round at last." I don't know exactly what the sickness is (and even today can't be sure), but I believe it has been here before in different guises. Coalescing among the gulf war vets, it is looking for a language in which to express itself, so that society can recognize and respond to it. It cannot use the language of psychology, which is alien to the patients and distasteful to their supporters. It has to choose another mode.

January 16, 1992, marked the first anniversary of the hostilities, a year since the start of the bombing campaign. A group called the Military Families Support Network held a vigil outside the White House. By its own count one hundred people attended. The war was not over, the speakers said, not over for the families of America's dead and wounded. The country must not forget the ongoing casualties, including problems of adjustment. A veteran spoke of his frustration over poor medical treatment. He had been going from doctor to doctor with an undiagnosed skin disease.

The founder of the group, according to its newsletter, "expressed concern about what he called the 'witches brew of chemicals' given to the troops to stave off disease and/or counteract potential biological and chemical agents. He stressed the need for the Department of Defense to establish a central registry of who was given what drugs in case dangerous side effects develop."

The protest got some press, not much. But now it was here.

3

Carol Exposed

> Every journalist who is not too stupid or too full of himself to notice what is going on knows that what he does is morally indefensible. He is a kind of confidence man, preying on people's vanity, ignorance, or loneliness, gaining their trust and betraying them without remorse. Like the credulous widow who wakes up one day to find the charming young man and all her savings gone, so the consenting subject of a piece of nonfiction writing learns—when the article or book appears—*his* hard lesson. . . . [H]e has to face the fact that the journalist—who seemed so friendly and sympathetic, so keen to understand him fully, so remarkably attuned to his vision of things—never had the slightest intention of collaborating with him on his story but always intended to write a story of his own.
>
> *Janet Malcolm,* "The Journalist and the Murderer"

Cheerful and forthcoming, anxious and aching, Carol Best was quite unlike my first sick veteran, John Cabrillo. Because she did not follow the politics of "gulf war syndrome" closely or care much about them, she lacked an armor around her condition that might deflect my questions.

Earlier I gave you a snippet of Carol, when I derived her risk of contracting cancer from exposure to the oil smoke during her posting to the Gulf. I might have left it at that; I didn't have to get personal. I do not excuse myself. When the right and wrong of a dispute are unclear, usually a journalist will take the side of the individual against the system, the little guy against the establishment. Not this time, I'm afraid to say.

For I have an agenda for Carol, and I must push ahead with it. To me not only is she a story—a narrative blending her facts and my impressions—but she also represents a medical case, an epidemiological statistic helping fuel a political controversy, and an exemplar of the murky class of illnesses that have emerged in fin de siècle America. In other words, I have asked Carol to do a lot of work.

On May 8, 1997, Carol Best arrived at the West Los Angeles Veterans Affairs Medical Center, a referral patient from her home VA in Washington State. Her medical records, chock-full of test results and professional opinion, had not been sent ahead of her. Along with the transfer letter there came only a three-page form, which was her enrollment in the Persian Gulf Health Registry in 1993, and even that slim paperwork was incomplete. Moreover, the West L.A. VAMC was not ready for the veteran. The admitting office had Carol wait for hours in the emergency ward, where she didn't get to eat lunch, and as a result, she said, "my hypoglycemia kicked in." In the early evening, by now quite upset, Carol was admitted and given a room on the third floor. She is a trouper, and she soon recovered her cheerfulness.

The next day a nurse practitioner conducted the initial assessment. Carol's main complaints, which she said had begun with the war and gotten worse, were "loss of fine motor function [she was concerned about the coordination in her hands], chronic back pain, depression, migraine headaches, insomnia, hypersomnia [a more serious sleep disorder than insomnia], extreme fatigue, blurry vision, trouble ambulating [she often used a cane], joint pains and shortness of breath."

The director of the Persian Gulf referral program, Ronald Hamm, examined Carol. He ordered a round of tests, which would take several weeks to complete. He had a good feeling about her because she seemed open to his help. "She's an ideal candidate," he told me. "She's had a good relation with her treating physician, and she's not into blame or conspiracy thinking."

"Will you find anything?" I asked. I was on my way to her room to meet her.

"With her we expect to diagnose depression or chronic fatigue syndrome. I say 'or' because chronic fatigue syndrome is a rule-out diagnosis. One of things we have to rule out is depression, which can cause the fatigue."

Referring to her joint and muscle pain, Hamm continued, "I wasn't that impressed with her arthralgia symptoms. But she is already comfortable with the diagnosis of fibromyalgia given by her doctor at home." Fibromyalgia, a pain syndrome, has many features in common with chronic fatigue syndrome. As an afterthought Hamm said that Carol reported having "an MCS reaction" when she was exposed to certain paints.

Later I realized that the doctor had floated three conditions—chronic fatigue syndrome, fibromyalgia, and multiple chemical sensitivity—in regard to a patient whose own preferred view of her case was "gulf war syndrome." Although I did not understand yet how the four conditions overlapped, it must have been then that I fastened on Carol as a means to explore the question, Carol to be my workhorse if she would cooperate. Vulpine John, I already knew, was too private, his condition too extreme.

You may wonder at my approach. Having established opposing frameworks for the emergence of the gulf war illnesses, represented by Agent Orange and the oil fires, on the one hand, and by PTSD, on the other hand—rival expectations of illness before any illness existed—now I trot out a person named Carol and introduce three new entities, in shorthand CFS, FM, and MCS. But I am simply extending the same line of argument using different terms. The constructs that oversaw the birth of the gulf war ailments had also shaped the medical debate over chronic fatigue syndrome, fibromyalgia, and multiple chemical sensitivity. The same dichotomy applied. Three nebulous conditions, arising in the 1980s, having nothing to do with war: Were they primarily psychological in nature? Or were they based firmly in the body and aggravated by chemical exposures, as the majority of the patients maintained?

Because of their similarities to the veterans' illnesses, CFS, FM, and MCS drew a lot of attention in Washington in the early years of the gulf war health mystery, suggesting a direction for understanding the problem, if not for immediately resolving it. However, because they were tenuous too, struggling, as it were, for their own foundations in medicine, the three guideposts could not stand up to the mounting political pressure and were swept aside. Louder and less instructive arguments hijacked the veterans' illnesses, although CFS, FM, and MCS were reinstalled as models when the controversy eased, five years later.

You see how much work Carol has ahead of her.

ARRIVING ON THE third floor, I saw her coming down the hall. Hamm had told me Carol had Native American blood, and such is the power of suggestion that I observed foremost her tanned skin and smooth face, her centered bulk, and her single braid of long gray hair. Earth mother, I thought, trying to place her. Later, when I asked her, she was not clear about how much Indian was in her, so I stopped thinking of her that way, but the aura of serenity—or was it stolidity?—remained.

She was leaning on her cane and being escorted toward the elevator by a very tall, very thin physician. The doctor bent over her solicitously but possessively. The various specialists of the medical center, each assigned a portion of the gulf war protocol, sometimes had to compete for the patient's time.

Carol exhaled audibly. "I've been going nonstop," she said. Two hours later the doctor escorted her back.

The first thing she told me, when she had got onto the bed, was "I'm not in it for the money." Her bed was cranked up like a lounge chair. "I don't know *what* happened over there," she added, implying that something untoward had happened to her. "All I can say is, My health is bad."

Carol said that she was sent to the Gulf in July 1991, several months after the fighting was over. She worked first as a clerk in Dhahran (living at Khobar Towers) and then ran an art center for GIs in Kuwait City. An army reservist, she had volunteered to go, over the objections of some of her family. Carol had been in the military before, and she liked to travel. "I like excitement, I like strange things," she said. "If someone tells me I can't do something, that just makes me want to do it more."

Placidly braiding her hair, Carol needed no coaxing to talk. I pointed out that her nail polish, which was two-toned, mauve and turquoise, matched the colors of her shirt. She said that it wasn't intentional but that others today had remarked on it. When I asked her age, she fiddled with the clasp on her bracelet and answered, "I'm forty-five. I only *look* sixty-five." She didn't seem embarrassed, though. According to her chart, her weight had gone up since she'd been sick, from 135 to 210 pounds.

Her motive for giving me her story, Carol said, was that "it might help someone else. I know what it's like to be out there and wondering what's going on." I sensed she also wanted validation for herself. "Since this happened to me," she added, "I've been made to feel—not by people at this hospital, but at some others—that I'm faking it or stupid or that I'm in it for the money or the pills."

I nodded: a noncommittal nod, a reassuring nod. On the wheeled table next to her bed Carol had set out bottles of pills. When I inquired about them, she said, incongruously, "I don't take medications," and then she proceeded to name them: "Excedrin extra strength for headaches. Ultram—

that's a painkiller. Melatonin to help me sleep. Magnesium oxide to keep my food down. I have acid reflux." She was demonstrating to me that her regimen was lighter than it looked. "That one's Zoloft for depression. I call it my happy pill. I'm on a reduced dose, only a quarter of a tablet, because I really don't like pills. We are trying to go more with the natural stuff. These here are my vitamins."

Next I asked her about her experiences in the Gulf. "I went all over the place," she replied. "One day [in Dhahran] there was a weird rain. It was so clear and fine, and it never hit the ground. . . ."

"Was it mist?"

"It didn't *act* like a mist. Now I wonder, Was it chemicals?

"Another time I was going to store some supplies, boxes of stuff, in a Conex—that's what we called those huge transport containers—and I found it had chemicals in it. So I wouldn't use it."

She was picking the bracelet apart and putting it back together, and I must have called attention to it, for she said, "I'm just a nervous person, I guess." She wasn't a nervous person on the surface.

"I flew around in a helicopter. I visited many places in the combat zone. I remember once I climbed on an Iraqi tank. They gave us medication and insect repellent."

"I see," I said. "Are you giving me a list of possible exposures?"

She paused. "Yes. But I don't know what the chemical might have been. I can't say, 'Here's the chemical sitting there.' All I know is—well, I injured my neck and back; that was one thing. But when I got home, I was weak and tired, and sick to my stomach. I thought it was the traveling, but the weakness and the tiredness stayed. It got worse and worse. At the VA hospital all they asked us was 'Did you inhale [oil] smoke?'" Then they told me, 'Oh, you're just tired and depressed.' "

Carol was shortening the time. Returning home in April 1992, she didn't go to the VA for the Persian Gulf Health Registry exam for another eighteen months. Immediately on her return, however, while still on active duty, she saw an army doctor about her neck and back. Her back had been bothering her since December, and the neck injury had occurred in March, as she was lugging heavy boxes, closing up her art center in Kuwait.

"Then the pain started," she continued. "I had headaches every day. Some days I've had blurry vision and some days it is tunnel vision. There are days when I can't remember my kids' names or my *dog's* name. When

I'm really tired, I slur my words and I can't think what I mean to say. I used to enjoy hiking and white-water rafting, and now I walk with a cane. My hands are so weak that a jar of Gatorade is hard for me to open. I called Gatorade to complain.

"Today is one of my better days, but if you hug me like this"—she squeezed her upper arm—"it hurts." This was an allusion to her fibromyalgia, whose symptoms are tenderness and a sharp sensitivity to pain—without swelling or inflammation—at numerous points around the body. A year before, fibromyalgia had caused her to take a disability retirement from her civilian job. Fatigue characterizes the condition too, but when I mentioned that Dr. Hamm suspected CFS, Carol said, "I never heard about chronic fatigue syndrome until I got here."

"Do you think you are sensitive to chemicals?"

"I'm more sensitive than most people. I never had a problem when I worked around jet engines in the seventies, but since then I'm allergic to ether and to cleaning products, like the stuff they use on the printing presses where I worked last. I have had asthma attacks. Today, if someone comes into the room wearing Gloria Vanderbilt perfume, I get a headache, and if I'm exposed to it too long, I'll have an asthma attack.

"But I don't get hay fever at all. And when I was in the Gulf, I only had to use my inhaler twice. What I mean is, I didn't have asthma over there. So that's not it. Something else happened. It started with the tiredness, and now it's causing me to lose the use of my hands and have trouble walking."

Clearly Carol was more than "more sensitive than most people." Although the condition called multiple chemical sensitivity could account for all the health problems she reported, she would not receive the diagnosis of MCS, not at this hospital anyway. The VA, like most government agencies, thought the MCS criteria too vague. The credibility of this condition was not in the league of CFS and FM, which only lately had achieved a doctors' consensus. Besides, Carol herself never broached multiple chemical sensitivity. It was not a diagnosis she was pursuing.

"At home I teach art two days a week and I'm totally exhausted," she was saying. "I take care of my seventy-five-year-old mom, and it turns out she has to take care of *me*. I can't do the construction or the electrical work around the house that I used to do.

"About a year and a half ago I got to where I was suicidal. I thought, *No one* can help me. I was going to take some pills, but my daughter walked in and stopped me. She knocked the pills out of my hand."

I was taken aback by this turn in her story, which she conveyed in the same matter-of-fact tone.

"So I sought psychiatric help, first through work and then later through the VA. I mean I went to see a headshrinker."

"What was the thrust of the therapy?" I asked. "What kinds of things did they have you work on?"

"The idea was to help me to cope, at first. Then it was trying to figure out what in my life may have contributed to my illness. But I didn't learn anything from that part of it."

"You don't think that has anything to do with it."

"I don't think my disease is psychological at all," she said firmly. "Before I left, I had a breathing problem. They call it occupational asthma. But otherwise I had only a hysterectomy and normal illnesses. When they diagnose depression, I say, 'Yeah, I'm depressed all right—because I have the headaches and the tiredness.' "

Carol returned to the loss of her physical activities. "I used to like to garden. A few weeks ago I was out in the yard, and I was only able to plant five flowers. I had to call up my son to come and help me. . . . All this stuff I'm used to doing I can't anymore, and so I break down, and I cry, and then I get angry."

Her eyes flashed; no more playing with the bracelet. "What went down over there? Let us know! Somebody *knows* what went down! Tell us so the doctors know what to look for and they can help us get our health back. They're making a game of us. I'm not some little small-town person, you know. What about Agent Orange? They *knew* about Agent Orange."

I didn't say anything.

"It wasn't just reservists who got it, you know. A lot of my boys have kept in touch, and I know of active duty people who are sick."

"Boys?"

"That's what I called them. The young GIs who'd come in to my art center. They called me Mom. They'd come and talk with me, the Special Forces guys, who were shook up. I let them cry on my shoulder."

After a moment she said, "This may be the last resort. These guys are the expertise, and I can't go any further. In my heart I feel I won't get better. But I came here because I prayed that I'd be proved a liar.

"Dr. Hamm said he'd do his best, but he said he couldn't promise me a cure. So I don't hope for that. My hope is to find out what's wrong with me. But if this doesn't give me answers, I'll have to cope and learn to live with it on reduced disability. Right now I live from paycheck to paycheck." She was already receiving disability payments from the VA for her service-connected neck and back injuries.

Carol got out of bed and went with bare feet into the bathroom. I was struck again by her frankness and unself-consciousness. After she came back, I asked if she had people she was close to at home.

"My kids are there. My daughter is married and lives in town. And I have two good friends, male friends, Doug and Rick. Rick will bark at me."

"Bark at you? Like he's telling you to snap out of it?"

"No," she said pleasantly, "he does funny voices. He barks like a dog, or sometimes he oinks like a pig."

"Ah, I get it. To make you laugh."

Carol nodded. "And I meow at him, like a cat."

Well, that was our introduction. I hung out with Carol for stretches over the next several days. Sometimes we were alone; sometimes she let me sit in as she was examined by the specialists. The doctors accepted me as they might a concerned friend or relative, except for the crusty neurologist, Dr. Gray, who refused to have a journalist in the room while he worked. Ronald Hamm paid several visits, once to offer to take Carol's laundry because she was having trouble getting it done at the hospital.

I learned much more about her. For example, I learned that when she was tired, sometimes her fingers "froze up." Other times she had the sensation that objects were lurking just outside her frame of view. Carol worried about paralysis, but her greater fear was that her illness might be causing her to go blind. Her eyesight was vital to her, she explained, because an artist—she'd earned a community college degree in fine arts—"needs to see the beauty of the world."

She combated her insomnia by listening to audiotapes of a science fiction show called *Red Dwarf*. She liked dragons, images of dragons in any setting because the dragon was the sign of her birth year. She kept a stuffed animal, a purple bunny, on her hospital bed and used it as a head and neck rest. As she lay chatting, her iron gray braid looped over the bunny and dangled off the head of the bed. "Ask my friends," she said with a pleased smile. "They'll tell you I'm a weird person."

Carol didn't smoke and was a spare drinker. She hated greasy food and bell peppers but loved enchiladas ("I don't care if they tear up my stomach"). She was still able to hike in the woods a little, loved how nature made her feel, but the effort cost her body afterward. Though she knew she ought to exercise more than she did, she was caught in the bind that is common to sufferers of chronic fatigue syndrome and fibromyalgia—namely, that exercise, if not done gradually, provokes the very symptoms of exhaustion and pain it is meant to alleviate. But more than that, Carol had a hard time hewing to anyone's prescriptions.

She'd endured painful passages in her life, including physical abuse by ex-husbands, which she referred to as calmly as if they had befallen someone else. Notwithstanding the hard knocks, Carol, you could tell, liked to laugh. I made her laugh just once. Dr. Hamm was describing a diabetic uncle who, when Ron was a boy, sterilized his insulin syringe in the same pot of water that he boiled for his tea. I said, "So that's when you decided to become a doctor?" Carol whooped. Apart from that, the relationship was one-way.

Carol wanted a "multitude of people to come together" to decide her case, and in due course the Wadsworth specialists issued their reports. Here is how they broke down the elements of her health: She was not diabetic. Her eyesight was suffering only from the normal effects of aging. Electronic monitoring of her sleep did not identify an organic basis for her insomnia. Lung function tests suggested she might have mild asthma.

According to radiological scans of her spine and head, there were signs of disk degeneration and sinus damage that might be responsible for her back pain and headaches, respectively.

The neurologists found that the fingers of Carol's left hand were weak. Her gait was slow but normal. The neuropsychologist found that because of her difficulty in concentrating, Carol did poorly on a word recollection test, which made her tearful, and poorly on a test of her fine motor function (manipulating pegs on a board), which Carol attributed to pain and cramping in her hands. She did much better on tests of nonverbal memory, like replicating shapes.

In the purely psychological realm Carol was found to be given to "feelings of self-criticism, worries about the future, feelings of worthlessness, and frequent crying." Sometimes she suffered panic attacks. There was ample evidence in her profile of a person who was anxious and depressed, but the pattern was not unyielding. One examiner, not a psychologist, described her affect as "happy." There might be "a significant somatic component" to her psychological symptoms, offered the psychiatrist.

The rheumatologist confirmed that Carol had fibromyalgia, because designated points on her body proved painful to his touch. Fibromyalgia was therefore one of two diagnoses given on Carol's discharge form from West L.A. VAMC.

The other diagnosis was "Persian Gulf War Syndrome." Yes, "Persian War Gulf Syndrome," dogging each of Carol's procedures like Hamlet's ghost and showing up explicitly at several stages in her paper work. The term is introduced on her admission form and it exits the hospital with her too. "NOOOO! Say it ain't so," moaned Hamm in an e-mail, when I pointed the specter out. "Can't believe (or don't want to believe) we actually diagnosed Persian Gulf Syndrome!"

A mistake? It had also happened with John Cabrillo. For reasons that no one could explain or defend, Carol Best had got from the medical center the diagnosis that she wanted. Yet she recognized that there was nothing of substance behind it, no connection articulated between the consultants' piecemeal findings and "Persian Gulf War Syndrome."

Hamm's own summary of her test results, which scrupulously avoided the term, displeased her. She criticized his evaluation as "wishy-washy" because it listed the many little things wrong with her but endorsed nothing major. And even her FM peeved her now. "If it's fibromyalgia," she said, "how come it started with the Persian Gulf War?"

MORE OFTEN THAN not I have put quotation marks around "gulf war syndrome," keeping it at arm's length. I have treated the term not as a ghost in a high drama but rather as a thing pulled up from the deep by a native fisherman, a type of monster, neither fish nor fowl. I have wondered with you about its origins. Now I will take it to the visiting scientists (epidemiologists, actually) for identification because the creature is beginning to smell.

On April 10, 1992, on the very day that Carol returned to her home in eastern Washington, tired but full of stories about her foreign adventure, the first official investigation of the gulf war illnesses got under way at a military hospital in Indianapolis. Then it was known only as a mystery illness affecting a number of units within Indiana's 123d Army Reserve Command (ARCOM). What had prompted the high-level investigation was not the miscellaneous symptoms themselves but their momentum, cutting through a swath of reservists who were noncombat veterans of the war.

Epidemiologists investigate epidemics, of course. The task implies a disease that is infectious, rapidly enlarging, and dangerous. In the Hollywood version of epidemiology, white-coated detectives scramble to the scene, set up a quarantine, and make cautious probes. But chronic, slow-moving illnesses that are not infectious, such as heart disease and cancer, also occupy epidemiologists. Such illnesses may be studied for years, without the researchers ever leaving their laboratories or their computers. "Gulf war syndrome" in time became just this sort of illness, the emergency drained out of it. In April 1992, however, the specialists arriving in Indiana were led by a field epidemiologist, Major Robert DeFraites, a doctor who was trained to act urgently.

The team came from the Epidemiology Consultant Service (EPICON) of the Walter Reed Army Institute of Research in Washington, D.C. Besides DeFraites, the team consisted of an occupational medicine physician, a psychiatrist, a dentist specializing in oral diseases, and a technical aide. Assisted by the reserve unit's doctor—he who had called for help from army headquarters—the investigators evaluated seventy-nine soldiers of the 123d ARCOM in two days. Three-quarters of the subjects were men, and 95 percent were either enlisted personnel or noncommissioned officers— that is, at the rank of sergeant or below.

Passing from station to station, the sick reservists filled out questionnaires, had their vital signs checked, sat for the dentist, gave blood and other samples for lab analysis, and met with at least two of the doctors to talk about their physical complaints, their frames of mind, and their environmental exposures in the Persian Gulf. The investigators returned to Washington to analyze the results.

EPICON's report, "Investigation of a Suspected Outbreak of an Unknown Disease," was issued two months later. Many official reports on the gulf war illnesses have been produced in the years since, but none has been done faster, and none, I submit, done better. I shall tell you about the EPICON study in detail and mention the others only as I come to them. Experts in and out of government may sputter at this, for surely much useful information was gathered after the spring of 1992, gobs of statistics and analysis, no less, packaged in the tomes of hardworking panels. The trouble is, except for one important finding, regarding the incidence, or rate, of these peculiar illnesses, the epidemiological work done after Indiana did little to resolve the conditions. "Suspected Outbreak of an Unknown Disease" remains an apt title.

The outbreak itself appeared genuine. Scores of people, from several locations in Indiana, had come forward with unexplained symptoms. Before the investigators could hope to control the outbreak, they had to learn its defining characteristics and its biological cause. The nature of the illness, its targets within the veterans' bodies, the measurements of their normal functions turned abnormal ought to provide clues to the germ or virus or toxic exposure that was responsible.

The classic example of a successful outbreak investigation is the one that identified Legionnaires' disease in the late seventies. As in the 123d ARCOM, the veterans who precipitously fell ill in the summer of 1976 had an experience in common. All had attended an American Legion convention at a hotel in Philadelphia. Their conditions, some swiftly fatal, involved a high fever and pneumonia, but the patients didn't respond to conventional antibiotics. Tissue samples were taken from the victims' lungs because the symptoms suggested that the pathogen or toxic agent might be lodged there.

An outbreak investigation is making progress when it is able to convert illnesses that are plural into a condition that is singular. In short, a syndrome is established. A syndrome is a collection of signs and symptoms pointing to a unique disorder. Less discrete than a disease, a syndrome is a disease waiting to be clarified, but even if the cause is never discovered, a syndrome remains a medical entity that can be differentiated from others. One way it stands out is by affecting a special population. Thus the Legionnaires' maladies quickly advanced to the stage of a syndrome. Likewise AIDS, when the epidemic started in the early eighties, immediately qualified as a syndrome because of the unusual diseases afflicting people who had the common experience of homosexuality.

The sick persons in Indianapolis shared the special history of the Gulf War, but the clinical picture of the outbreak was cloudier than it had been for AIDS or Legionnaires' disease. Trying to put together a formal description of the reservists' conditions, the epidemiologists found themselves juggling a lot of symptoms but not many signs.

The difference between these two elements is crucial. A symptom is something that the patient reports to the doctor, like pain, feverishness, coughing, or fatigue. A sign is something that the doctor can determine independently, by a thermometer for fever, say, or an X ray for pneumonia or by firsthand observation of the patient's cough or rash or swollen glands.

Symptoms are no less true, no less real than signs. Without the guidance of symptoms, the doctor wouldn't know where to look for the signs. However, because signs don't need symptoms for their verification, the former are more valuable to the physician in making a diagnosis. If the illness is a new one, signs are needed for formulating a case definition that will be used to make future diagnoses. Signs therefore are the lingua franca of epidemiology, enabling doctors at different places and in different times to translate the babel of illness into categories of disease.

To repeat, the EPICON team garnered a raft of symptoms but few signs. The symptoms most frequently reported by the veterans were fatigue (claimed by seven out of ten), followed by sleep disturbances, forgetfulness, joint pain, feeling "easily irritated," difficulty concentrating, depression, headache, abdominal pain, diarrhea and on down the list to fever (one person in eight). Also reported, more or less in the middle of the list of frequency, were rash, dental problems, and hair loss. These were signs, for objectively they could be observed by the doctors. Still, the rashes, dental problems, and hair loss didn't appear to be manifestations of an unusual or unique disorder. Instead what the researchers recorded were jock itch, gingivitis, male pattern baldness, etc.—unrelated conditions that could be found in the general population.

The laboratory screens of the veterans did not produce any breakthroughs either. The people with joint pain had no signs of acute inflammation. Twelve men had high blood pressure, not a common enough sign to suggest anything. The general blood work of the group, their liver enzymes, thyroid function, rheumatoid factor: all pretty much normal or negative. The scattered abnormal findings bore no relation to the number and diversity of the symptoms.

Diarrhea, which bothered a third of the study group, was perhaps the most worrisome of the chronic symptoms. That and back pain had cost some of the veterans time from their civilian jobs. The back pain, it was learned, was due to injuries and so was dismissed as a feature of the illness. As for the diarrhea, seven stool samples shed no light on its causes. There were no parasites found. The EPICON report had no explanation for the diarrhea but noted that cases had been common in the theater of war and had carried over to the States.

You begin to appreciate the predicament of the epidemiologists. The mystery illness will not come into focus. Symptoms reside in bodies without making much of a mark. So far there are not enough signs—abnormal findings, congruent from patient to patient—with which to formulate a case definition for a new syndrome, let alone carry the research forward to the cause of the signs and symptoms. Most critically, the investigators hadn't found the master sign, the linchpin of the illness, the prime mark of the morbid agent.

In the case of Legionnaires' disease, a new bacterium at last was identified in the tissue samples of victims. Today the *Legionella* bacterium is known as the cause of the disease as well as its diagnostic marker. AIDS research yielded two markers, one a new virus, HIV, the agent of the disease, and the other, indicating the mechanism, the decimated CD4 cells of the immune system. Knowing the agents and their markers and mechanisms opens the way to treatment, you realize, but my purpose here is to show that Legionnaires' and AIDS have passed beyond being syndromes. They graduated and earned their full nosologic diplomas.

It almost goes without saying that a biological marker for the gulf war illnesses has never been discovered. The DeFraites team was just the first to try and the first to fail. Repeated failures, even as the illnesses multiplied, led the Department of Defense to argue that the gulf war health complaints were not a syndrome after all. They were symptoms, said officials, known symptoms for the most part, belonging to other conditions. To be strict, "gulf war syndrome" did not exist. But Congress, the press, independent researchers, and the veterans thought that "syndrome" suited the erupting phenomenon perfectly well. What else were you going to call it while you tried to figure it out? Syndrome took the upper hand. Nobody, I should add, used quotation marks around it, and hereafter I won't myself.

The semantic dispute obscured a terribly important fact that all sides agreed upon: The veterans truly were ill. In racing to identify a disease, the DeFraites team, and many researchers coming after it, skipped over the living, breathing authenticity of the illnesses. Any person experiencing symptoms severe enough to require a doctor's attention is sick, whether or not the doctor is able to establish a disease or its markers. Any person who has pain and who worries over the pain is ill and probably impaired to some degree as well. Epidemiologists know this full well, but to acknowledge it is not part of their job description. Told there was no syndrome, the veterans assumed they were being told they were not ill.

When I met with Bob DeFraites five years later, he said he never would have predicted that he'd still be discussing and defending his investigation. He recalled that as he and his colleagues left Indiana, "we didn't have a good feeling about it. Usually in these things you know within three days what's up. For example, you find what the infectious agent is. But this was more like a sick building syndrome."

"Sick" buildings are a late-twentieth-century phenomenon. Freshly built or renovated structures, they cause allergic reactions and other health complaints among office workers, who blame chemical odors in the canned air or the new carpeting. Afterward a few of these people cannot tolerate chemical smells in general—they develop multiple sensitivities—and their health is permanently degraded. Indeed an early theory about the 123d's reservists was that the critical exposure had taken place in the armory where some of the units drilled and not necessarily in the Persian Gulf months before. For the Gulf itself offered no nexus. The symptomatic veterans were from twelve units and had served at different times and places throughout the zone of the war. Their support jobs were various—they drove trucks and fork-lifts; maintained fuel, food, and water supplies; and, after the fighting, hosed down and boxed up equipment.

"Everything was subjective," DeFraites continued. "The exposure was wrapped up in the outcome." He meant that everyone who was sick claimed to have been exposed to something. As many toxic agents were being reported as symptoms, and it was impossible, without better information on each, to match a substance from column A with a symptom from column B. "It would have been easier if we'd had either the exposure known or the disease known," he explained. "You need at least one to make headway."

Like Carol, the reservists didn't think it mattered what the agent was, whether it was stuff they had got into at their jobs during the war or something more widespread in the air or the water or the sand. In their interviews they spoke of microwave radiation, fuel oil, poorly ventilated heaters, oil smoke, spray paint operations, Scud fragments, pesticide-laced fish, anthrax vaccine, endemic viruses, any and all of which were hazardous, right? The point was, they were sick. Interestingly, poison gas did not seem to have been a concern for this early group of sufferers.

The EPICON researchers, unable to construct a case definition, were stymied on multiple fronts. For one thing, they could not measure the extent of such conditions among other veterans. "We went round and round on it—should we get controls?" DeFraites recalled. A control group is a parallel population that is studied for perspective. The idea would be to survey other units of the 123d ARCOM, units that had not been deployed to the Persian Gulf. Did these reservists attest to the same health complaints, in kind and number, as the seventy-nine who presented themselves in Indianapolis? In other words, how typical of the whole was the self-selected sample?

With no case definition, DeFraites held back. "I said, If there was only something objective to hang our hat on, then we might go get controls. How do you control for the self-reported nature of the fatigue?" He did not believe that asking other reservists whether they had fatigue or rash or forgetfulness would be helpful to the inquiry. The terms were too loose, "nonspecific."

(DeFraites did use rough controls to check one part of his study, the most specific part. The basic blood work and blood pressures of the sick veterans were compared with data previously collected from healthy, active duty soldiers who hadn't gone to the Gulf. DeFraites concluded that the two sets of biomedical profiles were similar. That is, the war had not produced changes that he could detect in the laboratory findings of the veterans.)

Buttoned-down and direct, his precision of speech accentuated by his uniform, DeFraites struck me as rationalism personified, not a hair or thought out of place. I sensed how Carol must have felt when she got her test results from the West L.A. VAMC. Medical science had taken all her nonspecific symptoms, the whole messy picture of her health, reduced them to biomedical fragments, and given them back to her in a bag. She peered into it. Was that really Carol in the shards?

I asked DeFraites to elaborate on "nonspecific" symptoms.

" 'Fatigue' is nonspecific," he said. "It's a path with many possibilities. But if you have fatigue on the heels of a fever and you are sleeping thirteen hours a day, that suggests a specific kind of fatigue and a diagnosis. If everyone in the group describes the same fatigue, then you'd say it's a phenomenon and you can begin to define it."

Another nonspecific condition, rash, had been claimed by 35 percent of the veterans. The EPICON report minimized its importance: "Skin rashes were representative of dermatological conditions found in general population."

I said to DeFraites, "Isn't thirty-five percent a lot of rash?"

"Some of the rashes we saw were unimpressive," he replied, and to demonstrate, he pointed to a small blemish, almost inconspicuous, on his wrist. "But yes, it would have been a good idea to have examined a control population for rash, to see what the normal incidence was."

I thought he'd left me an opening. "What *is* the incidence of rash, or fatigue, or some combination of the symptoms that you found in Indiana, among the people, say, whose cars are parked outside? Shouldn't you have considered that?" I was using the parking lot, which served a large mall in the suburbs of the capital, to get at the question of prevalence. Although the symptoms of the gulf war vets might not be unusual, didn't the vets suffer more of such symptoms than other Americans?

"To test this story of yours properly," he said, "you'd have to pre-suggest to your comparison group that they might have been exposed. You'd have to say to them, 'Remember when you went to the movie theater a couple of months ago? We're not sure but something may have happened in there. . . . Now take this questionnaire about your health and fill it out.' "

DeFraites believed that any group of people given reason to worry about their exposures in a particular place would tend to express physical symptoms as a result. The 123d had been given a reason to worry. In the months before the outbreak, having heard that some people in her battalion were unwell, a female sergeant passed around a survey asking about thirty-six particular symptoms. It was a bit of homegrown epidemiology, which she followed up with faxes and phone calls. Many of the questions would have drawn yeses from Carol: "Have you suffered from nervousness for no apparent reason/how often/to what degree? . . . Have you suffered from a stiff neck/how often/to what degree? . . . Have you suffered difficulty with your depth perception/how often/to what degree? . . . Have you suffered from eye sensitivity to indoor or outdoor light/how often/to what degree?"

Some of the reservists acknowledged that they hadn't been very concerned about their health until they received the sergeant's questionnaire. In any event, in March of 1992, when handed the results of the survey, the lead physician of the 123d ARCOM became concerned. He examined dozens of the veterans and came away puzzled. The local press got hold of the story. By the time the EPICON investigators arrived in April, it was too late to observe what I have called the pure cases of the gulf war illnesses, such as were glimpsed in 1991, the people untainted by expectations and quietly feeling rotten. Pure cases had existed in Indiana, some dating to the period of the homecoming. I don't mean that these later cases were inauthentic, but they were harder to assess.

Recall now that DeFraites had brought with him a psychiatrist and a specialist in occupational and environmental medicine. According to my scheme, the two doctors ought to represent rival hypotheses about the illnesses, but in Indiana there was no argument, the illnesses being too new. Working in concert, the two specialists helped DeFraites to interview the reservists after their medical exams.

Major E. Robert Wanat was the expert in occupational and environmental medicine. His cautious opinion, written in an appendix to the EPICON report, was that if the toxic agents named by the vets had posed a health threat, it should have been noticed by them right away—at least within days of exposure, a few weeks at the outside. The agents were recognizable for their acute signs and symptoms, unlike the delayed complaints of the 123d. This was the first phrasing of what became a saw in the debate, grinding back and forth: no acute health effects observed of agent X, therefore no likelihood of long-term effects from agent X.

Major Ann Norwood was the psychiatrist assigned to the team. There had been a hunch from the start that the outbreak might be psychologically created, and DeFraites himself went to Indiana with that "bias," he admitted, insisting it did not deter him from pursuing all the organic explanations. Norwood, whose job was to test the suspicion head-on, administered a psychological survey called the Brief Symptom Inventory, and then talked with each of the veterans. Specifically she was after evidence of either posttraumatic stress disorder, the prewar favorite, or psychological contagion, which she defined in her section of the report as "the spread of fear about a powerful element or agent which, when added to existing high levels of stress, causes involuntary psychosomatic reactions among the affected."

"They were a nice group of people," she said of the reservists. "They were candid and concerned. Some were focused on conspiracy and government cover-up, and I just let them talk. The one who had circulated the survey was a very angry person—or I should say, an active proponent."

Norwood ruled out posttraumatic stress disorder except in a handful of people. PTSD wasn't causing the group's physical symptoms, she declared. About psychological contagion, she didn't reach a firm judgment other than to say that the climate was conducive. This condition most often takes place among young people, who all come down with the same thing, fainting and gasping, for example, after a frightening incident at school or camp, and it has been suggested that sick building syndrome is an example of psychological contagion among adults. When people are overcome by sudden symptoms, usually they have witnessed others being overcome too, or to put it another way, the group is exposed simultaneously. But the 123d reservists, based throughout Indiana, lacked both the triggering incident and the critical mass of fear. If they were "contaminated" by the sergeant's questionnaire and then induced to a full-blown sickness by rumors and news reports, it was a slow-motion process, impossible to gauge afterward. The contagion scenario was very unlikely, it seemed to me. Although this thing's transmission was guided by many factors, as I have argued previously, I believe it effloresced of its own.

Norwood's main contribution was to have unearthed psychological distress among the reservists. She recorded it both in the individual interviews and on the Brief Symptom Inventory (BSI). According to the formal survey, symptoms of anxiety, hostility, depression, obsessive-compulsive behavior, somatization, even psychoticism were prevalent in the group. Norwood cautioned me that the BSI does not produce psychiatric diagnoses and that few of the reservists were psychiatrically ill, but she said it was correct that their psychological distress was very high.

I questioned her about the measurement of somatization, the tendency to express emotional distress as physical symptoms. As the most prevalent psychological feature, applying to two-thirds of the women and more than half the men, it seemed to throw cold water on the reservists' belief that their illnesses stemmed from their bodies.

"That's not a diagnosis," Norwood warned me again, "only an indication that they worried more about their physical health than most people do."

What was the Brief Symptom Inventory anyway? The version that Norwood administered consists of seventy-four items. It asks about fear, anger and many other stressful feelings and situations but also, at intervals, about bodily symptoms. By the end of the survey the respondent has told whether or not he or she has had problems during the previous week with faintness or dizziness; pains in the heart or chest; nausea or upset stomach; hot or cold spells; numbness or tingling in parts of the body; feeling weak in parts of the body; and trouble getting his or her breath. For each symptom the individual marks down the amount of discomfort, ranging from "not at all" to "extremely."

The health questions, you will notice, are not too different from those put to the reservists by the 123d's amateur epidemiologist. Both surveys educe conditions that are fuzzy, nonspecific, not the kinds of things that your doctor would ordinarily quiz you about, yet the results of the one suggested an outbreak of physical illness and of the other a psychological manifestation. Why should the BSI be right?

The professionals' defense of the inventory is that it has been "validated." It is held to be proved because its scoring system has been tested and confirmed on large populations of patients. But the sergeant's unvalidated survey had a private strength, which was the endorsement of the individuals who participated in it. Uncannily the questionnaire captured their strange and diverse bodily sensations. Although it asked them to rate their psychological states too, the queries in that regard were as few as the BSI's questions about physical health.

When DeFraites came to write up the EPICON study conclusions, he was guided by Norwood's psychological assessments, calling them "the most striking positive findings of our evaluation." He noted that the timing of the illnesses supported the stress argument. Ninety percent of the reservists said they had started feeling tired following their homecoming from the Gulf. Some had come back very early in 1991, and some as late as the following January, but whenever it was, their symptoms appeared to attach to that date, not to the period of their exposures in the theater. DeFraites wrote:

> The results of our investigation suggest that stress may be significantly contributing to, if not the major cause for a large proportion of the symptoms reported. Insomnia, lassitude and fatigue, lack of motivation, forgetfulness, mood changes, irritability, feeling depressed, and diarrhea are classical physiological manifestations of stress. The timing of the onset of most of these symptoms in association with redeployment may be a reflection of the stress of homecoming more than that related to specific events in SW Asia [the war zone].
>
> Soldiers in this group told us about considerable emotional difficulties

they faced during the mobilization, during the deployment, and since returning from ODS/S [Operations Desert Shield and Storm]. Many spoke of strained or broken marriages and relationships, financial setbacks, and the adjustments that return home has demanded. . . . We hypothesize that the adjustments demanded by these stresses may have been especially difficult for Reservists, many of whom may not have been prepared for the abrupt transition from civilian to military life when mobilized, and the equally sudden return to their homes and families when released from active duty. . . .

DeFraites summed up bluntly. Since the investigation had been unable to arrive at a unified diagnosis or a case definition for the symptoms, there was "no objective evidence for an outbreak of disease." The recommendation to the unit commanders was to address psychological needs. This was bitter medicine to the 123d reservists, and to veterans elsewhere, the clusters forming at bases and armories around the country, the networks starting, the dendritic connections of advice and alarm, the letters to the editor and to Congress, mothers writing about their sons, wives about husbands, veterans going onto the radio call-in shows and soon onto the fledgling Internet, like blood vessels advancing from a tumor. Or tumors, there being many metastases, already, of the gulf war illnesses. It was June of 1992.

CAROL BEST DID not hear about the mystery illness, for a lot was going on in her life in the months after her return from the Gulf. The main thing, she got divorced.

Carol had known she was coming home to a marital problem. While she was in Kuwait, her mother had warned her "to watch her back." Now she discovered that during her absence her husband had taken up with her best friend.

"He was *living* with her, my best friend," she said. "He spent eighteen hundred dollars of my money. The house was a mess. . . . I gave him the house, and I paid for the divorce."

This was the take-charge Carol, cutting her losses and moving on with her life. She couldn't have been too surprised, on the one hand, because the marriage, her third, had turned rocky and she had left for the Gulf partly to escape the tension. On the other hand, this divorce was inescapable proof of her failures with men. When, a few years later, a psychotherapist asked her to write down her marital history and tell how the relationships had affected her, she filled out three terse lines: "1971–1976—Div.—Made me stronger. /1978–1979—Div.—Made me stronger and afraid of marriage. /1981–1992—Div.—Hurt."

"Do you think you have bad luck in your choice of men?" I asked.

"I think so," she replied. "I've tried all ages, one older, one younger, one about the same age. The main problem is that I'm not the docile female. I was independent, or I used to be. I supported two husbands. But they were abusive and they had girlfriends. . . . Still, with my last husband I thought it was pretty good, it was going to work."

It seems that men were attracted to Carol because she was more capable in their realm than other women, but then they turned against her for the same reason. "How we met"—she told me, about her last husband—"he pulled over to help me with my truck, which was broke down on the highway. We decided it had to be towed, which meant the drive shaft had to be dropped [disconnected], and so I crawled under it and did it. That's when he knew what kind of woman I was." On breaking up, however, he told her she was "too powerful a person."

Carol's daughter, who was twenty-five, admired her mother's strength, as she remembered it in a letter supporting Carol's disability application to the VA:

While [I was] growing up, my mother was always on the go. Mom was the world's greatest "Super Mom." She did everything a mother and a father would do. . . . After coming home from work from a long hard day at work my mom would clean house, cook dinner, help with our homework, and get us ready for bed. On the weekends when she was not at work, she would plant gardens, weed, can vegetables and make jams. Wow the energy she had. That's not all though. Mom also would make our clothes and take us wherever we needed to go. For fun she would take us hiking, camping, bike riding, dancing, swimming, teach us arts and crafts, and many more things. Mom was also the handy man of the house (and you thought I was done). She fixed the plumbing, was our mechanic for our cars, and the list goes on and on. There is so much more I could tell you about the things my mom did for us and for others. Well I think you get the idea of how things were. You notice I said how things *were*!

Carol's friends attested to her dynamism before she got sick. She was a hospice volunteer; she taught arts and crafts at night. Weekends in her army reserve unit, she served as an illustrator, a typist, and a mechanic. At her regular job she was the tireless organizer of the annual company fair. "She was the person that spearheaded everything," wrote a coworker, "even getting her family involved. She spent days and nights organizing, painting, drawing. . . . At work she was always full of vim and vigor and the first one in line to push a broom or lift a paint brush. . . . At least she still has a big heart. You can't break that."

Reading the testimonials, I was reminded of the puzzlement of the doctor in Indiana who first reviewed the sicknesses of the 123d ARCOM. He knew the reservists in question, and they were the last people he would have expected to complain about their health. "These were Type A individuals," said the doctor, Norman Teer, "people who worked two jobs, coached Little League, were active and aggressive people." Jim Simpson, one of the most outspoken of the Indiana reservists, also referred to himself as a Type A, the archetypal hard driver. Moreover, if you go through veterans' statements to the fact-finding commissions and congressional committees over the years, you find a preponderance of individuals describing their superb prewar energy and physical prowess. Men and women alike, they appear to have been high achievers—now stunned and angered by their declines.

Carol worked as a "visual information specialist" in a printing plant. Her job was to design and illustrate brochures. The work, right on the floor of the plant, was well-paying and creative, but it had one major drawback: chemical vapors. The ventilation in the place was inadequate. There were vapors from the inks and blanket washes of the presses, from the ammonia in the big copying machines, and also from the spray glues, paints, and thinners that Carol used at her desk. Although she had tolerated industrial chemicals in previous jobs, the mixture here disagreed with her, it seems, from the start of her employment. A former boss recalled that she was "sensitive as soon as we pulled her into the printing plant in 1984." He added, "Some of those *were* strong chemicals."

Ether caused her the strongest reaction. Carol had reported to a doctor that an incident with ether had caused her to "go blind for two weeks." In 1989, two years before the Persian Gulf War, she put in a claim for workers' compensation benefits because of her breathing problems and headaches. The plant managers evidently opposed the claim, but Carol prevailed. She established that she suffered from occupational asthma.

Occupational asthma is no different in its signs from ordinary asthma, being characterized by wheezing and constriction of the bronchial passages. When an attack is ongoing, a physician can measure the patient's reduced intake of air with a device called a flowmeter. There are treatments for asthma, inhaled or ingested medications, such as those Carol began to use at work. But what makes occupational asthma intriguing is that it is a bridge to the novel condition called multiple chemical sensitivity. In the late 1980s, as Carol was pursuing her workers' comp claim, occupational physicians in industries around the United States were seeing cases of asthma they couldn't understand. Even after the initial symptoms, the allergic reaction to a chemical, had died down, the worker would come back and complain that far lower exposures, barely noticeable, were making him or her ill. And now it wasn't only shortness of breath. Patients got headaches; they had memory problems; their joints hurt, their bowels were out of kilter. A few of these people, unable to deal with any strong odors at home or at work, slid rapidly into disability.

The fact that no one diagnosed MCS in Carol, before or after the war, says more about her doctors than about her symptoms. MCS was and is a controversial label, and Carol's private physician, whom I'll name Dr. Brown, was conservative in these matters. He treated her often for occupational asthma and back and neck pain, according to her records, and spent a lot of time talking to her about her other symptoms as they developed, trying to help her through. But he appeared reluctant to diagnose the hazier conditions, such as fibromyalgia, adjustment disorder (a psychological condition) and Persian Gulf syndrome, labels that Carol later acquired from her caretakers in the VA medical system.

Carol liked and trusted her doctor. Since her health insurance at work covered her visits, at first she had no need of the VA. She went to Dr. Brown in May 1992, a month after her return to civilian life. Carol, who had turned forty in Kuwait, was having night sweats, fatigue, insomnia, and dry skin. Doctor and patient agreed that the symptoms were probably menopausal, and lab tests subsequently indicated a change in her female hormones. In June, after the two had met to discuss hormone therapy, Dr. Brown wrote that "her fatigue and other symptoms . . . may relate to menopause or may relate to situational changes returning to this country."

In addition to the trouble at home, Carol's situation at work had changed. With the printing plant under new management, downsizing was in the air. Out of the loop for ten months, she found the pace of the work faster, the demands on her greater. She had new software to learn on the computers. A coworker remembered that when a brochure had to be updated, new text and illustrations put in, Carol was given just one day to produce the layout, whereas before, her deadline had been two weeks.

In October her breathing got worse. She saw Dr. Brown three times that month. Confirming "scattered wheezes" in her chest, he adjusted her asthma medications. (Is it relevant, is it not part of my job also to report that she had gained 10 pounds since her visit in the spring? Divorced Carol now weighed 190 pounds. And that she was fighting with her stepdaughter? That her dog had just died, much to her grief? Her medical files spread in front of me, I am sifting for information in the doctors' notes that has nothing to do with gulf war syndrome. Are you getting the sense of the journalist's betrayal?)

One morning in early November she was standing at a printing machine and had a full-blown asthma attack. Leaving work, she suffered two more frightening episodes at home before she was able to get to the doctor. Two days later she returned to work, only to leave again, gasping. On the phone to Dr. Brown's nurse, Carol said that she had had it with the conditions at the plant, that she had demanded a medical release, that she was enlisting an attorney. Apparently she was persuaded to give the job another try. However, at the end of the month she was back in Dr. Brown's office, racked with a headache, clutching her inhalers. She asked him to write a letter that she be given a leave until the chemicals were reduced in her work area and the ventilation improved.

"I sense," Dr. Brown observed, "that seeing how this request is coming from her lawyer via the patient that we are leading down the road to a work-related disability and early retirement. She apparently was good friends to Chuck Richards who had similar symptoms that resulted in early retirement for occupational asthma."

Who was Chuck Richards? I found out about him too. He not only couldn't tolerate the chemicals in the printing plant, but was also affected by vapors outside, especially the pesticide sprays on the wheat fields. He got very sick and died a few months after winning his medical retirement— which management had resisted. According to their ex-supervisor, Chuck and Carol represented two mystifying cases of chemical sensitivity, the first two in his experience at the plant.

Earlier in his career in the printing industry the standards were looser, the supervisor added. People didn't wear respirators and gloves. No training sessions and posted warnings, as now required by the government, about the toxic hazards. Poor ventilation in the work areas? "Some people got used to it, and some people were bothered by it," he said, not defending the practices.

Times change, and the construction of illness changes. Until labels were sanctioned for the adverse reactions, the workers who were bothered by their exposures simply had to quit their jobs. If they raised objections, you didn't hear about it. Certainly they didn't sue over symptoms.

Carol Best went on medical leave for the month of December, while her employer had her evaluated for occupational asthma. This was the time, late 1992, that she first learned about the gulf war illnesses. "I had all the symptoms *before* I heard of the Desert Storm syndrome," she told me. Yes, she did.

It took awhile for the military health authorities to grasp that the phenomenon of the gulf war illnesses was serious, and growing. The first outbreak, in Indiana, was like a brushfire that the army and its investigators had attempted to put out. I don't mean that the DeFraites team denied the reservists' symptoms, only tried to rationalize them, but the effort seemed to fuel the problem rather than resolve it.

In August 1992 ABC's *20/20* program aired a story about sick veterans in Indiana and elsewhere. Some people were shown to be struggling for their lives. Multiple toxic exposures were alleged. DeFraites's idea about the stress of readjustment after the war was "unacceptable to the vets, even ludicrous," said the correspondent, Lynn Sherr.

Brushfires started in other regions of the country, each flaring a little differently until the flames were joined nationally. There were ill reservists in a naval mobile construction battalion, the 24th Navy Seabees, based in the Southeast. During the war they had been stationed in and around the Saudi city of Jubail, and several incidents, including a Scud missile attack, convinced many that they had been exposed to chemical warfare agents. In the Northeast the toxic substance of concern was depleted uranium (DU), a mildly radioactive constituent of American armor and munitions. Members of an Army National Guard unit in New Jersey, the 144th Service and Supply Company, claimed to have been exposed to DU dust while working on damaged armored vehicles. They were brought to the Boston VA hospital for tests. Boston became a hotbed of the illnesses.

The Department of Veterans Affairs announced it would establish national referral centers for war-related conditions that were difficult to diagnose. Originally called environmental medicine referral centers, they were located at VA facilities in Los Angeles, Washington, D.C., and Houston. As I detailed earlier, the special units were no help in solving the mystery. But their mandate to consider the health effects of agents in the environment was meant to offset the perception that the VA considered the problems purely psychological. Clearly a split in thought was deepening. Though I have no polls to cite, I don't doubt that the majority of VA clinicians tended toward the psych camp initially, following DeFraites's analysis or simply because they could not figure out or fix the vets' symptoms. Sooner or later the patient would be sent down the hall to see the psychologist. This was a dismissal, be it done coldly or kindly, and like Carol, these patients were not about to be dismissed.

The Pentagon did not feel the same pressure as the VA, because the active duty veterans of the war were not coming forward in the same numbers as the demobilized reservists. The overall problem was still a matter of hundreds, not thousands, of cases. Since the Pentagon, however, was ultimately responsible, at the end of 1992 a top army physician, Major General Ronald Blanck, came front and center.

In the history of the gulf war illnesses as projected from the Washington stage, Blanck commands an important early part. He moves into the wings in 1994, when the heavy artillery starts, being too smart, politically, to become a casualty in the battle over what happened in the Gulf. Blanck also was a quick learner of the medical dynamics. Unlike others in the military health establishment, he sensed that conventional medicine and epidemiology were not going to solve the problem because the illnesses drawing the most attention were unconventional. As long as he had influence, he tried to steer the issue of the unexplained illnesses away from the dueling paradigms—out of the line of fire, as it were, between the toxic hypothesis and the stress hypothesis, knowing that the argument over the cause of the problem was harmful to the vets' health.

Blanck was the newly appointed head of Walter Reed Army Medical Center. His army résumé listed impressive posts at home and abroad, rungs on the ladder of a twenty-five-year career. The one unorthodox part of his background was that he was a doctor of osteopathy, D.O., not a doctor of medicine, M.D. An osteopath, contrary to the opinion held by some

M.D.'s, is not just a souped-up chiropractor. Four years of graduate study are required, after which the osteopath must pass the same state examinations as the M.D. But once licensed, the osteopath indeed practices a different style of medicine, emphasizing the integrity of the muscles and bones, communication with the patient, and holistic care. The American Osteopathic Association says that ten percent of the doctors in military service were trained as osteopaths, twice as many as in civilian practice.

At first Blanck did not find the illnesses remarkable. He saw no reason to question the EPICON findings in Indiana. Rejecting the possibility of "another Agent Orange," he predicted in a newspaper interview that many veterans would file health claims in the future but that their conditions, like heart disease and cancer, would be due to aging, not to the war.

The army commissioned a panel of experts to review all research having to do with the Kuwaiti oil fires. The panel assured Blanck that the symptoms being reported were "unlikely to have been caused by exposure to petrochemicals or other environmental chemical exposures in the Gulf region."

Having directed the medical preparations for the Desert Shield operation and studied the infectious diseases of Gulf region, Blanck keyed next upon leishmaniasis, which he thought might underlie the cases that were resisting diagnosis. It didn't.

The cases kept building. Blanck met with some of the veterans during their evaluations at Walter Reed. "They were ill, but their tests were normal," he recalled. They were angry and upset, but most didn't have PTSD. With the best medical staff in the army stymied, Blanck looked about for new approaches. "Maybe it's my osteopathic background," he said, "but you're not locked into one way of seeing the patient. You have to be willing to admit that you don't know what you don't know.

"I started hearing about multiple chemical sensitivity. I was only dimly aware of [the condition] at the time. Anecdotally I heard of maybe three or four veterans being treated under these regimens, avoiding fragrances and strong smells, and they were feeling better. It seemed we might learn something by exploring MCS."

In September 1992 Blanck and other health officials were called to Capitol Hill by the House Committee on Veterans' Affairs. The subject of the hearing was "The Possible Adverse Health Effects of Service on the Persian Gulf." Also discussed was the establishment of a VA health registry. It was a contentious session, the first of many. Dr. Lewis Kuller, an epidemiologist advising the Pentagon, clashed with Representative Joseph Kennedy of Massachusetts, a strong believer in the toxic hypothesis.

Kuller said, "It's a bad mistake to suddenly create a new disease called 'environmental disease,' which is what we're doing here, and which is wrong, which we can't define, we can't measure, and we can't measure the environmental exposure."

"I just feel this is right out of *Dr. Strangelove*," Kennedy replied. "This is an indication—it almost verges on a cover-up of the difficulties that people face when they have environmental problems and they run into this mentality by their government. . . .

"This is the struggle of our generation," the forty-year-year-old congressman continued. "Our generation is the generation that has been exposed to all these chemicals. Then it is put on us, by people like Dr. Kuller, to have to prove to him in some unquestionable manner that the disease is directly related [to the exposure] or else he just doesn't want to deal with it."

Blanck when he spoke avoided taking sides. He said it was possible a connection existed between the hazardous exposures and the veterans' illnesses. The possibility required study, he said.

"Wouldn't you say there is a *probability* of a connection?" Kennedy demanded. "Why do you presume that this is in these guys' heads?"

"I absolutely don't think it's in their heads," Blanck said. "I think they have real illness, and I will be happy to tell you some of the things we found when we have looked at this. . . ."

Blanck informed the committee that he was being advised by Dr. Claudia Miller, "one of the foremost environmental physicians, whose work is firmly based on science and who wants to do some further studies on exactly these patients."

Claudia Miller: another pioneering figure. She was the coauthor of a 1991 book, *Chemical Exposures: Low Levels and High Stakes,* and a consultant to the new VA referral center in Houston, having interested the medical director there in her ideas about chemical sensitivity. Blanck soon became Miller's champion. She appealed to him because she was one of the most scientifically conservative of the active medical proponents of MCS, a qualification that is going to take some explaining.

Had Claudia Miller worked for Carol Best's employer, she would have been responsible for responding to Carol's asthma attacks because her experience was in occupational medicine and industrial hygiene. In the late 1980s she shifted her focus from industrial workplaces to sick building incidents and the health complaints of people living near hazardous waste dumps and tainted water supplies. In this work she came across individuals whose sensitivity to chemicals was sparked not just by pollution but by modern consumer products, including food items, medications, tobacco smoke, cleaning fluids, plastics, and perfumes.

Miller began to think that different groups of patients were linked: the factory workers, office workers, and housewives, all reacting to concentrations of chemicals that ought to be innocuous. These people, the women outnumbering men, had become hypersusceptible. Their symptoms waxed and waned under invisible prodding. The instability in their states of health had most often developed in the wake of an acute or frightening exposure, though it was not always a chemical exposure.

Conventional medicine had not helped these people. The family doctor would send them to see an allergist. The allergist wouldn't be able to detect an immune reaction, an antibody response, in the blood tests or skin-prick exposures. Substances in their environments were prompting symptoms, no doubt, but they did not cause inflammation or the other signs that the allergist recognized. If the allergist suggested to the patient that the next stop should be the psychiatrist, she or he would take offense. At that point, or after going around the medical mill several times, the chemically sensitive person would be drawn outside the mainstream, into the orbit of, how shall I say, the flakier practitioners, well beyond the sphere of osteopathy.

The alternate practitioners, some of whom had been trained as M.D.'s, called themselves clinical ecologists. Later they changed their name to environmental physicians. Their vision of the body under siege from environmental substances had been gaining adherents since the 1960s. (Thus the plaint by Representative Kennedy, a child of the sixties: "Our generation is the generation that has been exposed to all these chemicals.") Many of the environmental physicians faulted chemicals not just for their patients' respiratory troubles, poor concentration, headaches, and fatigue but also for hypertension, arthritis, and cancer, which they proceeded to treat with megavitamins, saunas, restrictive diets, stringently detoxified housing, injections of "neutralizing" allergens, etc.

Unproved remedies, unsubstantiated diagnoses, inadequate studies—of course the conventional doctors were hostile to the advocates of environmental illness. For years the excesses in the field of chemical sensitivity permitted the entire field to be ignored. But as more patients put pressure on government and business through the filing of disability and compensation claims, medical researchers with better credentials became interested. Claudia Miller, for one, reviewed the problem of chemical sensitivity for the New Jersey Department of Health in 1989. The term multiple chemical sensitivity (MCS) was coined by a researcher at Yale Medical School in 1987, and it stuck.

But the extra attention only aggravated the divisions among doctors. Several state and national medical associations repudiated MCS, while conceding the need for further study of patients. Typical was the statement in 1991 by the American College of Occupational Medicine: "Multiple Chemical Hypersensitivity Syndrome is presently an unproven hypothesis and current treatment methods represent an experimental methodology. The College supports scientific research into the phenomenon to help explain and better describe its pathophysiological features and define appropriate clinical interventions."

By the early nineties MCS had arrived at a stage of crisis. It had passed through the inchoate period of its puzzling new symptoms and was striving for formal recognition in the high court of medicine, to which the courts of law usually looked for guidance. Was MCS truly a new syndrome? If so, how did you define it? And if a new syndrome, was it a new disease as well? What were the biological markers?

In spite of the insistence by one side that the symptoms of MCS were riveted to the tissues and organs, the lack of agreed-upon signs precluded the creation of a new disease. But to establish the validity of an MCS syndrome was a somewhat less demanding procedure. The condition could be considered a unique entity when all other explanations for the symptoms had been ruled out. Having done that much, the advocates of MCS, and even some who questioned it, suggested case definitions. The goal was to give the epidemiologists something to try out on various groups of patients, something that might distinguish MCS and offer clues to its origins.

The case definitions referred to numerous environmental triggers, low levels of exposure, and chronic symptoms throughout the body. Yet no one research criterion captured the condition better than any other did. Sure, the surveys turned up people who said they had MCS, however defined, but without laboratory tests to verify that the illnesses were not only the same but also unique, the epidemiology meant little. One thing of value to come out of the research was the profile of the typical MCS patient. She was female, in her forties, and had at least two years of college (vide Carol).

The role of psychiatric disorders in MCS was a complicating factor. The more skeptical of the researchers had found that people who met their definitions of MCS also had more emotional problems, especially anxiety and depression, than people who did not meet the definitions. You could argue over whether the emotional problems had precipitated their MCS or vice versa. Still, diagnoses of psychiatric illness in chemically intolerant patients were the most consistent of the medical findings.

Against these obstacles the drive to legitimize the syndrome was stalled. It didn't trouble the majority of environmental physicians, continuing to treat patients, that their concepts of MCS were not scientifically certified. It did trouble Claudia Miller. When I said that she was a scientific conservative among MCS proponents, I meant that she refused to give up the effort to validate the condition by mainstream standards of proof.

Miller, who had moved to the University of Texas Health Science Center in San Antonio, believed that MCS represented a whole new family of diseases. Her term for the condition was "toxicant-induced loss of tolerance." The reason that its many symptoms and signs could not be fitted into a case definition, she said, was that the mechanism of disease was too new. Consisting of subtle irregularities in both the immune and nervous systems, it lay beyond the realm of current knowledge. Nevertheless, Miller argued, an MCS syndrome could be verified by default.

Since the patients got better by avoiding certain chemical and then got worse when they encountered them again, an experiment could be conducted to measure the effect. Hence her proposal: MCS patients would be put into a specially controlled environment, a sealed unit in a hospital setting that was devoid of synthetic materials. With their food strictly managed, their cotton clothing laundered but not dry-cleaned (the same for the attendants), their air filtered, and their water unchlorinated, even the water in the toilets, the patients would be allowed to withdraw, over the course of four to seven days, from the toxic exposures of the outside world. Only then, after the subjects had been "unmasked," Miller's term for the ridding of chemical influences, would the offending substances be brought back in controlled amounts, the doses of the "challenges" to patients so low at first that anyone in the unit who didn't have MCS should not be bothered or even notice.

The catch for the patients would be that they wouldn't know when a certain chemical was in the air or not. If they were told it was but it really wasn't and then they suffered a reaction, the experiment would indicate that their symptoms were behavioral responses, not organic. Alternately, if they failed to react to a covert substance in their food or water, the claims of hypersensitivity would be undermined. Miller expected that the MCS patients would respond exquisitely to the string of challenges, unlike the control subjects, who would be tested in the unit separately.

At the time of the Persian Gulf War, Miller had been shopping her proposal to federal health agencies without success. It would cost a million dollars to build the environmental medical unit, as she called it, and though she had letters of endorsement from the National Academy of Sciences and the National Institute for Environmental Health Sciences, there didn't seem to be a fund to pay for such a facility. As she well knew, the political implications of MCS made officials nervous. If her tests on MCS patients corroborated the physiologic basis for the condition, the patients would acquire powerful ammunition in civil actions against business and government for their incidental but health-damaging exposures.

When she saw the television pictures of the oil fires burning in Kuwait, Miller had an inkling that some of the troops would have reactions. The war with its welter of chemical exposures represented "an unfortunate opportunity for people to get sick," she said. When she interviewed sick veterans at the Houston VAMC eighteen months later, she saw "striking similarities" between their conditions and MCS. One vet, for instance, reported that his symptoms started when he moved into a new house. The house was tightly sealed, with new carpeting. Another patient told her, "I have fifteen deodorants in my medicine cabinet. I can't find one whose fragrance doesn't make me sick."

So Claudia Miller, a doctor on a mission, got together with General Ronald Blanck, a can-do guy who was open to new ideas. Blanck decided that the Defense Department should fund Miller's environmental medical unit and that gulf war vets should be the first subjects for testing. The project would need a congressional appropriation, which they pursued in 1993. The competition to define the gulf war illnesses, to rewrite, rather, the definition that was implicit in the DeFraites report, was under way.

CAROL WENT BACK to work at the printing plant in January 1993. Her boss had promised to reduce her exposure to fumes. She was told she would not have to use any substances that bothered her. Certain machinery was moved farther away from her desk, and she was given permission to leave work whenever her symptoms recurred.

The changes may have helped. Carol's visits to Dr. Brown were less frequent. She went just a couple of times in the spring for a sore throat and bad cough. Bronchitis was diagnosed.

In the late summer and early fall she saw the doctor for pain in her abdomen. Her neck and back were hurting too. Some of the pain was caused by injuries in a rafting accident, she told him. She'd also been bumped lightly by a car. But the pain in the lower right side of her abdomen was mystifying. The area was tender to the touch. Dr. Brown arranged for a gastrointestinal exam, ultrasound, X rays and an evaluation by a surgeon. He thought the pain might be due to scarring from her hysterectomy or perhaps to a hernia. For Carol, pain heretofore had not been a symptom as regular as her fatigue and respiratory distress, but it would be in the future. I should point out that MCS sufferers often have diffuse pain.

In October 1993 Carol bought a house. It was a fairly large house with a fairly substantial mortgage. She had her mother move in with her—her mother was recovering from cancer surgery—as well as her son, who needed to save on rent. As head of the new household Carol tried to be strong, the way she'd been in years past.

"I'm the rock in the family," she said to me. "If I have to depend on anyone else, you might as well shoot me. Every time I ask for help, I feel guilty. If I go to start something, no matter how hard it hurts, I try to finish it." She remembered the days when she was self-sufficient. "When you're in a man's job—a jet engine mechanic—you can't ask men for help, or they say you shouldn't be in the job."

In mid-November Carol was overcome at work. She went straight to Dr. Brown's office. She was "in considerable distress," according to the nurse's record. She told the nurse she had hyperventilated because of the fumes; during the attack she was lightheaded and couldn't think clearly. Carol wanted the incident documented for her workers' comp file.

Carol hadn't been taking her asthma medications because she'd decided they were making things worse. Overruling her, the nurse helped administer the inhaler, relaxing the constriction of her airways, and Carol, though teary-eyed, felt better for it. Had she been under the care of an environmental physician, she might have been applauded for stopping her meds, since MCS doctors believe that you have to eliminate all possible chemicals in order to identify the triggers of your symptoms.

Carol had a friend at work whose husband was a Persian Gulf vet. He too went to the Gulf in the aftermath of the fighting and was chronically unwell since coming home. Carol's friend kept her posted on the controversy over the illnesses, occasionally passing along clippings from an army newspaper. It happened that November was the busiest month yet for news about gulf war syndrome. Whether it was the news coverage that spurred her, her friend's husband's situation, or the latest crisis at work, Carol went to the local VA hospital on November 29. She signed up for the VA's Persian Gulf Health Registry (PGHR), which had been established the year before.

Recall that at the end of 1991, before there were recognized illnesses, Congress required the Pentagon to establish a registry of troops that had been exposed to the oil smoke. The registry actually had been conceived while the fires were burning, in anticipation of soldiers' health concerns. In late 1992, the illnesses having come to pass (though not the kind expected, except perhaps by Claudia Miller), the law was strengthened. Congress called for an additional registry and medical exams by the Department of Veterans Affairs. The VA medical program got going before the Pentagon's.

To enroll in the PGHR was simple. The veteran's portion of the paper work consisted of a one-page form with fifteen questions. The first twelve were biographical basics, and the last three addressed environmental health.

"#13. Were you exposed to Environmental Contaminants while serving in the Persian Gulf area?" Carol marked the box for "Not sure" but then crossed it out and put an X in the box for "Probably." Only by answering "Yes" or "Probably" could she continue to the last two questions.

"#14. How were you (possibly) exposed?" Initially she checked "Enveloped in smoke," and then she switched to "In a smoky area, but not enveloped." She also noted, on the line next to "Other," food that was greasy, undercooked, and burned.

"#15. Generally, how would you describe your overall health?" Carol indicated "Good" but changed it to "Poor."

Then she took a medical exam. I didn't obtain the full record from her, only the summary page.

"Nature and Duration of Complaints." The examiner had scrawled "Depression" and "tired."

"History of Present Illnesses." Here the examiner noted: "recurrent episodes of depression, tiredness, & weakness. These symptoms have materialized aprox 1 MO [month] following return from Gulf area."

Carol Best was unhappy with the conduct of the exam. She thought the VA had minimized her health problems. Regardless, she was now a national statistic. Of what it wasn't clear.

IDENTIFYING A NEW syndrome or disease is not just a medical process but also something of a social negotiation. The patients provide symptoms, signs, and opinion, and the doctors provide expert analysis and opinion, until a judgment is reached that satisfies both parties. Here it looked as though the patients were doing their part, but the doctors were dragging their feet.

The VA and Pentagon always maintained that the majority of the veterans' symptoms merited conventional diagnoses and treatments. Disease being part of the human condition, you would expect people to contract cancer, hypertension, and assorted disorders whether or not they had been to the Gulf. Indeed, the more specific the problem, the less likely it belonged to the gulf war syndrome. But even the vague ailments could be labeled. Come in with a headache, and your diagnosis would be the type of headache that you had, usually a tension headache or, less often, a migraine. If you also had chronic diarrhea—you probably had irritable bowel syndrome. Say that you were feeling depressed and also scored high on a screen for depression—you would be diagnosed with depression. Some people had nothing wrong at all but went through the registry process just to be reassured. Thus the bulk of the gulf war cases could be explained (or explained away, if you will) by the proper scrutiny, after which the proper care and medication could be administered.

It was the veterans with multiple complaints and unclear diagnoses who made the doctors hesitate. These men and women came back for help repeatedly, in pain that didn't relent. "They were the group that was left," observed General Blanck, "and they were clearly ill."

They represented roughly a fifth of the gulf war cases—at least twenty-thousand individuals by the end of the inventory. Classified by the VA as "undiagnosed," they might be offered intensive evaluations in the referral program, as John Cabrillo and Carol were. If they were on active duty and had enrolled in the Defense Department medical system, they would be placed in the category "Signs, Symptoms and Ill-Defined Conditions." This tautologous heading gave a label to conditions that couldn't otherwise be labeled. The most common symptoms in the SSID diagnostic category, according to a 1998 report, were "fatigue, headaches, memory impairment, dyspnea [shortness of breath] or cough, chest pain, lightheadedness or dizziness, digestive complaints such as nausea and numbness." Which is to say the classic gulf war symptoms, unexplained.

Two groups of veterans, those who were undiagnosed and those dissatisfied with diagnoses they had been given, were behind the political controversy. Even in 1993 they made a sizable force, a thorn in the side of the clinical database, and General Blanck was anxious to extract them—i.e., figure them out. Although signs of disease were missing, he believed enough information had been collected about their symptoms to support a case definition. He asked Dr. Jay Sanford, an infectious disease specialist and epidemiologist, to devise a definition, the first step toward a possible new syndrome.

Blanck went up to the Hill in early June 1993 to be queried on his efforts. The House Veterans' Affairs Committee was, as before, aggressive on the question of chemical exposures, putting forward sick veterans to testify and also environmental physicians, who explained the vets' symptoms in terms of chemical sensitivity.

Claudia Miller, with Blanck's support, lobbied for her environmental test unit. She received an enthusiastic response from Representative Kennedy. She even had to rein Kennedy in a bit. Disparaging the stress hypothesis and invoking the Agent Orange precedent, Kennedy declared that the illnesses should be presumed to be chemically related, should they not? More cautious, Miller said that her test unit offered a way to settle the arguments over whether such symptoms were physiological or psychological, "arguments that have been going on for the last thirty or forty years."

"Somebody said earlier in testimony today that, you know, they felt like a guinea pig," Kennedy continued, referring to the anti–nerve gas pills and anthrax vaccinations, which the military had never before tried on a broad scale. "Well, the fact is," he said, "that our whole generation is a generation of guinea pigs. . . . Nobody throughout the history of the world has ever been exposed to the kind of chemical contaminants of our generation. And so it is a very different set of sciences."

I keep citing Congressman Kennedy because his deeply felt ideas reached far beyond gulf war syndrome. The pathology he believed in was plausible, but it was not yet verified by science. Science? Kennedy, like Claudia Miller and several others you will meet, envisioned a new science that would comprehend the chemically derived ailments.

Note also that faultfinding and extreme ideas have begun to color the health mystery. While epidemiology groped about for a case definition of the illnesses, various toxic agents, each with its own backers, vied to be considered the likely cause. Initially it was the oil fires, an apolitical agent—not the government's doing, that is—and by the same token psychological stress was an apolitical agent. By late 1993, however, the harder-edged stuff was gaining: the pesticides, depleted uranium, special paints, and medicines, which were produced or dispensed by U.S. military commanders. Moreover, the characterization of the veterans shifted away from the vulnerable individuals, who may have been unlucky in their genes or makeup and susceptible to the exposures of war, toward a large class of people said to be carelessly treated.

Faced with a scientific complexity, the political system usually does not commit itself until the experts have thrashed out an agreement. But the gulf war syndrome wasn't like global warming or human cloning or genetically modified food, whose consequences for the nation could be debated at length. This was more like the controversy over silicone breast implants. The lives of ailing and angry people were on the line, and voices were being raised in every congressional district. A democratic system must act, even though it didn't know how.

General Blanck would not concede to Kennedy that the illnesses must be due to toxic exposures. But he told the committee, "[W]e recognize this as a specific, distinct entity that is due to some cause and that is more than stress. Stress is not the explanation for this illness in these affected individuals. . . .

"I think we must look at other kinds of perhaps more controversial but, I think, as real disease entities . . . one, chronic fatigue syndrome; the other, multiple chemical sensitivity. . . . I think chronic fatigue syndrome and multiple sensitivities may be the same kind of thing, perhaps on different points in a spectrum."

This, so far as I can tell, was the first official suggestion that chronic fatigue syndrome might be a factor in the veterans' illnesses. Formally recognized in 1988, CFS put a different spin on the matter, a domestic spin, because whatever it was that caused chronic fatigue syndrome, nobody believed it was chemicals encountered during a foreign war. Why did Blanck think of CFS? And how did he know to connect CFS to MCS? I need another digression to explain his thinking.

CHRONIC FATIGUE SYNDROME is an illness characterized by a tiredness so pervasive that the sickest patients may become disabled. The cause is unknown, and treatment is difficult. CFS is not brought on by exertion, nor is it relieved by rest. Typically it starts after a bout of flu, which is fatiguing in itself, but the exhaustion becomes chronic. Other problems soon accumulate: cognitive difficulty, disordered sleep, muscle pain, headache, weight gain, depression.

In its modern manifestation CFS dates to an outbreak of symptoms in Incline Village, Nevada, in 1984. A sickness in the town that was like mononucleosis didn't resolve, and dozens of people were left helplessly tired and muddled. Government and private health investigators thought a virus was responsible. Epstein-Barr virus, one of the family of herpes viruses, was an early candidate, being found in the blood of many of the patients, until it was found also in people who were not ill.

Similar cases were reported about the country in the latter half of the 1980s. The pattern of the fatigue became more random than epidemic. More individuals were affected than groups, which set back the hunt for an infectious agent, since it was difficult to speculate how contagion might occur among unconnected people. At the same time researchers in the United States and Great Britain revisited past episodes of the symptoms described in the medical literature. Some episodes had been local outbreaks, as in Nevada, dissipating without explanation. One very widespread illness, called neurasthenia, seemed in hindsight to have been the chronic fatigue syndrome of the late nineteenth century. The precedents gave heart to the researchers, who had biomedical tools that their predecessors lacked. They bored in on the immune system as the probable seat of the problem.

Ronald Blanck was commander of the U.S. Army Hospital in Berlin during this period. In 1986 the wife of a pilot came to see him. She had been one of the original patients in Nevada. Her ailment was new to Blanck, but he made inquiries, talked to her doctor back home, and took over her treatment.

"I ordered gamma globulin for this patient," he said. "It was expensive, but I had the means to do it." Gamma globulin, a concentration of human antibodies, is known to boost the immune system. The intravenous therapy costs several thousand dollars a month. The evidence that gamma globulin allays CFS was spotty, and few endorse it today; but Blanck's philosophy was that "the patient is the primary focus, not the medical process." The woman seemed to improve, he recalled.

In 1988 a case definition and a name for the new condition were hammered out. That chronic fatigue syndrome achieved the benchmark denied to MCS was probably due to the fact that mainstream doctors were involved from the beginning; they did not cede the problem to alternative practitioners.

However, the diagnostic description of CFS was an ungainly thing, jury-rigged by many authors and bereft of a unique marker. Chronic fatigue syndrome was said to be identified by two major criteria: one, fatigue that reduced the patient's daily activity by at least 50 percent, and two, the exclusion of all other illnesses, including psychiatric conditions. There were eleven minor criteria besides, consisting of signs and symptoms apart from fatigue. The patient had to attest to eight of these eleven, as well as meet the two main criteria, in order to qualify for the diagnosis. Hillary Johnson, the author of *Osler's Web*, a scathing history of the CFS investigation, called the case definition "a Chinese menu." It was modified in 1994, with fewer restrictions and some of the minor criteria made major. It still lacked a biological mechanism at its core.

The case definition at least quelled some of the confusion in the field. It enabled patients to claim a bona fide illness. It permitted epidemiologists to estimate the extent of CFS in the American medical population; four hundred thousand is the figure that has been put out. But the definition did not advance understanding of the CFS etiology or treatment, so the familiar split opened between the mind and body camps. When researchers holding the latter view compared CFS patients with healthy controls, they found immunological changes, subtle abnormalities in the brain, increased allergies, irregular hormones, and lower blood pressures, among other measures, but these signs were inconsistent. Not all CFS patients exhibited them, and not all healthy people did not. In other words, the signs that have been proposed to firm up the case definition of CFS do not predict who has the illness and who doesn't.

Depression was found to be tightly entwined with chronic fatigue, the two conditions feeding off each other, too blurred to allow the physician a clear shot at either one. (Recall that Carol's VA examiner had summarized her complaints in two words: "depression" and "tired.") According to Benjamin Natelson, a neuroscientist who runs the New Jersey Chronic Fatigue Syndrome Center in Newark, "The only symptoms of CFS that are not found in depression are the infectious symptoms of feverishness, sore throat, and swollen and tender glands. All the other symptoms—pain, confusion, weakness, sleep disorder—can be seen in depressed people." Medications for depression may help with CFS, but not reliably.

Natelson's 1998 book *Facing and Fighting Fatigue* is a Herculean melding, in my view, of the mind and body aspects of chronic fatigue syndrome. "Without a definite laboratory test for CFS," he writes, "we simply cannot disentangle the relationship between depression, disease, and the demoralization that may accompany being chronically ill for those patients who have depression, either as part of their CFS or preceding it." One of the first to recognize the connection between gulf war syndrome and chronic fatigue syndrome, Natelson was awarded a research grant by the VA in 1994.

Why are women more prone than men to develop CFS? The organic camp doesn't know; the psychological camp points out that depression is more prevalent among women. In medical surveys Americans who report mild everyday fatigue, the kind of tiredness that might be called normal because it's so common, are relatively even in terms of gender, but as the symptoms become more intense, the sex skew increases until, for crippling cases of CFS, the predominance of women over men is five to one.

The imbalance is one reason why CFS didn't spring to mind when the gulf war phenomenon began, for the ratio among the ill veterans was the opposite. Sociologically, too, the two medical populations were very unlike, the vets tending to be men of modest means and education, the CFS group tending to be women who were upscale and informed. But as I intend to show you, if you boil down the demographics of the sick gulf war veterans and select the most representative individual, you get Carol Best.

To return to General Blanck, who was on the hot seat in the summer of 1993. He wished to define the unknown illnesses so that he could measure and treat them. What the vets were expressing, he thought, was a gulf war version of MCS or CFS, for which approaches were available. Yet even as Blanck's adviser Jay Sanford was working up a definition for a gulf war syndrome, using major and minor criteria, per the CFS format, events occurred that would overrun their plan.

For months the *Birmingham News*, in Alabama, had been running stories about the sick veterans of the 24th Navy Seabees. Many of these reservists believed they had been exposed to chemical warfare agents. Alabama Senator Richard Shelby brought some of them to testify in Washington at the end of June.

Officials from the Pentagon maintained that chemical warfare attacks had not occurred in the theater. However, there was a report that Czech technicians, who worked under contract to the Saudi forces during the war, had detected nerve gas with their instruments on two occasions. The Pentagon wasn't disputing the finding. Blanck's office had already looked into the medical ramifications of the Czech report and had told Senator Shelby that "even under the worst case analysis, the very low levels of agent detected would not be expected to produce significant long-term effects in exposed persons." When the Birmingham paper broke the story of the detections, however, the news started to snowball the other way. The veterans' assertions about their exposures had gained an element of support.

Michigan Senator Donald Riegle assigned a staffer to work on the issue full-time. The staffer, an ex-Secret Service agent named James Tuite, has been mentioned before. Tuite produced an investigative report, which the senator released in September. Titled "Gulf War Syndrome: The Case for Multiple Origin Mixed Chemical/Biotoxin Warfare Related Disorders," it explored the incidents and allegations of hazardous exposures. The report said nothing about CFS or MCS. Tuite produced other reports, but after this first one, though I may give him too much credit, the questions turned irrevocably. They changed from, What is wrong with the Persian Gulf War veterans' health? to, What were the veterans exposed to during the Gulf War?

The VA announced that its Birmingham facility would test veterans for possible neurological damage from possible exposures to chemical weapons. Under pressure, the Pentagon conducted an internal investigation of the Czech findings and briefed members of Congress in November. While minimizing the health risks, as Blanck had done, John Deutch, the undersecretary of defense, would not provide details about the detections, citing intelligence concerns. To the other side this was stonewalling, the embryonic phase of cover-up.

Blanck shifted too. As anyone in his position might do, he attempted to reconcile the new information with what he had espoused previously. When he went up to the Hill, he still talked about CFS and MCS and the need for an environmental test unit, but he also agreed that the illnesses of the veterans were due "to some kind of exposure to something or some combination of things in the Gulf." As he explained the adjustment to me later, "This little bit has got to be brought into the equation."

The bit about the Czech detections was not so little, for it had opened the door in his mind to a synergy of effects encompassing sarin (nerve agent), oil smoke, insect sprays, pyridostigmine, diesel fuel, etc. The chemicals may have been at harmless levels by themselves, but perhaps they acted together as the MCS trigger. To Jim Tuite, the Czech detections suggested there had been theater-wide exposures to nerve gas.

You might object that I've given short shrift so far to the effects of the chemical exposures. Do I imply that the argument about their health consequences was just rhetoric? Couldn't this stuff have made at least some of the veterans ill? I'll cover the biomedical basics later, but the short answer is yes, I do think the talk at that time was rhetorical. I have the advantage of writing my history from the present state of inconclusiveness about the gulf war illnesses. Neurotoxic, synergistic exposures? Nobody has demonstrated that they occurred or that they caused the chronic ailments that occurred. Nobody has yet demonstrated that psychological stress was the cause either. The science is still out—permanently out perhaps, since science is exacting about determinations of cause and effect. But if the talk was rhetoric, it was not mere political rhetoric. In 1993 what you had were hunches and hypotheses about chemical illness doing battle with other ideas about illness, the ideas soaring and seizing the facts with which to construct themselves, and it was still possible that one idea would acquire the mass necessary to shoot the others down. That type of rhetoric.

At the end of 1993 General Blanck and Senator Shelby went abroad on a fact-finding mission. They visited all the U.S. allies in the campaign against Iraq, trying to find out from their counterparts what had happened in the Gulf. The answer to the troops' illnesses was over there, probably. Sanford's case definition was put on hold. This was the time that Carol, at home, went to her VA hospital for the Persian Gulf medical exam.

THE PERSIAN GULF Health Registry consisted of case information collected at the local level, thousands of Carols bringing their symptoms to the VA for diagnosis and treatment. Although the statistics of the PGHR and of the smaller registry started by the Defense Department, the Comprehensive Clinical Evaluation Program (CCEP), were sifted like tea leaves, they revealed little about the cause of the problem. With a narrower ailment such a broad intake of information would have generated clues to pursue, but the registries by themselves were not designed to resolve anything. They were catalogs, raw databases, not epidemiological tools.

Even as the PGHR was being established, Dr. Lewis Kuller, the epidemiologist advising the Pentagon, criticized its shortcomings. He told Congress in 1992: "The basic problem that I see here is whether you want to commit your resources to doing a very refined study, using modern technology, which is very expensive, in a relatively limited number of individuals, to try and get an answer, or whether you want to have a very large registry which will basically be very useful in following a large number of people that will get you no answers, I guarantee it."

After the registry had been up and running for two years, the Institute of Medicine, an arm of the National Academy of Sciences, had this to say about its performance: "The VA Persian Gulf Health Registry is not a population database and is not administered uniformly, therefore, it cannot serve the purposes of research into the etiology or treatment of possible health problems."

In 1998 Dr. Robert Haley, an epidemiologist and prominent independent researcher of the gulf war illnesses, said that the registries "provided no useful insight over and above what was known" and "drained away energy and resources that might have gone into case control studies."

Why do epidemiologists knock health registries? Let me illustrate the reason, using figures from Carol's VA medical center.

Between the fall of 1992 and the fall of 1997 the hospital in Carol's community enrolled 135 veterans in the PGHR. At my request the hospital broke down the 135 cases according to the primary diagnosis, or the primary health complaint if the veteran hadn't got a diagnosis.

"Fatigue"	36
Myalgia	22
Headache	19
Dermatitis	16

Depression   12
Memory loss   11
No complaint   8
Lymphoma   8
Graves' disease 3

Carol is on this list, filed either under depression or "fatigue." The category called myalgia, or muscle pain, probably includes joint pain as well. At any rate, the top six categories typify the features of the gulf war illnesses, and the seventh category, "No complaint," contains about the right number of people too, although it's a little low in the context of the entire database.

Context is the key point—the missing point. Consider the veterans having the top six complaints. Coming forward of their own will, they are known in epidemiology as a self-selected group, or patients with self-reported ailments. But how many of the Persian Gulf veterans *don't* have these problems? How many veterans with the same problems *haven't* come forward? How many people who *aren't* veterans experience these same problems? To count up symptoms is well and good, but to understand the extent of an illness, especially an unfamiliar illness, you have to know, Compared with what? Bob DeFraites, investigating the outbreak in Indiana at the start of the controversy, was unable to address the crucial question of context, and for years afterward no one else managed to either. The prevalence of the gulf war symptoms (a separate item from whether they constituted a new disease or syndrome) was as vague as the symptoms themselves. "All those numerators," as one scientist ruefully put it, "in search of a denominator."

The condition that is most startling on the list above is lymphoma, a cancer of the lymphatic tissue. Eight lymphomas occurring in a group of 135 people qualifies as a cancer cluster, and it is a short step to infer that exposures in the Gulf caused the disease in veterans. Likewise for the three cases of Graves' disease, a not unusual thyroid condition. But as is almost always true, clusters of disease appearing in a given community lose their significance when they are put into a larger context—when a town's spate of illness is compared with a state's, for instance, or when the vets with lymphoma at Carol's hospital are compared with the population of vets as a whole. Because chance causes random phenomena to bunch up, in time or in space or both, only by backing off from the close view and increasing the perspective can you observe the true pattern of events.

The rate of lymphoma in Carol's group was 6 percent, very high. But the rate of lymphoma in the VA registry as a whole was just eight-hundredths of 1 percent. Moreover, Persian Gulf veterans in the VA medical system had less of the disease than the population of the United States, whose incidence of lymphoma is not quite two-tenths of 1 percent. Viewed in context, Carol's cluster was a run of bad luck in eastern Washington not duplicated elsewhere.

Across both gulf war registries, the incidence of *all* cancers was less than 1 percent. Several epidemiological studies mounted by the government found that the cancer risk of those serving in the war was no greater than that of military personnel who didn't. You could find faults in these studies that weakened their conclusions, but considering all the evidence, cancer did not appear to be characteristic of wartime service or excessive among the veterans. Most important, because the latency period for cancer developing from a chemical exposure is ten to fifteen years at the shortest, it was too soon for the vets' wartime risk, if there was one, to express itself.

Yet I was not surprised that the vets who were cancer patients attracted an outsize notice. For one thing, there was no argument about the case definition: Here was a disease that might kill them. An Alabama veteran named Nick Roberts, who served with the 24th Navy Seabees, was diagnosed with non-Hodgkin's lymphoma two years after his return. He had been complaining of swollen glands, which he attributed to a chemical attack near Jubail. His local VA missed the signs; a biopsy by a private doctor led to the diagnosis. Roberts then collected reports of cancers among gulf war vets and publicized the numbers of cancers in congressional testimony and interviews. He became a cluster all of himself.

At about the same time the Institute of Medicine, following a mandate of Congress, impaneled a Committee to Review the Health Consequences of Service during the Persian Gulf War. The committee may be described as scientifically conservative. According to its final report, issued in 1996: "No matter how well documented an illness may be, or how moving a personal story, unexplained illnesses also occur in the civilian population and in troops not deployed to the Gulf. A basic question regarding the connection between illness in veterans and their service is not whether specific illnesses or adverse health experiences occurred, but whether the frequency or severity of such outcomes was increased over what occurs in otherwise similar populations that were not in the PG [Persian Gulf]." Such questions, the committee said, could be decided only by rigorous epidemiological study and use of control groups, work that was late in starting, as I have indicated.

Unless I have misread, the committee took a shot at the news media for the heart-tugging personal stories about the illnesses. You might not appreciate the similarity between journalistic enterprise and epidemiology, but the scientists and the reporters were competitors for the truth of the issue. A formal investigation of an outbreak of illness is but one step up from the anecdotes collected by the delving reporter. But where the epidemiologist tries to supply a denominator, or statistical context, to the case reports, the journalist has only his or her judgment as a corrective. Deciding which experts to cite is a major part of the reporter's judgment.

Were the sick veterans who told their stories to the press representative? The more accounts that journalists put together, the more they believed they had confirmed the frightening validity of the gulf war syndrome. It was not science guiding them, but human nature. They had put their finger on *something* that was valid, but was it the rampant condition that they described?

"I've tried to make my stories consistent with the science," said one reporter, whose articles on sick veterans had helped launch the issue nationally. "But I do science in the context of the person, not the person in the context of science—because the science can be twisted."

He was right about the manipulation of science. When uncertainty about a hot issue creates a flexibility in the facts, scientific partisans may twist the facts toward their point of view. But I am working up to defending my own choice of Carol as a subject. Why would you trust that she stands for anything other than my own prejudices about the gulf war illnesses?

Carol fell into my book out of the universe of veterans, like the apple onto Isaac Newton's head. Provided to me at random, she presented almost all the germane symptoms. If the evidence I took from her was anecdotal, meaning unscientifically derived, not generalizable, she was more instructive than the media-tested subjects that were also available. I liked it that she hadn't gone before Congress or joined a gulf war veterans' organization.

I have depicted her in the context of MCS and CFS, two of the domestic precursors, if you will, of her gulf war condition, but there is another way to render Carol, and that is by using risk factors. As it happens, Carol embodied most of the risk factors for the Persian Gulf illnesses.

Risk factors are measures of statistical association. They compare frequencies. The Alsea study, the example I cited in the last chapter, found an association between a woman's risk of miscarriage and her residence near forests in Oregon that were sprayed with a herbicide. Proximity to the spraying was said to be a risk factor for miscarriage. Whether a risk factor signifies a cause and effect must be determined by other research, more arduous than a simple match.

Some risk factors may be due to chance. For example, in my experience, journalists tend to wear corrective lenses and also to vote on the left side of the political spectrum. These two characteristics of journalists are prevalent, I think. If I were to survey the field properly and analyze the data with a computer program that epidemiologists use, I might be able to show a positive association between poor eyesight and the "risk" of becoming a journalist. Alternately, I might show that being a liberal puts one at risk of being a journalist. But I would be mistaken to maintain that the risk factors had caused the choice of career.

Epidemiologists who do this kind of work are sometimes faulted for data-dredging—for running their computers overtime in a search for associations between chronic diseases like cancer and risk factors in the lives of the patients. Scientists justify the practice by saying that the correlations open up new avenues for investigation. In the meantime, though, if the report has moved from the scientific literature into the news media, the public will have had its scare of the week, as the link between chemical substance X and disease Y engenders confusion, occasionally alarm, and eventually cynicism.

Cautiously, then, what are the risk factors for the gulf war conditions? What was different about the sick veterans compared with the majority who kept their health? Since the illnesses themselves evade definition, the fallback is to make the registry rolls represent the conditions. Demographic distinctions can be made between the veterans who sought government health evaluations and those who did not.

The sharpest distinction is by service type. Although reservists made up only 16 percent of the 697,000 people deployed to the Gulf, they contributed about twice that number to the registries. Conversely, active duty forces were 84 percent of the deployment but only 69 percent of the registry population. You may infer that reserve troops are overrepresented with the gulf war illnesses and that being in the reserves was a risk factor. One explanation is that reservists went off to the Gulf older, less fit, and less focused than the regular forces, making them more vulnerable to the chemicals in the environment or to the stress. But many have argued it's the other way around: Active duty soldiers, having more to lose if they reported chronic conditions, are sadly underrepresented in the databases. Regardless, veterans in the reserves were at greater risk of reporting symptoms.

Another factor was gender. More women served in this war, 7 percent of the troops, than in any previous American conflict. Like the reservists (and substantially overlapping them), females show up in greater number in the health registries than they did in the deployment. Is there something here to explore, gingerly? The disparity is much less than the skew in gender for CFS, FM, or MCS patients, however. Males make up 90 percent of the gulf war cases.

A navy epidemiologist named Gregory Gray has crunched the demographics further. In a study published in 1998 Gray and colleagues examined the characteristics of some seventy-five thousand veterans who took the registry health exams. The size of the sample was large enough, Gray wrote, to illuminate small differences between risk factors. Among the variables analyzed were age, sex, race, home region, marital status at the time of war, education, rank, branch of service, type of service, and period served (whether the veteran was posted before, during, or after the heavy fighting). In ranking these, the study identified the characteristics that posed the highest risk. Again they were not things that perpetrated an illness, but were factors associated with it, as footprints and fingerprints are associated with a crime.

The strongest risk factor was being in the army, as opposed to the other service branches. Next, reserve status was a better predictor of sickness than active duty status. People who were older than thirty-one were at higher risk than younger troops. Enlisted personnel and females were at higher risk than officers and males. All the high-ranking attributes apply to Carol. In only two respects was she less typical than other vets: in hailing from the Northwest (people from the South were slightly more likely to be ill) and in having served after the fighting (the combat period put veterans somewhat more at risk).

Maybe you are not impressed by this epidemiological card trick, pulling one individual out of the deck of thousands of sufferers. Let me offer you an additional risk factor, which was noticed by Gray's team and by other researchers. The people who had used medical services in the year preceding the war, as hospital inpatients or outpatients in doctors' offices, were a little more likely to sign up for the registries afterward than people who hadn't needed care earlier. The implication, cautiously: The vets who registered may have been less healthy to start with. Or as medical consumers they knew what it was like to be sick and to seek help for it. Or both.

IN 1994, THOUGH she had registered with the VA, Carol still did not use the VA medical services. Trips to her private doctor increased, however. Carol saw Dr. Brown or his assistants more than a dozen times that year.

Early in the year she experienced pain in her left shoulder, from an old injury of the eighties, and pain in her back, from her injury in the art center in Kuwait. Both conditions improved after a course of physical therapy, an approach that was new to Carol and remarkably successful, she stated, but unfortunately she reaggravated the injuries. She fell on the bad shoulder when she was out hiking in February, possibly cracking a rib besides. Her back went out when she lifted a child at a picnic.

The MRI scan of her shoulder was unclear. If the rotator cuff was torn, said the doctor, she might need surgery to fix it. Carol didn't want surgery, but her insurance company was balking at further rounds of physical therapy. As for the back pain, anti-inflammatories were prescribed, but they caused a reaction that was serious enough for her to be advised to go the emergency room.

At work Carol continued to have respiratory problems, and she continued to have Dr. Brown document them for a workers' compensation claim. She became allergic to Mylar, a polyester film used at the plant. The printing operation was slated to move to a new building in the fall, with improved ventilation, but right now the work environment was unacceptable to her. She maintained she was still being exposed to too many chemicals.

One spring Sunday, out for a "strenuous" hike, Carol was frightened by chest pains and a rapid heartbeat. There was a family history of heart disease. Her electrocardiogram the next day was normal, but to be sure, Dr.

Brown scheduled a second EKG on the treadmill. He also found a tick embedded in Carol's right shoulder and took it out.

The treadmill test came back normal. While not ruling out organic explanations, Dr. Brown suggested that the heart incident was due to stress and anxiety, and Carol seems to have agreed. More than once during 1994 she talked to him about her feelings of depression. Unhappy with her weight, she wasn't dating, not that she wanted a romantic involvement. She had hot flashes, hypoglycemia, and attacks of stomach pain. She soldiered on with her irritable heart.

In February 1995 Carol decided to go to the VA for a full workup. At her first appointment she detailed her medical history, focusing on the occupational asthma. A lung function test confirmed a "mildly reduced diffusing capacity."

Scheduled to come back to the hospital for more testing on the following Thursday, Carol appeared instead on Wednesday, in acute distress. The staff put her on a stretcher in the ER. It was her breathing, Carol told a nurse. "I'm a Persian Gulf veteran. I have this terrible fatigue syndrome. I'm an active person, but I want to just lay down and die. I'm not faking it. I also have swelling in my fingers and in my ankles. I can't even open a jar. They said it was depression. Well, of course I'm depressed. I can't do what I want to do."

Carol's newly assigned doctor, Dr. White, was paged. He observed the swelling she spoke of and recorded her complaints of pain, fatigue, weakness, and respiratory difficulty. "Multiple symptoms," he concluded for the record, "no obvious cause." So now Carol had two doctors on the case.

Dr. White was more passive than Dr. Brown, it seemed to me, but he did one thing that the other physician did not do, which was commit to an overarching diagnosis. Carol, he decided, after seeing her again and reviewing her (negative) test results, suffered from fibromyalgia. Dr. White ordered a neurological consultation just in case he was missing something, but having diagnosed a number of patients with FM, he was confident that Carol Best qualified. The two talked about treatment, and he prescribed oil of primrose because Carol preferred a natural medication.

What exactly is fibromyalgia? Dr. Frederick Wolfe, a rheumatologist well known for his work on FM, has defined it as "chronic fatigue in people who get sent to the rheumatologist, or whose joint pain is worse than their fatigue."

In practice a stricter definition is used, but Wolfe's point is that fibromyalgia and chronic fatigue syndrome are overlapping disorders with hallmarks so similar that whichever label the patient comes away with depends upon the background of the physician. There are no good tests to tell the conditions apart.

CFS, you will recall, was delineated within the sphere of infectious disease and immunology because researchers suspected a viral cause for the fatigue. The rheumatologists got the patients with fibromyalgia because they treat pain in the muscles and joints. Traditionally such conditions were due to arthritis. Here the telltale inflammation of arthritis was absent, although soreness and tenderness were easily confirmed, the patients wincing as the doctor's hands pressed upon their bodies. Their pain was exhausting, the patients reported, yet they had a terrible time sleeping. This too was Carol's experience.

Just as chronic fatigue syndrome was formerly known as neurasthenia, so fibromyalgia used to be called muscular rheumatism and fibrositis. The patients with unexplained aches and pains have always been difficult to treat. In the 1970s rheumatologists sought to clarify such conditions. As a substitute for organic signs, they mapped the areas of patients' musculoskeletal systems that hurt. They found, in what was to be FM, that the pain resided on both sides of the body, above the waist and below, and in the neck, and back and down the spine.

But how to measure the *amount* of pain, a notoriously subjective question? Doctors came up with the concept of the tender point to distinguish fibromyalgia patients from those less sensitive. A tender point is a spot that shows no physical damage but that when pressed with about nine pounds of force elicits discomfort. An instrument can deliver the pressure exactly, or the physician may approximate it with his fingers. Healthy individuals will describe the sensation as pressure only, not as pain. Eventually eighteen tender points were identified in fibromyalgia, from the neck to the knee, on front and back, nine on each side.

Biologically real, FM nevertheless needed a social consensus to come into being. The American College of Rheumatology assigned a committee to put together a case definition. Led by Fred Wolfe, the committee published criteria for fibromyalgia in 1990. Wolfe is sometimes referred to as the "inventor" of fibromyalgia, in a wry acknowledgment not that he made up the syndrome but that he was most responsible for its reification.

To qualify for the syndrome, the FM patient must attest to diffuse musculoskeletal pain and respond to at least eleven of the eighteen tender points. Unlike the Chinese menu approach to chronic fatigue syndrome, which offset the vagueness of the symptoms by listing a lot of them, the FM definition rooted itself in the objectivity of the tender points. The definition was simple for doctors to use once they had ruled out other disorders. Thus Carol's Dr. White, seeing nothing in her lab work to direct him elsewhere palpated her tender points and diagnosed FM.

Yet hardly had the new syndrome been constructed than its builders began to pick it apart. Diagnosing fibromyalgia is all very well in practice, quipped Wolfe, at a meeting in 1997, but does it work in theory? The biological rationale still was not there. In search of biochemical abnormalities, scientists have looked at serotonin, a neurotransmitter, which appears to be deficient in FM patients; at a protein in spinal fluid called substance P, involved in the transmission of pain signals and found at high levels in FM patients; and at a new type of antibody in the blood. Such markers do not apply exclusively or consistently to fibromyalgia, and even if they did, they would not reveal its mechanism.

The eighteen tender points, upon close review, fall apart. If you exert pressure just about anywhere on a FM patient's body, she or he will find it painful, specialists say. For example, the VA neurologist who examined Carol at Dr. White's behest reported: "There is no specific tenderness to very light touch, but to very light pressure she is diffusely painful, with a touch-me-not avoidance maneuver at times." Conversely, if you take a random sample of otherwise healthy people and test them for tender points, you will get a spectrum of positive responses, from zero up through the eleven locations required for fibromyalgia.

A consensus viewpoint that is gaining ground is that the FM syndrome is a problem of sensory amplification, a disturbance of the central nervous system. Patients have a low threshold not just to pain and pressure but to bodily turmoil in general. The symptoms that accompany FM are fatigue, sleeplessness, stiffness, chest pains, heartburn, irritable bowel, headache, failings of memory, poor concentration, and depression. In view of the extensive complaints and the difficulty of treatment, other scientists simply believe FM to be a psychiatric disorder.

Armed with the FM case definition, epidemiologists have surveyed Americans and estimated that fibromyalgia is the most common rheumatic condition in people under the age of sixty. (In older people osteoarthritis afflicts more.) About 2 percent of the U.S. population is said to have FM, not all of them seeking treatment. That's a huge number, millions of people, for an illness certified only a decade ago. Women with fibromyalgia outnumber the men seven to one. For the other risk factors, the FM patient is more likely to have been divorced, to be less educated, and to have a lower income than the average American. She is also more likely to frequent the doctor's office than other patients.

Fibromyalgia is not curable. If patients improve, it is not from any one treatment. An exercise program helps, especially if it is supplemented with cognitive-behavioral therapy, a kind of counseling that encourages patients to take control of their illnesses. Because about half the patients meet the criteria for depression, medications for that condition are tried. The pills may be effective at first, but after six months the patients are back where they were. Oil of primrose? Clinicians have prescribed it on the say-so of its advocates, but FM researchers don't believe in it. Primrose oil might work for some people, but not Carol Best, who tried it off and on for several years.

Wolfe has observed that having a patient with FM or CFS wears on a physician. "You have to sit there for a long time and talk to people," he said, "and they are unhappy with what you tell them, and the medicines do not work." Often the doctor will put a conventional label on the condition, osteoarthritis instead of FM, say, in order to get them out of there with a conventional prescription.

The information is not all discouraging. As with CFS, the formal diagnosis gave the sufferers of FM a shield against the unfair criticism that their pain was all in their heads, that it was nothing, that it could be willed away. They also had a basis, in the more disabling cases, for compensation claims.

It is more than a coincidence, I believe, that fibromyalgia, chronic fatigue syndrome, and multiple chemical sensitivity should have established themselves as medical entities at the same time in the late twentieth century. The researchers of the respective conditions certainly noticed the coincidence. They have shared clinical records and compared one another's case definitions. Picture three circles, each one overlapping the other two by half. This is the extent to which patients in one diagnostic category meet the criteria for the others. By shopping around, patients can easily acquire all three diagnoses.

Politically fibromyalgia has kept a lower profile than its two cousins. The patients representing this portion of the complex seem to be less angry, or less empowered, in the modern parlance, in their attitudes toward chronic illness. It has helped that the rheumatologists embraced fibromyalgia ungrudgingly, precluding charges of neglect or inaction. Finally, the gist of the condition was more familiar than the other two. Corporeal pain, you might say, is humankind's aboriginal complaint, and fibromyalgia its makeover for the millennium.

DURING 1994, CAROL'S year of pain, the issue of the gulf war illnesses caught fire in Washington. Hearings and conferences were held, investigative reports released, laws passed, bureaucracies formed, scientific studies begun . . . science bringing up the rear, as usual. The cases of the gulf war syndrome grew in number and also mutated in kind, encompassing unique neurological manifestations like John Cabrillo's, and a cluster of cases of deadly amyotrophic lateral sclerosis (ALS, or Lou Gehrig's disease). There was a cascade of reports about veterans' semen burning their wives and birth defects blighting their children. Illnesses were being transmitted, it was believed, from veterans to family members and even to pets. You could open up a box of clothing or equipment that had been shipped home from the Persian Gulf and become infected as well.

I refer you to the endnotes for further discussion of the more extreme signs and symptoms. While veterans and their supporters ushered them into the syndrome, the scientists asked, Were these odd or rare conditions products of the war or of chance? Were they, like the cases of cancer, expectable in a population of seven hundred thousand or were they bound to the veterans' unique experiences in the Gulf? The "burning semen," birth defects, ALS, and other extreme conditions were put to tests of epidemiology and in general were not found out of the ordinary. Since the core symptoms of pain, fatigue, headache, rash, diarrhea, shortness of breath, sleep disturbance, and memory loss continued to predominate, I am going to hew to those cases. They remained central to the mystery.

In early 1994 General Blanck of Walter Reed was still of the opinion that MCS and CFS could account for the undiagnosed cases. (FM came onto his radar screen a year later.) MCS and CFS were "real illnesses," he maintained, and though willing to posit that exposures during the war were the trigger, he still thought that the illnesses were part of a broader, domestic phenomenon. On his foreign trip he had learned that allied troops were not having postwar health problems, except for several dozen cases in Britain that looked similar.

Nevertheless, of the ten thousand–plus U.S. veterans who had been examined to date, only a smattering had received diagnoses of MCS, FM, or CFS. The first condition technically wasn't allowable, and chronic fatigue syndrome and fibromyalgia were too new to have impressed many doctors in the corridors of the military health system. CFS and FM were not even in their diagnostic codebooks, though they are now.

In April the National Institutes of Health held a three-day workshop in Bethesda, Maryland. It was titled "The Persian Gulf Experience and Health." For the first and only time in the controversy, all points of view were gathered under one roof. Government researchers and health administrators made presentations, as did veterans' advocates and outside investigators. Psychiatrists sat beside chemical-warfare experts. As the workshop convened, the headline in *USA Today* was AGENT ORANGE ALL OVER AGAIN, VETERANS CHARGE.

The proponents of multiple chemical sensitivity, not just Claudia Miller but some of fiercer disposition, demanded and got a major place on the workshop agenda. They were out to capture the veterans diagnostically. If the gulf war ills could be explained in terms of chemical sensitivity, then surely MCS merited recognition as a genuine syndrome, with consensus on a case definition to follow. A medical population that, to its detractors, was made up of neurotic women chasing chemical phantasms would abruptly be infused with a cohort of fighting men.

Blanck made several presentations at the workshop. Walking his fine line between rival views, he put forward the provisional case definition that Jay Sanford had worked up. It consisted of eight signs and symptoms, with weight loss and low fever rounding out the by now familiar list of complaints. Other known maladies having been excluded, a veteran must exhibit at least five of the eight criteria to be considered a case of gulf war syndrome. Yes, General Blanck was prepared to formalize the gulf war syndrome if epidemiologists, given a case definition, could now go out and corroborate it.

MCS proponents didn't like the Sanford definition because it was modeled too closely on the definition of chronic fatigue syndrome, and it didn't presume a chemical exposure. Mainstream physicians didn't like it, either, because it was too vague and had no organic underpinning. Sanford himself had no illusions that his criteria were definitive and called for more study.

When the workshop was over, its leaders issued a report. They agreed that a case definition could not be derived from the disorganized body of clinical data. The Defense Department and VA were faulted for their lack of coordination. Possible causes for the "unexpected illnesses" were reviewed, ranging from the many chemicals in the field to the many psychological stressors. Again not enough known. The strongest statement in the report was that "No single disease or syndrome is apparent, but rather multiple illnesses with overlapping symptoms and causes."

It is hard to believe that the conference did any good. Afterward, the battle of ideas about the illnesses increased. Research also expanded, but the cankerous irresolution at the heart of the problem seemed to propel the parties in different directions.

In May 1994, under the imprimatur of the Senate Banking Committee and its chairman, Senator Riegle, James Tuite produced an updated version of his report on chemical and biological weapons exposures during the Persian Gulf War. Tuite had compiled just about every incident that had come up in two years of hearings and news media accounts. His report connected the vets' illnesses to their alleged exposures and the exposures in turn to the prewar export of U.S. materials to Iraq.

Senator Riegle held a hearing concurrent with the report's release. When witnesses from the Defense Department were brought before him, Riegle said, "I want to know whether they can give an assurance here, based on their expertise and credentials, that there are no Desert Storm veterans that were exposed to chemical or biological agents during the war period that now account for their illnesses." Proving a negative: This the witnesses could not do.

The Pentagon officials insisted that alarms sounded by the automatic detectors must have been false because follow-up testing by more elaborate means hadn't confirmed the presence of chemical or biological agents. Impatient with the technical drift of the discussion, Riegle said, "When you talk to the sick veterans who were in the theater of operation where the alarms were going off, the ones who are now sick are overwhelmingly convinced that there is a relationship. Now maybe you're smarter than they are and maybe they're smarter than you are. The consequences for them are a lot higher than they are for you because you're not sitting here sick, with all due respect." Applause in the chamber, Tuite sitting at Riegle's ear.

One of the scenarios proposed by Tuite—how nerve gas might have been disseminated at low levels in the atmosphere—was plausible and is worth taking up in a later chapter. Moreover, Khamisiyah, the site where nerve gas undeniably was released as a consequence of U.S. demolition of Iraqi munitions, had not yet come to light. But even if troops had been exposed, to gas, as Tuite and others claimed, the medical link to their illnesses was a reach.

For the majority who were sick, a considerable period (months or years) had elapsed between the exposures and the development of symptoms. According to the prevailing understanding of neurological toxins, including nerve agents and insecticides, symptoms erupted soon after the exposure, and recovery occurred over time—opposite the pattern of the gulf war vets. Whether there remained any chronic damage depended on the severity of the incident, but full recovery was the general rule. In the cases where nerve poisons did have lasting physical effects, the warning signs were a tingling in the hands and feet followed by paralysis, again not like the suite of ills among gulf war vets.

For all its 151 pages plus appendices, the Banking Committee report had no room for the homegrown etiologies of interest to me. Tuite was convinced that the cause of the illnesses lay on the coast of Arabia. Even there he exempted the oil smoke, pesticides, and more mundane chemicals because "these types of exposures are not specific to the Middle East or to the Gulf War and the evidence for these hazards causing the large number of unexplained illnesses is less than compelling."

In June the Defense Department fired back with its own report. A Defense Science Board panel headed by Dr. Joshua Lederberg, a prominent medical scientist and Nobel Prize–winner, examined the wartime intelligence pertaining to chemical and biological warfare agents. Noting that their findings were dependent on the Pentagon's veracity, Lederberg and his colleagues took a hard line ("no evidence") against nerve gas and biological agent exposures, whether deliberate or accidental, and thus a hard line against Tuite's argument about the source of the illnesses. One mustard gas exposure was acknowledged, to a soldier mildly burned while he was searching an Iraqi bunker.

For that matter, this first in-depth scientific review minimized the long-term health risk from any toxic substance, because there had not been "acute injury at initial exposure." Lederberg pointed out in a cover memo:

In fact, the overall health experience of U.S. troops in Operation Desert Storm (OSD) was favorable beyond previous military precedent, with regard to non-combat as well as combat-related disease. This remarkably low background has probably put into relief the residual health problems that have instigated this inquiry.

We do recognize that veterans numbering in the hundreds have complained of a range of symptoms not yet explained by any clear-cut diagnosis—a number of cases in many respects resemble the "Chronic Fatigue Syndrome"; it would be advantageous to coordinate further research on veterans' illnesses in this category with ongoing studies of "CFS" in the civilian population. This is not to deny the possibility of service-connectedness, as severe stress, infection and trauma may well be precipitating causes of "CFS."

Like Blanck, Lederberg had known people with CFS. "I have friends who have suffered from it," he told me, "three close friends, in fact. True, one doesn't explain the other. The work on CFS has gone around in circles too, but why not at least coordinate it with the Persian Gulf vets?"

His instinct, like Blanck's, was to separate the illnesses from the political conduct of the war, but it was too late for that, too late. The Nobelist himself was speared by the politics, when it came out later that he had served on the board of directors of a company that had exported biological materials to Iraq. Lederberg had lent his name to the non-profit company after the shipments were halted and had never even attended a board meeting, but his critics said he should have disclosed the connection before leading the Pentagon inquiry. Tuite blasted him as "unethical." Thereafter Lederberg refused to speak about the gulf war illnesses except to the most persistent of interviewers.

In the fall of 1994 Tuite released another report for Riegle, "Chemical Warfare Agent Identification, Chemical Injuries, and Other Findings," expanding the list of wartime incidents. By now Tuite had either talked to or been told about some twelve hundred vets. He informed reporters that according to his survey, gulf war symptoms affected 78 percent of veterans' wives, 25 percent of their children born before the war, and 65 percent of those born afterward. From this Tuite concluded not only that the syndrome was transmissible but also that putative causes such as posttraumatic stress could be dismissed. How a chemical exposure might progress to an infectious disease, however, was a process that Tuite had not yet worked out. The immune system had to be involved somehow.

Meanwhile Congress provided funds for gulf war studies. Research institutions, public and private, sent proposals to Washington, and over the next several years nearly 150 projects were assigned by federal agencies. The cost of the work through 2000 was put at $160 million. The research fell into three areas: epidemiology and clinical studies (trying to define the illnesses and who had them); toxicology (investigating various agents that might have caused the illnesses); and nervous system research (looking at both psychological and neurological bases of the problem).

It is a measure of the government's incertitude that it would not put all its eggs in one basket. The scientific pie, to mix a metaphor, was sliced as many ways as there were theories about the illnesses. Short of starting another war and sending fresh troops into identical circumstances and watching what happened to them, the studies could not hope to be definitive. Laboratory animals and computer analyses stood in for human test subjects, in most cases, and environmental conditions and exposures had to be re-created as best as could be estimated. But if a breakthrough was a long shot, the scientists were not deterred, for the piñata of federal expenditures would help their laboratories stay in business, whatever they might find, and would hold a career-making prize if their ideas were on target. "All the researchers thought *they'd* be the ones to find it," said Timothy Gerrity, a VA official overseeing the research.

The "it" didn't have to be the mechanism of a chemical in the environment or body; it could be a new germ or a virus or an unusual breakdown of the immune system. At the Department of Defense Stephen Joseph, the new assistant secretary for health affairs, had a hunch that it was a pathogen, an undescribed infectious agent native to the Gulf region. Joseph had been health commissioner in New York City after the AIDS virus was discovered and was influenced by that experience.

Senator Jay Rockefeller, head of the Veterans' Affairs Committee and a rival to Senator Riegle on the gulf war issue, placed his bet on pyridostigmine bromide. PB, the nerve gas pretreatment pill, was standard medication for a muscle-wasting autoimmune condition called myasthenia gravis; patients took the drug for years. It was not an experimental drug, but its use on a broad scale by healthy military personnel was a kind of field experiment by the Pentagon, requiring special permission by the Food and Drug Administration. About one-third of the troops took the PB pills. The recommended doses were lower than for mysathenia patients.

PB posed the same difficulties for researchers as the other exposures of the war did. Since no records of the doses were maintained, there was no way scientifically to correlate the pill taking with the illnesses. Some soldiers did undergo the immediate side effects of pyridostigmine—nausea, abdominal pain, frequent need to urinate—and the number of complaints in the field, conceded a Pentagon expert, had been "unexpectedly high." Perhaps the acute signs of PB were markers in people's systems for symptoms to be expressed later, something you couldn't say about the other agents.

Rockefeller's staff put out a report titled "Is Military Research Hazardous to Veterans' Health? Lessons Spanning Half a Century." The precedents, in this view, for the administration of PB were the toxic exposures to military subjects as far back as the forties, when soldiers were ordered to test gas masks against real gas, to witness atomic explosions at close range, and to take new vaccines and even hallucinogens, all without their informed consent. After the Rockefeller report, pyridostigmine, whether acting alone or in league with other chemicals, moved to the top of the list of suspect agents. Jim Tuite was concerned about PB interactions too.

In the battle between the toxic hypothesis and the stress hypothesis, the former had the latter on the run. Veterans and their representatives, led by Riegle and Tuite, were scornful of the stress argument. A favorite Riegle line was: "This is not a mental problem with the veterans. It may be a mental problem over at the Defense Department. This is not a mental problem with the veterans." One researcher, looking back on the contentious period, told me, "People had to back off from psychological explanations for political reasons."

The third path, the middle way of CFS/FM/MCS, was not entirely neglected, but the three ailments were not much of a draw to the research community. Stuck in their own etiologic morass and hard to treat, they would not produce a quick fix for the veterans, nor would they put a feather in the cap of any investigator who drew the connection to them.

In the end General Blanck's and Claudia Miller's special test unit for chemical sensitivity was not funded. That slice of the research pie went instead to investigators who were more ambivalent than Miller, not nonbelievers, necessarily, but, like Benjamin Natelson, doctors willing to entertain psychological sources for the overlapping conditions. The VA established what it called environmental hazards research centers at its Boston, East Orange (New Jersey) and Portland (Oregon) medical facilities. Under Natelson, the East Orange group studied the incidence of CFS and MCS among the veterans, and the Portland group studied fibromyalgia.

Several physicians to whom I talked said they thought Blanck had gone too far out on a limb promoting Miller's project. Natelson's methods, by contrast, didn't involve exposing patients inside purified environments. When you got down to it, the federal research managers did not want to be told that gulf war vets would feel better if they could live their lives within high-tech bubbles. Who could pay for that kind of therapy?

By late 1994 Blanck was managing the illnesses only as they pertained to patients at Walter Reed. He set up a small treatment program, which I describe at the close of the book. Higher-ups in the Defense Department relieved him of the larger medical investigation. That was fine by him because the pressure was increasing, and so was the criticism.

At a scientific conference on chronic fatigue syndrome in Florida, Blanck gave the keynote speech, in which he noted the similarities between CFS and the gulf war illnesses. Chatting with several doctors afterward, Blanck confessed, "I think gulf war syndrome *is* CFS, but if I come right out and say that, it will seem as if we've solved the problem and we can all go home. But we haven't solved the problem—we still don't know what chronic fatigue syndrome is."

Here was the main reason why health officials did not make more out of CFS and the other two syndromes. "It is a circular exercise to define one mystery in terms of another," said Timothy Cooper, an infectious disease specialist who treated gulf war vets for the U.S. Air Force. "You don't gain very much that is scientifically worthwhile." Cooper, a believer in CFS, added, "Politically, yes, it might have been helpful. We could have said, 'You guys are part of a twentieth-century process.' "

Had the researchers and clinicians followed Blanck's lead and made CFS, FM, and MCS their models for gulf war syndrome, they probably would not have cured the vets' problems, but I think they could have warded off the worse illness—the one that was virulently under way in 1994, the syndrome loosed from the laboratory and assuming a sociopolitical form. When institutions become infected, it's beyond the scientists to do anything.

The vehemence of the sick, their impatience with the agonizing slowness of the medical investigation, triggered the disease that I bemoan. Paradoxically the investigation distracted the VA and Defense Department from the needs of the people who were complaining. "The care message was perceived as secondary," admitted John Mazzuchi, the deputy assistant secretary of clinical services for the Pentagon, in an interview. "It was a mistake to leave the clinical aspect to General Blanck. We were cold, fact-based, scientific-medical types and we should have been healers first." Mazzuchi said that the authorities should have done more to validate the illnesses by emphasizing to the veterans that their illnesses were real, regardless of whether or not the gulf war syndrome was real.

"Our society demands answers NOW," Blanck observed in an e-mail, "and when those answers are unsatisfactory (stress, don't know, not fully compensated, etc.), particularly with an undercurrent of distrust of the Government, politics take over and the issue is used often by well-meaning people to further their own agendas. The result is that there is further distrust, more demands for non-existent answers and a flurry of shallow reviews, reforms and, all too often, the sacrifice of a scapegoat or two."

Ronald Blanck, no scapegoat, was promoted to surgeon general of the Army. "It's the veterans who paid the penalty," he concluded. "They fell into the hands of people with private agendas. They are *still* focused on what they got in the Gulf."

THROUGH THE NEWS media Carol learned more about the nature of her illness. She came to the "perception," Dr. Brown noted in 1995, "of being afflicted by a neurological process that she believes was precipitated by her tour of duty in the Middle East and her understanding that chemical warfare was indeed used during that period of time. . . ."

The neurologist at her local VA agreed with Carol that she had the gulf war syndrome, although his understanding of the condition was a bit different from hers: "Carol Best shows no objective neurological or diffuse signs that would explain her diffuse sensory and perception symptoms. The presentation, their timing and nonspecificity suggests that this might be the so called Gulf War Syndrome. This is similar to the agent orange syndrome. Fibromyalgia is basically a similar diagnosis. Any one of these three terms would be equally applicable." From this blithe judgment Carol concluded that Dr. White's diagnosis of fibromyalgia was more or less an alias.

There was more to the neurologist's report: "She notes that in 1968 or 1969 or thereabouts she had at least one serious head injury from a car accident and she had had other car accidents as well. . . . She has also fractured her left forearm and she has fractured her nose eleven times."

"You broke your nose eleven times?" I said to Carol later, trying to hide my amazement.

"It was thirteen times," she replied. "one less than my brother—we counted." Growing up, she and her brother had competed in athletics. Her broken noses occurred on the trampoline, on the baseball diamond, etc., and later in motorcycle accidents. Carol by her count had been "in five or six motorcycle wrecks."

"So you were a tomboy who never stopped being a tomboy," I said.

Carol, leaning on her cane, was pleased at the description of her old self. "I'm just accident-prone," she said with a shrug. The broken arm happened when she was eight, and the car accident, which fractured her skull and caused double vision temporarily, when she was a teenager. Two of her thirteen broken noses had not been accidents, though, for Carol was counting the two times she had surgery to repair the cartilage from her mishaps.

This extraordinary series of injuries, each one imprinting a memory of pain, Carol had been able to withstand because of the ebullience of her youth, but the pain caught up with her when she got older. According to the experts, a history of regional pain, in specific parts of the body, is a good predictor of the risk of developing fibromyalgia, which is chronic pain felt all over. It is rare that a fibromyalgia patient or for that matter a chronic fatigue patient has been completely healthy beforehand. Often she can name a specific accident, in the case of the FM patient, or an episode of flu, for CFS, that started her symptoms. The persistent new illness has not sprung out of the blue.

Carol soon swung Dr. Brown, her private physician, around to the VA diagnosis of fibromyalgia. One reason he acceded was that the condition was covered by her health insurance. He and her government physicians also began to share notes. Since she hadn't been tolerating her natural medications very well, the doctors got her started on amitryptiline, an antidepressant medication that sometimes helps with FM.

Her medical files bulging, Carol put in for a disability retirement from her job, which if granted would qualify her for a pension. Although the printing company had moved into a new, cleaner plant in the spring of 1995, Carol still had reactions to the chemicals.

"We took her out of everything that was bugging her," her ex-boss told me. "She was working with oil-based paints, and we went to watercolor. The spray mount stuff, I had her quit using that. When she was dizzy, we kept her away from the machinery. I wanted her to work with a respirator. It didn't help."

Carol also filed a disability claim with the VA. In July of 1995 she took the VA's compensation and pension exam at the hospital. The doctor was tough. He issued two rather narrow diagnoses: degenerative disk disease, the reason for her back and neck pain, and depression, "due to her work stress and also her pain and weakness." Carol was granted a partial disability compensation because the agency agreed she had hurt her neck and back in Kuwait. Believing she deserved more, she appealed the finding.

Depression—it was the first time a formal assessment of Carol's mental state appeared in her files. It was recommended too that Carol have a psychiatric examination. If you are skimming through my story, you may say aha, I was waiting for the part where the VA shunts the sick veteran off to the shrink. No doubt this happened arbitrarily in many cases of the gulf war illnesses, but at Carol's hospital the psychiatric option was hardly the only one that her caretakers pursued.

Dr. White kept ordering tests, the most invasive of which, a bone marrow biopsy, produced a result that might suggest a lymphatic cancer. The very opposite of minimizing Carol's symptoms, the VA doctor, in expanding the investigation, maximized the possibilities of her illness, much as the government's overall research plan was to "leave no stone unturned." But the full-tilt, open-ended approach has a drawback. There is a rule of thumb in medicine that the more tests you run on a patient, the greater the likelihood of a result that will erroneously identify a disease. Similarly, if you fund scores of researchers to beat the bushes in different directions, most of the answers that you get back will be wrong.

Carol, if anything, was overmedicalized. As she herself put it, "I've been picked, probed, pinched, stuck by needles, had every kind of test." But when Dr. White sent her to the VA hospital in Seattle for a consultation, the specialists there dismissed her bone marrow results and declined to do a second biopsy. Carol was angry. Perhaps she hoped—perverse corollary of being overmedicalized—that cancer lay at the end of her painful quest. Instead the Seattle doctors confirmed that she had fibromyalgia syndrome, about which they could do little. "She seemed to have little insight into her illness which will make her therapy difficult," noted the rheumatologist in his report to Dr. White.

Back home the patient vented her frustrations upon her two doctors. She stopped taking her fibromyalgia medication; she didn't see the point. One night in October 1995 she came close to collapse. This was the suicide attempt, or cry for help, that she told me about in Los Angeles, the time when her daughter knocked a bunch of pills from her hand.

Carol sought counseling. On the one hand, she was not ashamed to have emotional problems, nor did she belittle the physical role of psychological stress, as some of the sick veterans did. On the other hand, she would never allow that her psychological problems could be the cause of her poor physical health, only that they were among the consequences. To her, chemical exposures in the Persian Gulf had instigated the miserable sequence of her decline.

In an evaluative session with a VA psychiatrist Carol denied having health problems prior to the war. Mainly she talked about her worries for the future. Although she expected to win a medical retirement from her job, she would then become disabled, not only by official designation but also, she feared, in her daily life. She had so much pain walking that at home she had to go down the stairs backward. How could she pursue a new career as an artist or art teacher if her hands hurt too much to hold a paintbrush? When she put her pencil to her sketch pad, for God's sake, she couldn't even *draw*.

In the fall of 1995 Carol had sessions with a psychologist recommended by her private doctor. The therapist tentatively diagnosed "Adjustment Disorder with Mixed Emotional Features (depression, anxiety)." Full-blown clinical depression didn't fit, he thought. It was the daily strain of her circumstances that brought her down.

"Carol is a sincere and very distressed person," the psychologist wrote, "who has been extremely independent all of her life and is now anxious that she may be experiencing progressively more loss of movement and of cognitive abilities. It should be recognized that she did apply for medical retirement in June of 1995 and that secondary gains may be operating in terms of hypervigilance about symptoms." Secondary gain is the term psychologists use for a conflict in motivations. The distressed person is suffering and wants to get better, but there may be a reward or benefit in the distress that acts to prolong it.

The therapist tried to get Carol to accept her physical impairment. "She has been in military all of her adult life and has attitudes consistent with 'never saying die.' " He said it was all right for her to grieve for the loss of the old Carol, the gutsy woman who could fix a jet engine, hike ten miles, run the company picnic, crash a motorcycle, go off to war . . . and get up and do it all over again. That Carol was gone, and she had to learn to live with the new one, who was disabled. With the help of friends and family she could do it; she could still have a rewarding life.

At this period American troops were about to be posted to Bosnia, to manage the peace agreement between the warring Yugoslav parties. A fellow reservist called her up, a guy she knew from the Gulf. "Mom," he said, "I'm headed over to Bosnia. You coming?"

Carol was tempted. "My health won't let me," she said.

MORE ON THE national story: In early 1995 President Clinton appointed the Presidential Advisory Committee on Gulf War Veterans' Illnesses. Its mandate was to make an independent review of the problem. The committee traveled about the country, taking testimony from experts and from veterans.

CBS's *60 Minutes*, whose correspondent Ed Bradley was an archadvocate of the toxic hypothesis, aired a hard-hitting segment, "Gulf War Syndrome." The focus was the chemical warfare alarms and the Pentagon denials of their significance. If U.S. troops had been exposed, maintained John Deutch, the Pentagon official, it was not in "any widespread way."

Riegle's former aide James Tuite served as adviser to the CBS program. Having dug deeper into Defense Department documents, Persian Gulf weather reports, and the general medical literature, Tuite was more convinced than ever that the illnesses were "the result of either the immediate or delayed toxic effects of exposure to chemical, and possibly biological, warfare agents."

A toxicologist at Duke University reported that a combination of pyri-dostigmine bromide and insecticides caused more damage to the nervous systems of chickens than did the chemicals administered singly. The report—aired in the news media before it was presented in a scientific jour-nal—caused a surge in enrollments in the Pentagon health registry.

Timothy McVeigh, a gulf war vet, bombed the federal building in Okla-homa City, killing 168 people, and the unsolved illnesses were briefly implicated in his crime.

The VA and Defense Department continued to accumulate undiag-nosed cases. Even so, the issue of the illnesses lost momentum in 1995. The press did not relax its interest; but the thrust of the stories, anguished patients versus unresponsive government agencies, was getting familiar, and the number of stories diminished. Congressional legislation had enabled research teams to get started and the VA to pay compensation for undiag-nosed conditions. In the absence of anything new, there wasn't much more that Congress or the White House could do. Three years after the outbreak of the mystery illness in Indiana, medical opinion remained divided, and the political controversy had hardened into a kind of scab, under which the sicknesses festered. It was the calm before the Khamisiyah revelation, the ex post facto nerve gas exposure, which broke open the controversy the follow-ing year.

Probably the most interesting event of this period was the Persian Gulf War National Unity Conference, held in Irving, Texas, in March of 1995. This was a convention of veterans, veterans' advocates, and doctors who treated or studied the veterans outside mainstream channels. The organizers billed it as the successor to the 1994 National Institutes of Health work-shop in Maryland, which they said, correctly, had failed to accomplish its goal of clarifying the illnesses. If the NIH meeting was the Woodstock of gulf war research, a hopeful gathering, at least going in, the Texas confer-ence was Altamont, a darker affair.

Agreeing that the gulf war ills represented not a single syndrome but multiple disorders, each independent researcher put forward a candidate disorder, which, in concert with the others, might explain the collective symptoms. The biochemists Garth and Nancy Nicolson had evidence that mycoplasmas, a type of microorganism, had entered the bloodstream of veterans, possibly as a result of genetically engineered Iraqi weapons. Mycoplasmas had spread to the veterans' families, they believed, exhibit A being the Nicolsons themselves, for their daughter was a gulf war vet who was sick and they had gone through bouts of symptoms too. A New Orleans physician named Edward Hyman also thought that bacteria were responsible, but a different strain, which he had found in patients' urine. Hyman and the Nicolsons reported successes in treating veterans with antibiotics.

Other presentations told of an aggressive treatment for multiple chemical sensitivity, of the hazards of depleted uranium, of a rare and crippling allergy to the fine sand of the Gulf region. Howard Urnovitz, a molecular biologist from Berkeley, proposed a connection between the chemical exposures during the war and the activation of viruses in genetically vulnerable veterans, causing immunological and neurological breakdowns. Urnovitz's sketch of the disease process appealed to James Tuite, and thereafter the two became partners, Tuite providing the exposure scenarios and Urnovitz the biomedical consequences.

As a group the presenters criticized "the appalling lack of financial support for their studies and the failure of the Veterans Administration to cooperate with diagnostic and therapeutic clinical trials." Shut out from federal funding, they hadn't the resources to do the science that was necessary to validate their ideas.

Take a moment to appreciate the labor underlying scientific acceptance. It's fine to have a hypothesis, a new idea about a baffling medical condition, and it's right to collect facts in support of the hypothesis, as the doctors at the Texas conference had done in their work with small numbers of veterans. The scientific trial of a new idea is a whole other business, however. I've spoken of the problem of numerators without denominators. The numerators here were the preliminary clinical findings, but to obtain the denominators would take a lot more time and money. Corroboration of a hypothesis is gained through properly designed experiments, statistically robust sample sizes, verifiable case definitions, clearly specified outcomes, control subjects, all the arch stuff that the outside practitioners railed against because they had sick people in their care who had need of answers now.

Researchers such as Claudia Miller (not at the conference) knew they had to acquire this costly proof if they were going to break through, and many of the Texas conferees recognized it too. Good scientists challenge their own ideas—devise tests to disprove them, pitting their new medicines against placebo pills, for instance—so that if a positive finding holds up, the profession is more inclined to embrace it, improve upon it and put the idea to use.

It is something of a catch-22, though, to gain scientific acceptance. When the outsiders applied to the government for money to test their ideas on larger samples of veterans, the federal peer reviewers, who were scientists of established reputation, voted them down because their ideas were unorthodox and their track records slim. The outsiders couldn't prove their ideas without prior funding, and they couldn't get funding without prior proof. Nevertheless, by publicizing their hypotheses and their unfinished results, the mavericks might make headway in the press and in Congress, the two institutions favoring the individual over the mass, numerators before denominators. Transmitted through the press and Congress, the endorsements of veterans who'd been helped pressured agency officials to accommodate the outside researchers. After Khamisiyah, which upset the Pentagon's version of events and put scientists associated with the government on the defensive, the demands to consider alternate views became overwhelming. At that point several who were at the Texas conference got federal contracts to explore their theories.

In August 1995 the Defense Department released an analysis of ten thousand veterans who had enrolled in its health registry, the Comprehensive Clinical Evaluation Program. Stephen Joseph, the official presenting the CCEP report, argued once again that the veterans' illnesses were neither new nor unique. Support for this argument was taken from three civilian surveys, which showed that joint pains, headache, fatigue and sleep problems were common in the American medical population. People brought these complaints to doctors all the time. But just as the outside investigators were tempted to do, the Pentagon had pushed its data too far. The civilian surveys comprised mainly older Americans, people over sixty, including many more females than in the gulf war group. The comparison of symptoms was cast into doubt because it mixed apples and oranges. The data in the registries simply could not be utilized that way.

Out of the spotlight, government-funded epidemiologists did make progress during 1995. They drew rough boundaries around the problem. Taking the entire gulf war cohort, sick and healthy people alike, and comparing them with military personnel of the same period who hadn't been called to the conflict, researchers found that gulf war veterans were not dying from diseases at a higher rate than their peers. In addition, a review of the postwar hospitalization records of active duty veterans showed they weren't being admitted to military hospitals more often than their peers. The second study excluded the reserve complement of the original force and missed many who had since retired from service, a major shortcoming because reservists and retired veterans were more likely to be ill. But the two studies did confirm a general clinical impression about the gulf war symptoms. Whether the veteran was as vociferous as Job about his pain or just hobbling along like Carol, the group on the whole was not fatally or even gravely incapacitated.

State and federal epidemiologists also surveyed smaller groups of veterans and nonveterans in order to get at the question of prevalence—not the prevalence of the disease or syndrome, which still did not formally exist, but the rates of the most frequently reported symptoms. Did Persian Gulf vets have more headache, fatigue, pain, rash, etc. than other personnel? You would think that the answer must be yes and hardly worth pursuing. But until the increased rate of symptoms could be verified, researchers could not be sure that gulf war vets were not voicing complaints that other soldiers would voice also, if given the opportunity.

In 1995 the first results appeared, and they followed at an average of one per year, all in agreement. For veterans living in Hawaii and Pennsylvania; for Air National Guard units in Pennsylvania; for military residents of Iowa; for active duty Navy Seabees; for veterans in the Pacific Northwest; for reservists from New England; and finally for a national sample of twenty thousand deployed and nondeployed personnel, it was true that gulf war service carried with it an increased likelihood of health problems, both physical and psychological. Veterans were two, three, and four times sicker than their nondeployed counterparts. The comparisons were science's way of declaring that the illnesses were real—a phenomenon apart.

If the figures were rough, it was because the patients' accounts of their health were not tethered to a clinical marker. Time and again the researchers tripped over the lack of a case definition. The rickety structure of the symptoms, dragged from study to study, was a poor substitute for a fundamental understanding of the illnesses. Each team's arrangement of the symptoms was a bit different, like the competing definitions for MCS. No consensus, such as had been forged with CFS and FM, unified them.

Some of the researchers reinforced their papers with exposure data, even though information on toxic exposures was as subjective as the symptomatology. The veterans' exposures (self-reported) did not match up with the symptoms (self-reported), except in vague proportion. A veteran having a greater number of symptoms would tell of a greater number of exposures, but that was not much of a breakthrough.

Dr. Robert Haley tried hardest to construct a case definition for gulf war syndrome within the context of toxic exposures. Haley, an M.D. and epidemiologist at the University of Texas Southwestern Medical Center in Dallas, got involved at the end of 1994, thanks to financial backing from Ross Perot, the billionaire and ex-presidential candidate. Hostile to the idea that the illnesses were psychogenic, Haley developed an organic theory, and mainstream science took it seriously. Unlike other independent investigators I have cited, Haley was strict about his experimental methods and skilled in the statistical packaging of his results.

Measuring the prevalence of raw symptoms was a waste of time, Haley believed. The symptoms offered too many possibilities since the headaches, fatigue, pain, diarrhea, etc. occurred in other medical populations. The new illness he was after was a subtle thing, affecting only a minority, and he thought it had slipped through the broad mesh of the government epidemiologists. To catch it, a case definition was essential. Haley sought signs, not just symptoms.

For his study population Haley chose the 24th Navy Seabees, a well-probed reserve battalion, whose members had reported chemical warfare incidents during the war. He conducted a detailed survey of the unit. Filling out a booklet of questions, the reservists addressed the range of their symptoms as well as their chemical exposures. Haley and colleagues distilled the information with a mathematical technique called factor analysis, and three variants of the gulf war syndrome emerged, three main batches of symptoms.

According to Haley's case definition, syndrome 1 described those veterans complaining of faulty memory, fatigue, depression, and headache. Syndrome 2 involved disorientation, dizziness, and impotence. Syndrome 3 featured pain, muscle exhaustion, and the tingling that suggested nerve damage. In addition, Haley found three other syndromes, but they weren't as important.

Neurological damage was the master mechanism of Haley's gulf war syndrome; he held that the three variants of the syndrome were caused by different mixtures of neurotoxic chemicals. Although the Seabees had reported many exposures, Haley highlighted nerve gas, pyridostigmine, pesticides, and insect repellents because these compounds work in similar ways upon the nervous system.

Haley's theory was that the chemicals, none so concentrated as to have prompted acute responses in the Seabees, had combined at low levels to injure their brains, from which ensued a more general attack on their bodies. In support of the theory he was able to link different chemical combinations to his three symptom clusters. A veteran with a particular array of symptoms was more likely to report a particular exposure, unlike the blanket associations shown by other studies.

Haley then attempted to demonstrate there had been brain damage. He brought forty-three Seabees to Dallas for testing. Twenty-three of the group met the criteria for one or another of his syndromes; the remainder said they were healthy. Haley and his team put all forty-three through a battery of neurological and neuropsychological tests. The hypothesis was that the sick people would score lower on the test scales than the healthy people, owing to a deficit in brain function. Indeed the scores of the symptomatic veterans were lower.

The researcher had fashioned a plausible story about the delayed effects of chemical agents. He had strung together a chain of positive results, each piece lending substance to the others. In January 1997 the prestigious *Journal of the American Medical Association* (*JAMA*) published three papers by Haley in the same issue, one on each aspect of his work, immediately thrusting him and his theory to the center of the gulf war debate.

His critics—and there were many—said he hadn't achieved as much as he claimed. Haley was charged with recall bias and selection bias because he had confined his sample to suggestible, high-profile 24th Seabees. Recall bias occurs when subjects are asked about events in their past and their answers are influenced by their feelings at present. Selection bias occurs when a researcher has a sample of people who aren't representative of the whole. A way to guard against the latter is to use a control group, but Haley hadn't done so. Lastly, it was possible that the neurological differences between the sick and healthy subjects in the unit were due not to their toxic wartime exposures but to occupational factors, chemicals at their civilian jobs, say, or to personal habits antedating the war, if they were drinkers, for instance, or to anxiety and depression, which can impair performance on many of the tests that Haley administered.

The doctor rebutted the criticisms. The one point he conceded, because he had reported it in his paper, was that a panel of neurologists, reviewing the test results without knowing which veteran was which, had not been able to make diagnostic distinctions. The sick veterans had scored lower than the others, yes, but not so low as to fall beneath the normal range of performance. If the ill reservists' brains were truly damaged, they should have tested outside normal limits. Such limits are determined by examining populations that are far larger and more diverse than Haley's forty-three subjects. As it was, he had to build his case upon the "abnormal direction" of the test results.

My sense was that it was neurological hairsplitting. Haley had identified a gulf war syndrome, a new organic ailment, he said, but he had located it inside the boundaries of what most other doctors considered normal. Either the parameters of brain health were too loose or Haley's vets were not that ill.

Politically, however, Haley had fortunate timing. Having started his work well before the 1996 Khamisiyah revelation but having published it just afterward, he was given credit for prescience. The neurotoxic scenario again was riding high. The Defense Department awarded Haley three million dollars to try to extend his findings.

CAROL DECIDED SHE must change her life. At work at the printing plant she had been making mistakes. She was having trouble spelling the words on the brochures. She'd used up all her sick leave and felt her boss was harassing her and accusing her of faking. Early in 1996 she went to Dr. Brown. She told him, "You have got to help me." He wrote a recommendation urging that she be granted a medical leave from her job for six weeks. Carol got it and never went back.

Now that she was retired, Carol felt a bit better, although there were days that she had to use a cane to get about. She began to teach drawing and painting to students who came to her home. Adopting a different medical routine, she saw Dr. Brown for the bodily symptoms of her disability, and for emotional counseling she went to a psychiatric nurse practitioner, Nurse Jones, at the local VA hospital.

Carol's counseling sessions took place once a month. The therapist let her work through her anger at the agency. Talking rapidly and blinking back tears, Carol said that Dr. White must be hiding knowledge about the toxic exposures in the Gulf, the stuff in the air or the sand that had made her sick. Was Dr. White forbidden to diagnose gulf war syndrome? At the very least he and the rest of the VA doctors didn't believe her account of her illness, she said.

Nurse Jones's notes indicate that she kept an open mind about the gulf war syndrome and about fibromyalgia, neither of which she was in a position to evaluate. She trusted the diagnosis in Carol's file of adjustment disorder, however. Carol was a person bowled over by circumstances in her life, and over the next year and a half Nurse Jones tried to teach her the means to stand up to them. Primarily she used the techniques of cognitive-behavioral therapy, whereby Carol might learn to recognize and root out negative thinking. Jones gave Carol a self-help book, *Living through Personal Crisis*. She showed her how to relax her body and monitor her breathing.

Not a lot can be accomplished in one meeting a month, but Nurse Jones did get Carol to glimpse important issues of her personality, her need to be in control of situations, for example. "She is accustomed to being productive and powerful, and typically doesn't ask for help," observed Jones.

" 'I'm the type of person that's in total control,' " she quoted Carol as saying. "'I don't know what's happening to me. I'm one who's always been in control of my body.' "

Another time: " 'I've always been there for everybody. People thought I was superwoman, but to me it was just normal. I still want to be needed, but now I can't help people.' "

And: " 'My strongest feeling is being worthless.' "

Carol's disability pension from her employer came through in April, easing the financial pressure. She lost a little weight and started wearing earrings again. But if days that spring were brighter for Carol, she also had the feeling of being "on vacation" and that "reality" must set in soon.

It did. Carol's back pain returned, particularly to the area of her "tailbone," which reminded her, she told Dr. Brown, that her first husband had kicked her there and injured her twenty-five years ago. During the second half of 1996 Carol fell back into the cycle of ambiguous X rays, inconclusive blood tests, halfhearted physical therapy, and unsuccessful anti-inflammatory medication. She relied upon her cane more and more. Her depression got worse, yet she stopped taking her Zoloft.

Arriving for her August session with Nurse Jones, Carol had neglected to do her "homework," the worksheets examining her daily emotions. Having learned some of the jargon of psychotherapy, the patient said she accepted the problems she couldn't change, especially the problems of her physical health, but Jones wondered in her notes whether Carol was "calling suppression/repression 'acceptance.'"

Nurse Jones and Dr. Brown encouraged Carol to recognize the toll of psychological factors upon her body. Otherwise they could not help her fully. But Carol, who suffered at the time from insomnia, nosebleeds, headaches, and aching hands, clung to the idea of an organic explanation, if only the doctors could find one, if only they would reveal it to her. She learned about the VA's referral program for special cases of the gulf war illnesses and got on the waiting list to be sent to the West Los Angeles VA Medical Center for evaluation.

Carol was receiving disability payments both from her former employer and from the VA, but when she placed a claim with the Social Security Administration, it was denied. "[T]here is no objective evidence to establish a severe medical impairment," the adjudicator stated. Distraught, Carol in her next session with Nurse Jones talked about killing herself. Jones calmed her, and decided to try a bolder approach, something that might break the detrimental cast of Carol thinking.

When Carol came back a month later, the therapist proposed a mental exercise. She asked Carol to think of a negative response she'd had, a negative thought about a recent encounter, whatever first came to mind. Carol came up with "Nobody believes me," referring to the government's attitude toward her gulf war illness. Jones then led Carol to a deeper idea about herself, which was also pessimistic. She said, "I cannot protect myself." After further prompting, Carol began to talk about her first marriage, when her husband abused her.

Jones asked Carol to name other incidents in which she had been unable to protect herself. Carol acknowledged that these memories made her feel angry and afraid. At that point Jones introduced what she called a positive cognition, a concept that Carol could use to combat her negative reflex. It was " 'I can learn to take care of myself.' Say it, please, Carol: 'I can learn to take care of myself.' "

At the end of the session Jones suggested that the next time they got together they might work on the problem of powerlessness in Carol's first marriage. But all the probing had exhausted Carol. She didn't want any more of that kind of therapy. She missed the next two meetings with Jones, pleading fatigue. She said she was more concerned about the delay in her plan to go to the referral center in Los Angeles for testing.

In the spring of 1997, as Khamisiyah flared in the news media, the veteran got the call at last. Dr. Hamm and the specialists at the West Los Angeles VAMC would attempt to get to the bottom of her symptoms, her perplexing gulf war symptoms.

THE KHAMISIYAH INCIDENT was first reported on the front page of the *New York Times* and other newspapers on June 22, 1996. The *Times*'s story, by Philip Shenon, reads in part:

> The Pentagon disclosed today [June 21] that American troops may have been exposed to nerve gas shortly after the war in the Persian Gulf when an Army unit blew up an Iraqi ammunition depot that contained rockets armed with chemical agents. The announcement may help explain some of the mysterious illnesses reported by Americans who served in the gulf. . . .
>
> The announcement could mark the beginnings of a dramatic policy reversal for the Pentagon, which has insisted in the past that it knew of no reason for the array of medical and psychological ailments reported by soldiers who served in the gulf. . . .
>
> Dr. Stephen Joseph, the assistant secretary of defense for health affairs, said today that the Pentagon's initial review of its records showed "no unusual frequency" of illness among the soldiers who were nearest the explosion at the depot.
>
> "There are no reports that we have located of acute illness in that time," he said at a news conference. . . .
>
> "The issue really turns on were there any low-level, chronic health effects from the dispersion," he said. "There are some people who claim—and there's a debate about this in terms of medical fact—that it is possible to have long-term chronic effects in the absense [sic] of acute clinical illness."
>
> So far, he said, "we have not found that either."

My selections from the article emphasize the health questions raised by Khamisiyah, not the political questions, such as, Why had it taken five years for the government to bring the incident to light? What else might the Pentagon be guarding about the incident? The political and health ramifications of Khamisiyah were only thinly connected, and over the next months they increasingly diverged, the political questions leapfrogging ahead upon fresh revelations, pulling journalists and congressional investigators after them, while diverting the more cautious panels, such as the Presidential Advisory Committee, from the nagging health mystery.

In 1998, when the dust from Khamisiyah had settled at last (the health questions still up in the air), a report by the Senate Veterans' Affairs Committee summarized the affair: "The story of Khamisiyah is one of confused location identities, inaccurate records, conflicting personal recollections, possible chemical exposure health risks, and claims of Pentagon cover-up after the fact. It illustrates issues common to many other events during the Gulf War."

Some aspects of Khamisiyah were not universal. The exposures could not have caused gulf war vets who weren't in the vicinity to be sick. Some veterans, including Carol, were not even in the theater during March of 1991, when army engineers and demolition teams, arriving at the sprawling Khamisiyah depot in southern Iraq, blew up the bunkers and the unsecured munitions. Even the Pentagon critic James Tuite, an important voice on the political aspects of Khamisiyah, considered the incident a red herring in regard to health. In his view, the coalition bombardment of Iraq earlier in the war had caused more significant exposures.

Khamisiyah also overshadowed the relationship between the veterans' illnesses and chronic fatigue syndrome, fibromyalgia, and multiple chemical sensitivity—not that there had been a rush of recognition before then. With the environment of the Gulf once more the setting for the illnesses, the research apparatus of the Pentagon and VA swiveled its sights toward the long-term health consequences of nerve agents. Outside investigators who had been working on neurotoxic theories got a boost. I have mentioned Robert Haley and Jim Tuite, but there were also William Baumzweiger, who figures in my story later, and Tuite's colleague Howard Urnovitz.

Again I appear to neglect the substance of the neurotoxic theories. Again I assert that my object in this chapter is the war of ideas, the aerial battle, as I've likened it, that was fought above the heads of the veterans suffering in the trenches. Since the neurotoxic theories remain unproved, the power of the argumentation is what really mattered.

A brief history of the Khamisiyah incident: The fact that chemical weapons were stored at the depot had been known to the U.S. government before the war. The CIA warned the Pentagon, but the warning wasn't passed along. Almost everyone puts the prewar failure down to confusion over place-names, the one hand not knowing what the other was doing, etc. The differences of opinion begin with the period just after the conflict.

Two detonations at Khamisiyah, one on March 4 and the other on March 10, probably released sarin, a nerve agent. Deadly levels certainly were not attained, for no telltale symptoms were reported, no gagging or gasping by the U.S. troops on the scene or downwind of it, no runny noses or contracted pupils. The concentrations of nerve agent had to be low, but how low? At least one alarm went off during the first of the incidents, and some soldiers recalled others sounding during the time that they were working at the depot; but follow-up testing at the site didn't confirm the presence of chemical munitions. The day after the second and larger detonation men stood around the debris in shirtsleeves, oblivious, while the suspect plume wafted hundreds of miles to the south, this according to computer models that reconstructed the event years later.

United Nations inspectors learned from the Iraqis after the war that some of the rockets destroyed at the depot had contained nerve gas. American intelligence officers didn't believe it when they were first informed, and U.S. military logs recording communications about Khamisiyah and other incidents were either lost or destroyed. Even after the illnesses had become important, the Pentagon and CIA were less than eager to retrieve the facts about the rockets stored at Khamisiyah. External pressure finally shook out the truth.

Did the episode constitute a cover-up or just a persistent screwup? Bernard Rostker, the Defense Department official appointed to investigate the exposure incidents, told me that the failure was due to "a series of mind-sets reinforcing each other's point of view." He maintained there wasn't a cover-up of Khamisiyah, only a blind spot. Privately, and cynically, I agreed with him, for I doubted the military bureaucracy could be competent enough to bury an issue this hot for five years. Regardless, I would have more to tell you about missed warnings and missing logs if I thought they would shed light on the gulf war ailments.

As I've labored to show, the illnesses then and now were chimerical entities—not imaginary, but unfamiliar in their conglomeration of symptoms, intangible in their paucity of signs. The only way that Khamisiyah could be helpful to the doctors was if low concentrations of nerve gas would produce a batch of chronic ailments. This was not known to be the case, according to the majority of professional opinion. Yet because the unknown, even if unlikely, was scientifically not impossible, politically it could not be ignored. Allowing the assumption that some of the troops, inhaling the emanations from Khamisiyah, were somehow made sick, the Pentagon was compelled to estimate the number of people who had been exposed. And so a tangled exercise began, one with a déjà vu feeling in America, as health officials responded defensively to angry constituents who'd been subjected unwittingly to environmental chemicals.

When the Khamisiyah incident was first publicized, in June of 1996, up to four hundred veterans were said to be at risk. The threat was thought to be limited to those who worked at the site at the time. In August the number was raised to eleven hundred. In September it went up to five thousand, comprising all the troops within twenty-five kilometers of the depot.

In October, after estimates of the wind speeds and the amount of sarin had been fed into the equation, it was decided that all those within a fifty-kilometer (thirty-one-mile) radius, some twenty-one thousand veterans, ought to be notified of their potential exposures to low-level nerve agent. The men and women who received letters from the Pentagon were encouraged to go to the health registries and get checkups. They also were asked about symptoms that might be connected to a chemical exposure.

Obviously the wind in southern Iraq could not have been blowing sarin vapors in all directions simultaneously. The point of drawing a large circle around Khamisiyah was to ensure that no individual soldier in the area would be excluded from the possibility of contamination; he or she shouldn't be deprived of that information while the scientists worked up a closer estimate of the health hazard. Scientists refer to this practice as conservative thinking, the making sure that if you err, you don't err on the side of harm. Conservative thinking also poses "a wonderful opportunity for the miscommunication of risk," one scientist commented, because though its intent is to be cautious, its results can appear to be alarmingly liberal. To the ailing vets and their supporters, the ballooning Khamisiyah numbers suggested not only a health alarm but also a cover-up unraveling.

The agencies thereupon made it worse for themselves. Since the Pentagon had identified twenty-one thousand people in the circle around Khamisiyah, the Department of Veterans Affairs felt obliged to see how many of these people were in its care and what, if anything, might be wrong with them. Hurriedly, VA epidemiologists looked up the names of Khamisiyah veterans in the Persian Gulf Health Registry and from the Pentagon got their specific locations at the time of the detonations.

The hypothesis of the inquiry was that the vets who had been positioned closer to the site, ostensibly having incurred a greater exposure, might be sicker than those who had been stationed farther away. Therefore the VA researchers compared the health records of eighty-one soldiers who had been at Khamisiyah with the records of a larger number within the fifty-kilometer radius and beyond.

The veterans near and far turned out to be similar. The two groups reported about the same percentages of fatigue, rash, headache, sleep problems, diarrhea, and memory loss. However, in one category, that of joint and muscle pain, the vets who had been at the site had a higher incidence of symptoms. About 28 percent said they had pain versus 18 percent of the others.

What did the difference mean? Could you conclude from the survey that Khamisiyah was a cause of the vets' joint pain? When the results were released, the *New York Times* wrote: "For the first time, a Federal agency [the VA] acknowledged today that there appeared to be a direct link between the release of toxic chemicals in Iraq and one of the many different symptoms that have come to be called gulf war syndrome."

Bear in mind that (a) personal exposures to sarin had not been verified at Khamisiyah, (b) the exposures, if they occurred, were not necessarily harmful, (c) the vets reporting musculoskeletal pain were not necessarily the ones who had been exposed, and (d) the mathematical distinction between the near and far groups with pain might be a statistical artifact. Relevant too was that a unit of paratroopers was stationed at the site, men vulnerable to joint injury from having jumped out of airplanes. In short, the link that was reported was in no way good epidemiology. Nevertheless, many received it as a confirmation of the existence of the gulf war syndrome. Carol, distantly aware of the news, must have believed she was on the right track in going to Los Angeles.

The Pentagon and CIA expanded the Khamisiyah investigation. A tremendous amount of brainpower and months of work went into the modeling of the plume from the detonation on March 10. The Pentagon even tried to replicate the explosion at an army test range in Utah. Combining the most conservative estimates of five different computer models, experts produced a "superplume," a hypothetical cloud that they said transported sarin much farther to the south than previous scenarios had allowed, into the northern tier of Saudi Arabia. This superplume would have touched me personally had I stayed in the region a week longer.

The numbers got worse. Officials declared in July of 1997 that the veterans who might have been affected by Khamisiyah were up to 98,910. You can see why the controversy was able to last a whole year. Still, this figure, the most conservative to date, representing 1 in 7 veterans of the war, might increase, it was said, as the modeling was refined.

The number of the exposed was the bad news. The good news, claimed officials, was that none of the troops within the footprint of the plume could have absorbed a dangerous amount of nerve agent. Indeed the heading of the Pentagon press release in July put the best foot forward: "Troops Not Exposed to Dangerous Levels of Chemical Agent." The concentrations—assuming the sarin had dispersed in the air the way that the computers calculated—were too slight for anyone in the field to have felt them.

The *New York Times*'s headline was NEW STUDY RAISES ESTIMATE OF TROOPS EXPOSED TO GAS, and the article by Philip Shenon observed that nearly one hundred thousand veterans would be notified about the possible risks to them from nerve gas. I hope my point is clear. The worst-case scenario is no sooner been put forward than it becomes the basis for a debate over the health hazard, as if there was no question it existed. The *Times* story ended with an ominous prediction by Jim Tuite, his eye ever on the big picture: "When the assessments are done and the analyses are finished, we're going to find out that there was theater-wide exposure."

I must try to keep my account from veering into an attack on a sequacious press, always an easy mark when issues are complicated and emotions are high. In a sense the press only ran through the door that the Defense Department had opened for it. The public affairs officers at the Pentagon must have been tearing out their hair. Covering up facts was politically dangerous, but so too was laying out the facts as far as they might go, because of the danger of misinterpretation.

Was it possible to determine if the gas from Khamisiyah had made people sick? The epidemiological challenge was immense. After 1997 there would be no more back-of-the-envelope calculations. The plan devised by the government scientists was to correlate the health histories of all the troops in the area with the exposures at each of their locations, as estimated by the plume model. Slow to get going and complex to run, the study would not produce results until late 2001, five years after the incident was revealed, ten years after the incident happened.

Philip Shenon produced his own health study of Khamisiyah six weeks after the news broke. "After years of Pentagon denials," he wrote in the *Times*, "a group of veterans of the Persian Gulf War are offering the most compelling evidence to date that American troops were exposed to Iraqi chemical weapons, and say that nerve gas and other chemical agents have begun to ravage their bodies."

The reporter interviewed 37 of the 150 members of the battalion that had been involved in the demolition. Of these, 27 were said to have had health problems since the war. Shenon named 6 of these men and described their cases. One was Brian Martin, who was already known for his effusive symptoms and his commitment to the veterans' cause. Martin's recollections of chemical incidents during the war had been featured in Tuite's reports for Riegle in 1993 and 1994.

Having been steered to the most disturbing cases, Shenon was aware that his presentation lacked a denominator, or statistical context. Still, he was struck by what he had found: "While those interviewed are not a random sample, there still seems to a remarkable amount of illness among a group of young men who, as paratroopers in the war, were required to be in peak physical condition."

Whatever was going on with these men five years after the war, it *was* remarkable. Their experience had changed them, but how? The war had pushed a range of people through the same hard filter, people not representative of the whole but as diverse as Brian Martin, John Cabrillo, Carol Best. The war changed them in the way that a polarizing lens takes scattered rays and makes them vibrate in the same direction. But their intensity, their wavelength going in, hadn't changed when they came out.

IN MAY 1997 Carol was evaluated at the West Los Angles VAMC. I made her acquaintance there, as I have described, and gained her trust. After her latest round of testing she went home with renewed purpose. Although she was unsure how she had come by it, she had in hand a new diagnosis, "Persian Gulf War Syndrome," which she saw as the ace atop her existing cards of occupational asthma, degenerative disk disease, reflux disorder, depression, and several others.

"Persian Gulf War Syndrome" had been entered on her discharge form by mistake. This was perhaps fated to happen given that the patient was ardent for the diagnosis and her doctors had found no organic alternatives to it. In the same paperwork Carol's fibromyalgia had been confirmed, and from Dr. Hamm she got the idea that she also had chronic fatigue syndrome. She accepted those labels on the understanding that they were covers for her gulf war syndrome.

As her daughter put it, in a statement about her case: "She had many different doctors take a look at her and each one of them came up with the same conclusion. Carol Best indeed had Persian Gulf War Syndrome. Of course they can't call it that so once again they put it down as Fibromyalgia and now also Chronic Fatigue Syndrome."

Part of Carol's renewed purpose had to do with compensation. The VA already was paying her four hundred dollars per month for back and neck injuries, after rating her as partially disabled. She reopened her medical claim to the agency, citing the results from West L.A. and requesting a finding of full disability. She collected letters of support from friends, family, Dr. Brown and "those who've seen a change in my health," she said to me on the telephone.

"Dr. Hamm didn't tell me much about the test results," she continued, "but he told me to file for one hundred percent service-connected. He feels it *is* service-connected, since I got it right after the war." Though not endorsing the syndrome per se, often Hamm did urge vets like Carol to try for a full service-connected disability. Most in the referral program deserved it, he thought.

Carol was sounding peppy. One thing she had learned in Los Angeles was that she wasn't going blind, a great relief. She also had acquired some "tips for working around the house" from the occupational therapist. Occupational therapy is rehabilitative instruction. Carol was shown how to open doors without hurting her back and how to twist the caps off jars without straining her hands. She was given a tool for hooking the buttons into the buttonholes of her clothing and another device for pulling on her socks. She got a padded toilet seat, a cane with prongs for extra support, and rubber bands and balls for strengthening her wrists and fingers. Foam cylinders around her pencils and brushes permitted her to draw and paint with less pain.

The devices were a great help to a disabled person, and Carol was pleased to tell me about them. She was so pleased that on her return she had demanded to know why her local VA hadn't put her onto occupational therapy in the first place. Dr. White had no response. Following the lead of the Wadsworth doctors, White now prescribed both occupational and physical therapy for the patient, and he entered "Persian Gulf Syndrome" among Carol's diagnoses.

"I was at the stage of giving up," Carol was saying. "Now I'm not. I've got a new headshrinker, and I'm on a total health diet. I'm trying to clean the poisons out of my system. I'm using vitamins and natural painkillers."

"Carol, it sounds like you've made a change," I said hopefully.

"I feel a difference, even in two weeks," she said. "I still have pain, but there's more energy in me." She said she was able to put aside her cane temporarily. She was teaching three art classes a week. At the recommendation of a friend who was a psychologist, Carol also was going for walks with a young man who was retarded, lending him some needed company.

"I am changing my attitude," she averred. "This crap ain't gonna beat me. If nobody can help me, I'm going to have to help myself."

Great, I said. When I asked whether I could visit her in August, Carol unhesitatingly assented.

At the next phone call she had skidded back into depression. Couldn't sleep, worrying about bills and the appeals of her disability claims. Had a sharp pain in her leg, which prompted a visit to the VA emergency room, her daughter half-carrying her, and then "this jerk pulled on my leg, gave me a pain pill, and sent me home."

I called again a few days later. "My speech has been off today," she said thickly. "At physical therapy they could barely understand me. My left hand and left foot are weak."

But she was feeling better as I left for Washington State. A camping trip with her buddies Doug and Rick had cheered her up. "Carol, I'm on my way," I said, "and will call you when I get to town on Sunday night." Generously she offered to put me up at her house, but I thought a motel would be best because a journalist, I didn't say, should not get too friendly with his subject.

"EXPOSURE." IT'S TIME to deconstruct the term. If I am exposed to something, what does it mean to me? It means that something is close outside my body, trying to get in. A chemical exposure means that the chemical is in my air, water, food, backyard, wherever, but technically I am not affected by it until I absorb it, at which point it is a "dose" and may have significance for my health. Now, if I say that *you* have a chemical exposure, the connotations may be different to you. You may not want to be so analytical about it.

A bottomless topic, just the thing to make the miles pass on I-5, the highway connecting California to Washington.

Bernard Rostker, who after Khamisiyah was the Pentagon point man on exposures, went around the country in the summer of 1997 to face the veterans. In "town meetings" that were open to all, Rostker spoke of the government's new commitment to find out what had happened during the war. He met with a lot of skepticism. Some of the people asked him sharp questions about their exposures, and some told him wrenching stories about their health.

In San Francisco a veteran with a pale, restless face stood up. The man said he had been a member of the 82nd Airborne Division, which had helped secure Khamisiyah during the period of the detonations.

He started off by criticizing the account of the incident disseminated by Rostker's office. Then: "My body's getting worse and worse," and he described some of his symptoms.

Rostker listened impassively at the lectern, a stout, bald man, like a bowling pin that wouldn't be knocked over. It was hot in the room.

"This is about the modeled cloud," said the veteran, raising his voice. "I know I wasn't five miles out of the plume and I want the letter."

Rostker didn't understand. He let the man continue.

"I've had some go-rounds with your office about this. I've called—Hey, I *know* I was there! I could see the explosions when I was driving by on the road! I want that letter!"

Rostker began to get it. "Do you want the letter?" he asked cautiously. The letter to one hundred thousand telling them they might have been exposed to sarin.

Emphatically the veteran nodded.

"OK," said Rostker, making a small wave of the hand, as if he had a magic wand. "We will send you a letter." Poof, the guy was exposed.

The sick man's face relaxed; his shoulders sagged in relief. He wasn't finished, though.

"What about the others in my platoon? We want these letters because it's the first exposure you guys have admitted to. It's a step but more has to be done. . . ."

Exposure or illness, which came first? If you were exposed, were you bound to be ill? Certainly many veterans believed they were ill because they had been exposed.

In Berkeley I interviewed Dr. Joyce Lashof, former dean of the School of Public Health at the University of California there. Lashof served as the chair of the Presidential Advisory Committee on Gulf War Veterans' Illnesses. By 1997 the committee she headed had developed a split personality. Assigned in 1995 to investigate the illnesses, the committee took on the additional charge of investigating the allegations of chemical exposure. It issued reports critical of the Pentagon's handling of the exposure incidents, even as it played down the importance of exposures in causing the illnesses. (Stress was found to be "an important contributing factor" in the illnesses and, pointedly, the committee would credit no other factor.)

I said that the two missions of the committee were incompatible and confusing and even harmful.

Lashof disagreed. "We said over and over again you have to separate exposure from effects," she explained. "I said it to Shenon, to whomever. You have to separate it [the Pentagon's handling of the incidents] from the question of the illnesses. . . . 'Aha, there was exposure? So that's the answer?' 'No, aha, it's *not* the answer.'

"It disturbed me," she reflected, "that this was going to be misunderstood. In meetings we asked ourselves, Why are we pushing this? If there hadn't been those alarms going off, maybe the question of low-dose exposures wouldn't have been important. But by the time we got into the act, Congress and Tuite were going on about the exposures causing illness, and DoD was saying there wasn't any exposure, and then after [the report of] Khamisiyah the press jumped on the bandwagon. So we felt we had to restore the credibility of government. The veterans had a right to know."

The veterans had a right to know—or right-to-know, as the phrase sometimes is put. In the field of public health, right-to-know is shorthand for a law that gives citizens the right to know the types and amounts of toxic chemicals that are being released into the environment by factories and other facilities. The Environmental Protection Agency maintains a public database called the Toxic Release Inventory, which you can access for information. Really you cannot know much, because the information is presented as pounds of chemicals, and you are given no way to extrapolate from the quantities released to your own personal exposure, let alone are you able to figure how exposures to chemicals of differing potencies might result in a health risk. Right-to-know tells you only that stuff is out there, stuff that is bad.

The veterans had a special right to know because they were sick. Along with the Presidential Advisory Committee, the news media championed their right to know about their exposures, but the kind of information that the press passed along was, like the Toxic Release Inventory, too raw and remote to be useful. It wasn't any good for their health. Often it made them feel worse or, if not worse, angry and helpless. The reporters, however, were only messengers serving at the directive of the culture and cannot be blamed for the culture's insistence on the right to know.

As long as you are with me on the trip north to Carol's, you may as well have my short course on America's fascination with toxic exposures. This isn't about the gulf war ailments or their domestic analogs, but about the idea hovering over them all, the toxic hypothesis, linking chronic illness to low levels of chemicals and radiation in the environment. This model of sickness, this mechanism of how one may fall ill, is grounded in facts fifty years old. I am heading for their source at this moment. Driving east along the Columbia River, cutting deeply through the basalt plateau of eastern Washington, I come to the rolling region of America's first exposures.

The exposures were to radioactive gases from the Hanford atomic reservation. The public was unaware of them until after they had ended. Built during World War II, Hanford was the top secret complex that made the plutonium for the nation's first atom bombs. In the forties and fifties it regularly emitted plumes exposing ranch families to radioactive iodine (I-131), which can cause cancer. Of course hazardous pollution had occurred in the U.S. prior to Hanford, but these vapors were the first to combine high technology with government secrecy, the evil twins of the modern age.

In the 1950s the testing of atomic weapons in Nevada subjected many more Americans to radiation. It reached far beyond the "atomic vets." In addition to I-131, such long-lived elements of nuclear fallout as strontium 90 entered people's bodies. Revealed by its radioactive ticking, fallout could be detected in bones and teeth and soil and plants in infinitesimal amounts. The first toxic agent to be diffused globally, fallout created brand-new specialties in biology and ecology, which later were extended to the investigation of chemical pollution and pesticides.

Nuclear testing was no secret to the public. One of the citizens who was exposed to fallout and appalled by it was Rachel Carson, a biologist and writer whose interest had been marine science. The gestational period of *Silent Spring* is hardly remembered today. Barry Commoner and Linus Pauling, scientist-activists like Carson later, organized public opposition to nuclear testing in the atmosphere, and for years the government wasn't responsive, denying the hazard.

To Carson pesticide sprays were "a new kind of fallout." Her book, which appeared in 1962, is arguably the most important work of nonfiction to be published in America in the past century. It started a national movement that is still gaining strength. Right up front she states: "In this now universal contamination of the environment, chemicals are the sinister and little-recognized partners of radiation in changing the very nature of the world—the very nature of life."

Her eloquent brief had two parts. The first documented the acute damage to birds and fish caused by careless applications of DDT and related insecticides. Society could and eventually did control these abuses. Her second point about the pesticides—that there were harmful chronic effects, owing to their slow magnification in the food chain—had come as a scientific surprise. The bald eagle and peregrine falcon were nearly done in before the long-term threat was understood. Seizing upon the hidden durability of the new compounds, Carson drew conclusions for human health that scientists are still trying to verify. She predicted there would be genetic adulterations and widespread malignancies from people's exposure to chemical toxins.

In the 1970s it seemed that her dark scenario might come to pass. A number of cancer-causing compounds were identified, through both laboratory experiments on animals and epidemiological studies of industrial laborers. Tobacco smoke, a type of environmental agent, was linked damningly to lung cancer. Thus you commonly heard in the late seventies that as many as 90 percent of cancers were environmental in origin. Pesticides and industrial chemicals were said to be responsible for half of the cancer incidence. Today the most informed scientists gauge that industrial and agricultural carcinogens account for less than five percent of all cancers.

Congress passed a dozen major pieces of environmental legislation during the seventies. The EPA was established, DDT was banned, and occupational health conditions were tightened up. The Toxic Substances Control Act became law in 1976. However, the decade closed not with a recognition of the country's progress, the gross pollution of the air, soil, and water having been reined in, but with Three Mile Island, a frightening release of nuclear radiation, and Love Canal, America's first toxic waste crisis.

Both incidents led to health complaints by exposed residents. The releases from the Three Mile Island plant in Pennsylvania were too faint, insisted officials, to account for the diverse symptoms arising in their wake. Illness in the Love Canal neighborhood, in upstate New York, was attributed to the chemicals buried beneath houses, but the scientists for the health agencies would not certify the problems as disease clusters. Impasses like these have since become customary. Lois Gibbs, leader of the Love Canal citizens' group, said, "We just knew we were getting sick. We knew there were too many miscarriages, too many birth defects, too many central nervous system problems, too many urinary tract disorders, and too much asthma and other respiratory problems among us."

As many commentators have noted, a society must have controlled infectious disease and attained a high standard of public health before it can worry about subtle, slow-acting agents of illness. In the 1980s, notwithstanding the Republicans in the White House, the health consciousness of an affluent public and the conservatism of environmental regulators fueled a broad campaign against toxics. The technical capacity to ferret out chemical and radioactive substances in the environment made it possible to define ever-fainter exposures, ever-lower doses of concern. There were no national crises on the order of Love Canal or Three Mile Island, but locally, whenever there was a flap over a hazardous waste site or a sick building incident, a minority would come down with nonspecific ailments, and some worried that cancer and birth defects would hurt them next.

EPA's strategies to limit toxic exposures have included, as I described, the Toxic Release Inventory (TRI), alerting citizens to potential threats to their health. A more sophisticated tool brought to use in the eighties was quantitative risk assessment. Risk assessment takes a factor that is missing from the TRI—the estimated potencies of various chemicals—and puts it together with the estimated pathways of exposure. The procedure is used to calculate the number of cancers that might result from different levels of pollution. It's a powerful technique, extrapolating from the high chemical doses sustained by factory workers and test animals to the lower exposures incurred by Americans at large. The hazard is much less, but the population at risk is much greater.

If you will recollect, a risk assessment was used to figure the health damage that might result from the oil smoke in the Gulf. The computer crunched out one or two cases of cancer, depending on where U.S. soldiers were stationed. Of course these later-to-be-sick people, among the hundreds of thousands exposed, can never be identified against the background of disease. They can't be distinguished from those who will contract cancer from other sources. But the EPA's philosophy is that the toll of a carcinogen or a teratogen (a substance causing birth defects) need not be observed to be true and that no dose is so small as not to produce an effect. This unswerving calculation of risk is called the linear, no-threshold model of carcinogenesis. It is taken from studies of radiation victims, starting with the A-bomb survivors of Hiroshima.

You see I'm back in the shadow of Hanford, beneath the fallout from the bomb. When President Kennedy came out for an atmospheric test ban, in 1963, he said: "[T]he number of children and grandchildren with cancer in their bones, with leukemia in their blood, or with poison in their lungs might seem statistically small to some, in comparison with natural health hazards, but this is not a natural health hazard—and it is not a statistical issue. The loss of even one human life, or the malformation of even one baby—who may be born long after we are gone—should be of concern to us all."

The quote always sends a frisson through me like a burst of gamma rays. Kennedy is saying that the health rights of the individual are worth more than any rationalization erected by science. That is why U.S. policy makers can carry the flag against chemical exposures without regard to nuance or complexity. Because America treasures the individual, the prospect of one individual being damaged is all that need be established. You don't have to prove a population effect or a cancer cluster. For the sake of one person being harmed, the government may demand pollution control or a costly cleanup. Industry objects to the reasoning, but industry in this great country can afford to pay.

I really can't gripe either, inasmuch as the environment has been made cleaner since Rachel Carson's time and the process has taken place under full democratic scrutiny. It's the intellectual sloppiness of the process that irks me. Hypotheses about the harm of small exposures to chemicals and radiation are given as facts when their authority owes mainly to being repeated. More troubling, people have learned a way to be sick—a rationale for their symptoms now or in the future—that doctors and scientists cannot alleviate.

Edith Efron, a predecessor of mine, was so upset about the process that she wrote a book about it in 1984, titled *The Apocalyptics*. The book was too long and technical—Carson knew not to swamp her readers with data—and argumentatively it went over the top. But the author identified the source of the problem, which was first articulated by C. P. Snow. Efron wrote of " 'the two cultures'—the dangerous barrier which separates the scientific and humanist cultures and which may leave even the most educated layman incapable of differentiating between serious science and ideology in a white smock."

Patting myself on the back for my discrimination, no smock on me, I arrived in Carol's town in the evening. I arranged to meet her in the morning, when she would be overseeing an art class.

CAROL, HER MOTHER, and her son lived in a roomy two-story house in a modest part of the city. Welcoming me, Carol took me upstairs to see her studio. It was nicely lit by a skylight, with a worktable in the center, shelves of art supplies spilling from the corners, and posters and framed paintings on the walls.

The day promised to be warm. Carol wore paisley shorts and a gray sleeveless blouse that showed off the tan of her arms. She was bare-footed, and she walked fluidly.

Almost immediately her morning class of three arrived. I hadn't been aware that all of Carol's art students were developmentally disabled. They were cheerful young women in their late teens or perhaps late twenties; I couldn't tell from their smooth and smiling faces. Sarah and Jane looked older than Susan, who had Down's syndrome.

The trio trooped in and hugged Carol each in their turn and then got right to work at the art table. Today they were learning how to stencil. Billie, a little girl who was Carol's granddaughter, pulled up a chair beside them.

The room buzzed with scratchy sounds and little laughs, and occasionally there were breaks in the activity for hugs. Carol—glasses perched atop her gray braids, padding back and forth across the carpet—kept up a stream of talk. She coached and praised her students ("Cool . . . all right . . . I like that!") and at the same time told me about her job at the art center in Kuwait following the war.

Her students then were GIs, coming in during their off hours to sculpt, paint, crochet, and make tie-dyed T-shirts. On the blank shore of Arabia, Carol taught lonely guys how to draw mountains. Bold, blue-chalked renditions of their alpine scenes hung in the studio, next to her posters of dragons. There was also work from Kuwaiti kids she had instructed.

When the army found out that Carol could do calligraphy, she was asked to inscribe certificates of merit to the members of her battalion. She penned hundreds of names and also mounted and framed the awards for those who requested it. The military even had certificates for the husbands and wives at home, written with the same windy congratulations: "You measured the war in hours watching CNN, static filled telephone calls from Saudi Arabia, yellow ribbons, and lonely nights. We are grateful for your appreciation and steadfast devotion. . . ." Knowing that her marriage was on the rocks, Carol had inscribed her own relative's certificate to her mother, Beverly.

She'd had the time of her life in Kuwait, marred only by a clash with a supervising officer, who was jealous of her accomplishments, she believed. She also had a problem with a general who wouldn't provide her help in packing up the art center, leading to her neck injury.

Carol showed me another room, which she called her Desert Storm room, full of banners and medals and other memorabilia, not something that I expected from a person whose health was ruined by the military. "If I had to do it all over again, would I go back?" she said. "Yes, I would. If I lose the memories, I lose the wonderful people I met over there."

Passing by the bathroom, I noticed the padded seat on the toilet and the handrails on the bathtub. Yet my impression overall, in this second meeting with her, was of the competent, giving Carol, not the disabled, demanding Carol. Here was the "Mom" to those who needed her. Still, I wondered, who in the world was taking care of "Mom"?

Carol presented me with a stack of her medical records since 1991, and I sat in a chair across from Susan and thumbed through them. The young woman was working on a portrait of a girl, using colored pencils. "A little lighter under the neck," said Carol, leaning over her. "Here, you do it this way, with shading. . . ."

"Dealing with the VA has been a battle," she said to me, "and like all bat-
tles you get tired of it."

She told me about her reduced income, which she called pay, from her
two disability pensions. "I'm sitting here on the verge of what to do finan-
cially." A finance counselor had recommended that she file for bankruptcy.
When I mentioned the large house, wondering if she could keep it, Carol
flared. "If I had to sell the house, I'd have to put five animals to sleep—four
cats and a dog—'cause most places won't take pets. They're part of my family too."

Susan was painting a watercolor of a duck. "I'm in this because I love
teaching," said Carol. "The doctors said that if I exhausted myself, I should
quit. I said, 'What do you want me to do, die?' "

After the class, we went downstairs and I met Carol's mother. A frail-
looking woman in a dark wig, Beverly had had cancer, arthritis, high blood
pressure, stroke, diabetes, and a thyroid problem, all of this gleaned by me
from Carol's medical history, but she had a survivor's glint in her eye.

Carol took her cane, and we went to Burger King for lunch. We had an
appointment, the two of us, with Dr. White at the VA hospital in the late
afternoon. The doctor's comments on her case would be helpful, and I
hoped also that he would serve as a screen for my skepticism, the side of me
that Carol had never seen. In the early afternoon I made copies of the trove
of medical records.

CAROL AND I sat in the waiting room of the hospital. She told me more
of her life story. She was born in Corpus Christi, Texas, the youngest of
four. Her family moved all over the West because of her father's construction work. Travel, Carol always maintained, was the biggest plus in her life.
"I have lived in thirty-nine states and three foreign countries," she said
proudly, counting Kuwait, Saudi Arabia, and Mexico.

Switching schools frequently, Carol boarded with a friend's family in
1970 in order to complete high school. "I was seventeen," she continued,
"and there was Vietnam. I *fought* to go to Vietnam. I wanted to be a flight
nurse. But I was too young, and then I got married and got pregnant."

After having two kids, she joined the U.S. Air Force, but she was too late
for Vietnam duty. Carol was still regretful about the missed excitement, and
for another reason too: "Maybe I could have taken the place of a person

who didn't want to go." My place, for instance, I might have interjected, which was taken by someone else.

Some of what follows you already know. Moving about the country, Carol married three times, and there was physical abuse of her in all the relationships. She thought about suicide more than once. Moreover, she suffered an unusual number of accidents, the broken noses the least of them. As she looked back, Carol had only positive proclamations about her life, but to me her experience was riddled with pain and distress.

Now I will relate Carol to a finding that several MCS researchers have reported, which is an association between a patient's sensitivity to chemicals and physical or sexual abuse earlier in life. In the studies I refer to, the link to abuse is not found in all the cases, but it occurs far too often to be a curiosity. The finding doesn't come exclusively from researchers who believe MCS to be a psychological disorder. Those on the organic side theorize that a brain sensitized to pain may be vulnerable to chemical exposures by the same injurious pathway. Physical abuse also turns up in the histories of FM and CFS patients, who, like MCS sufferers, are preponderantly female. Indeed, if there is one factor in a person's background, male or female, that puts him or her at risk for developing unexplained physical symptoms, it is childhood abuse.

I *relate* Carol to this finding, cast her in its ominous light, without any professional insight or information. I have put two and two together anecdotally, and to this I add a biographical detail garnered just before Dr. White arrived. It is not about abuse but about exposures.

In the spring of 1979, while she was still in the air force, Carol's father had a serious accident on the job. He was working at a chemical plant in Texas when a leak of toxic vapor badly burned his lungs. He was hospitalized for a while, declared disabled, and sent home. "He could never go back to work," said Carol. He died of a heart attack within two months, at age fifty-seven. She got to see him once before he died.

"The accident could have been prevented," she said. "OSHA [Occupational Safety and Health Administration] could have prevented it. That leak had been reported earlier. . . . I'm still coming to grips with it. I was very close to my father."

So there you have my portrait of Carol Best, aching from fibromyalgia, chronically fatigued, sensitive to chemicals in body and mind. A trouper despite all. If you like, she had the gulf war syndrome besides.

DR. WHITE WAS tall, thin, and laconic. His eyes were bloodshot from a long day of seeing patients.

We went into a small office. He asked how Carol was feeling, since he'd treated her the week before for an upper respiratory infection. She said she was better, and then they both looked over at me.

I started by showing him the record of her vaccinations during the war. He said they seemed to be part of a standard military protocol.

"What about her other chemical exposures?" I asked.

"We haven't talked about chemicals a lot," Dr. White said uneasily.

"I haven't pressed him because he doesn't know," said Carol. "We inhaled smoke, I do know that. Something happened over there. . . ."

I kept my gaze on the doctor. "There are two ways to look at her case, aren't there?" I said. "You have a middle-aged woman, with acute episodes of back and neck pain, and then she develops fibromyalgia. Or you have a Persian Gulf vet who reports being exposed to unknown chemicals, and you say she has the gulf war syndrome. Carol's got both diagnoses from the VA. But why do you need to invoke the war when she perfectly well fits the profile for fibromyalgia?"

"Well, at our first meeting," he said, "I did tell her that if I'd seen her in my civilian practice, I'd have said that everything she's got is consistent with fibromyalgia."

"Why not just leave it at that?"

"Fibromyalgia is no wonderful diagnosis either. It's hard to say what it is exactly. Then of course there is the question of her exposures—well, the history of her being in the Gulf. That's what makes her different."

Although I think she agreed that her diagnoses were arbitrary, Carol did not like where this discussion was going. She broke in: "They don't know about the [effects of] the shots, and they don't know the areas where I may have gone where there was chemicals. The doctors are playing a guessing game."

"That's why I ordered the tests," said Dr. White. "I kept coming up with dead ends. I've tried everything. I was happy to have help from the doctors in Los Angeles."

"Persian Gulf syndrome was listed on her discharge form from West L.A. Do you agree with that?"

"I use the term. But I'm in no hurry to tell people that they have Persian Gulf syndrome because, then, how do you treat them?"

"It seems to me that it was Carol who got you to accept the diagnosis of Persian Gulf syndrome."

"No, I don't feel I've done that." Carol broke in again. "*He* came up with the fibromyalgia. . . ." Almost kindly she added, "He just doesn't know what the cause of it is." Then she veered into a criticism of Dr. Hamm, who had eschewed the gulf war diagnosis.

"Of the gulf war vets you've seen," I asked Dr. White, "how does Carol compare? Is her condition worse than the others'?"

He began to stroke his left arm, the fingers of his right hand reaching around his chest and moving lightly up and down. "Carol is one of the more significantly ill people," he said.

"She has filed a claim for complete disability. Do you think—"

"It was Dr. Hamm who told me to try for one hundred percent!"

"Do you think she's disabled?"

He cleared his throat. "That is the area that is the most difficult for me. I would say her illness has had a significant impact on her life."

"It was Dr. Brown who retired me! He put me out of work! Dr. Brown saw me getting worse and worse. And Dr. White saw me several times then too, crying, when I couldn't get a psych appointment at the VA, and I thought nobody believed me, and society was saying it's all in their heads. . . ." As the words spilled out, Carol's eyes were swimming.

"What about stress as the cause of her symptoms?" I asked White.

"Well, we know that your psychological state can affect things like your asthma . . . or your ulcers. To say that it's all in somebody's head isn't helpful, though. I never considered that it was *all* stress-related, but some of it's there. . . ."

"It did go through my mind," Carol, calmer, allowed. "I thought, Maybe it *is* the stress of my job, et cetera. I slowly ruled that out. I am sitting here now with pain in my joints. I feel swollen. I feel the pain *now*, shooting to my feet. I've been in high-powered, high-stress jobs before and this never happened. . . ."

She drew herself up. "In my opinion, my health is getting worse."

"What does 'worse' mean, Carol?" I said. "In my experience veterans with this have good days and bad days, and they measure their health by the number of bad days."

"Yes, I mean that the bad days are starting to get more frequent."

Dr. White was frowning, looking at her as if for the first time. "I asked her to keep a daily log [of her symptoms]," he said, "but it hasn't been revealing of a pattern."

"Do you think she's getting worse?"

"I can't *detect* that, but . . ." He nodded at her, implying that she was the one who knew best.

"Dr. White, what do you say to Carol when you send her out the door? What do you tell her?"

"I say, 'I understand your symptoms.' But I don't have a Gipper speech to give her or anything like that."

"But you don't understand her symptoms, do you? You're just saying to her that you sympathize."

He shrugged.

Carol took over the talk then—that was all I was going to get out of the doctor. She went on about her health and her life, concluding with a flourish: "I'm not going to let this beat me."

We rode back to her house in my car. On the way she was pleasant and forthcoming still, speaking of her childhood and chuckling, even, about being accident-prone. But her good-bye to me was short, and as she walked from the car to the house, her back was stiff and cold.

As 1997 ENDED, the political wrangle over the health mystery quieted, and medical investigators looked with fresh purpose to chronic fatigue syndrome, fibromyalgia, and multiple chemical sensitivity for a handle on the undiagnosed cases. A number of research teams measured the overlap of the gulf war symptoms with CFS, MCS, and FM. The conditions applied to a great many of the sick veterans, though in general the vets' symptoms were milder, less disabling, than seen in the civilian versions.

There was also a movement toward a taxonomic consolidation. "All of us are coming at these ill-defined conditions from a different perspective," declared Dr. Dedra Buchwald, an expert on chronic fatigue syndrome, "but we are probably all looking at the same elephant." The experts, not quibbling any more whether gulf war syndrome existed, placed it in a group they called functional somatic syndromes. The cardinal features of this protean creature were tiredness, pain, gastrointestinal difficulties, a heightened sensitivity to environmental stimuli—and a psychological component, whose contribution, whether ancillary or ascendant, was impossible to know.

Gulf veterans were sicker with this sort of illness than comparable military personnel, the studies plainly showed, but not to be overlooked was that non–gulf war vets also displayed gulf war symptoms. In 1998, for example, the Centers for Disease Control published a thorough study of Pennsylvania reserve units. Forty-five percent of the war veterans attested to the complex of symptoms, as defined by the researchers. So did 15 percent of the controls. The results suggested that the war had reconfigured a health problem, not created it: Carol's story in a nutshell.

At decade's end the Pentagon and VA enrolled hundreds of veterans in treatment trials of aerobic exercise and cognitive-behavioral therapy. These programs were designed not to cure the maladies but to test complementary methods for managing them. Exercise and cognitive-behavioral techniques shift the responsibility for improvement off the doctor and onto the patient. The approach has been shown to make headway against chronic illness, including FM and CFS.

I do not claim that my preferred models of illness finally had carried the day, not at all. For the government also launched a trial of antibiotic therapy, in case the illnesses might yet prove to be a cryptic infection. In addition, the adherents of neurologic explanations, led by Robert Haley, pressed forward with their attempts to demonstrate the markers of a toxic injury. Haley and his associates made some progress.

If at the decade's end you had conducted a poll of Americans on the question of the unsolved illnesses, the majority would have said they were unique to the experience of the Persian Gulf and were due to an exposure, some sort of elusive chemical exposure, incurred on the battlefield in 1991. But as I am in the minority, this chapter has nearly wrapped up my interest in an infirmity peculiar to a desert war. I am going deeper into the nature of chronic illness, so far as the patients will let me. I am going to try to be kinder as well.

"I GOT VERY depressed after you left," Carol said on the phone. "I just collapsed. I couldn't get out of bed, I couldn't function for two weeks. I got the feeling you were trying to disprove everything I said. I felt like I was being put through a ringer. I thought your job was to help out other soldiers—that's why I talked to you."

"Well, Carol," I said lamely, "that's the other side of being a journalist.

To ask the hard questions. Really, I was addressing Dr. White more than you, and he wasn't answering much."

"I thought he was kind of wishy-washy," she said. "But you, I felt like you were saying I was faking it. I got defensive because other people have said that about me, and after you left, I felt like I was this stupid person all over again. Yet I strive each day, I try to make it work every day. . . ."

She halted and collected herself. No more tears to be wasted on me. "It's got so that they've put a wheelchair in my house for the days that are bad."

"I'm sorry to hear that. . . . Carol, it's true I don't think your symptoms are due to exposures in the war. I think maybe it's the fibromyalgia. . . ."

"Then all of us got fibromyalgia at the same time! We all have the same illness! Something happened over there to me and my friends, and if you don't want to believe it, that's fine. You're just doing it [the book] to get attention and to get money."

4

Ron Loses One

Before Ronald Hamm went to medical school, he served for five years in the U.S. Army. He was a paratrooper in the Special Forces, the elite Green Berets. In Vietnam he won a medal for helping rescue a downed helicopter pilot. In another action, spraying fire from the hip "like John Wayne," he tried to take on a whole North Vietnamese squad. "Bravery?" he said, "No, I was just mad, because a buddy got hit. It was a reflexive action on my part." This was not modesty talking so much as his clinician's scrutiny, turned upon himself.

Hamm hurt his knee in Vietnam and was compensated while recovering from the injury. His experience as a soldier also aggravated a bowel condition. The Department of Veterans Affairs, for which he now works, ruled that the two conditions were service-connected. But he is not disabled, nor did he apply for monthly disability payments after the service.

Because of his Vietnam background, Hamm was named the environmental physician and put in charge of the Agent Orange Health Registry when he came to the West Los Angeles VAMC, in 1987. He examined veterans who were concerned that exposures to the herbicide had made them ill. After the Persian Gulf War, he was naturally assigned to the Persian Gulf Health Registry as well and to the hospital's referral program for difficult cases of those illnesses. In ten years Hamm examined and treated many hundreds of Vietnam and Persian Gulf vets for their respective, suspected conditions.

Ron had other duties too, the major one being to take care of the hospital employees within the Administrative Medicine section. Plus he was in charge of compensation and pension exams for veterans of all eras who filed claims at the medical center. Surprisingly, the Persian Gulf vets, their high profile notwithstanding, were being juggled at this major hospital by a single overtaxed doctor.

A couple of times I heard Hamm give speeches about the gulf war ill-nesses at medical meetings. He would introduce himself, rather daringly, as "chief of administrative medicine at West Los Angeles VAMC and a com-bat vet, exposed to Agent Orange." Then he would tell a joke to break the ice—he was fond of telling jokes, though not all of them went over—and he would launch into his overview of the illnesses.

Without having done a whole lot of research, Hamm said that 80 to 90 percent of the veterans without conventional diagnoses could qualify for either chronic fatigue syndrome or fibromyalgia. The men and women with these conditions represented about 4 percent of the total wartime deployment, he said, and that figure was close to the national incidence of CFS and FM. "So it is about what you'd expect from a population this size," he'd conclude. "There isn't any such thing as gulf war syndrome."

Breezy and pony-tailed, Hamm was not totally in tune with his col-leagues, but this opinion was medically safe. In private he was caustic. "CFS and FM are wastebasket diagnoses," he told me. "You can't extricate these syndromes from the process of somatization."

Likewise he had no respect for the Agent Orange health inquiry. "Pseu-doscience," he sniffed. He imagined writing his own book, which would be titled *Agent Orange, Gulf War Syndrome, and Voodoo.* "People do die in voodoo," he said, "when a curse is put on them. So if you can believe your-self into dying, you can believe yourself into getting sick. You probably can believe yourself well too."

"Gulf war syndrome," he said another time, "is a bogus diagnosis, like multiple chemical sensitivity. I'm afraid the medical community will be dragged into a position of accepting that which we know nothing of—the dark ages of medicine all over again. . . . It's a stress disorder, yes, and it's as service-connected as you get. But we have to be able to use the p word—psychological. They're [the vets] going to have to stop telling us it's other than a stress reaction. If the vets insist on there being a Persian Gulf illness, it may be hurting them. When they insist on that, they're put in limbo because there aren't treatments."

Hamm was prepared to accept that there had been low-level chemical exposures to soldiers during the war, perhaps even exposures to nerve gas. He conceded that more research had to be done on chronic health conse-quences "absent acute sequelae," a reference to the fact that veterans hadn't felt sick at the time of the alleged exposures. Maybe there was something to the possibility of adverse reactions to chemical combinations. But Hamm was very dubious.

You're wondering, How could a doctor whose mind was made up be of help to the veterans, resistant as they were to psychologizing their illnesses? In his interactions with referral center patients, Hamm disguised his true opinions. He reasoned that he and the veterans were on parallel tracks, each believing the illnesses to be genuine, connected to the war, disabling to some degree, and compensable. Therefore he was cheerfully vague. He opted for tolerance, kindness, and the provision of the best tests that medicine had to offer, knowing that the results were likely to be inconclusive and the patients likely be dissatisfied.

"Sometimes we doctors are not the most kind and gentle types," he observed. "We don't do things subtly. These patients are not faking their symptoms consciously, but we—some of the clinicians in the VA—come right out and tell them they're faking. Of the vets I've examined, I've seen one only who was an out-and-out fraud. We have some sensitivity issues to deal with."

Hamm sympathized with the veterans for another reason, since he too suffered from what he considered psychosomatic ailments. His bowels, for one, pressured him when he really didn't have to go. Irritable bowel syndrome, which presents itself in several forms, is diagnosed frequently in civilian practice. Millions of Americans have it. Some of the veterans with diarrhea had IBS, including twenty-nine-year-old Pete Timmons, whom Hamm was about to meet.

Irritable bowel syndrome has no specific cause that can be determined, and it is often accompanied by psychological illness, putting it in the camp of other syndromes I have described. But interestingly, researchers are sure that emotional ailments do not cause the bowel symptoms. Why? Because surveys have turned up people like Hamm, who have the syndrome without seeking medical treatment for it and who aren't depressed or anxious or otherwise disturbed. It seems that to be troubled psychologically, and to have bowel problems, make it more likely that the person will go to the doctor and come away with the IBS diagnosis. It doesn't mean the mental symptoms have prompted the bowel symptoms or vice versa. The two conditions simply coexist.

That said, psychological distress can irritate the bowel condition further. A psychological magnification, or exacerbation, of bodily symptoms surely bothered Pete Timmons, whom I also was about to meet.

In addition Hamm had bad insomnia, he told me, but like his bowel problem, it didn't bother him the way it used to. He'd learned to accept his health quirks. "Acceptance is the difference between pain and suffering," he said chirpily.

"I want to think my mind is too strong to get these hysterias," he added, "but now I know I'm subject to them. I had several psychogenic episodes when I was being treated for cancer."

What, cancer too? In 1996 Hamm had surgery for colon cancer, which had advanced more than it should have because he had dismissed the bloody warning signs, thinking them part of his IBS. So far as he knows the operation got it all out. Undergoing chemotherapy afterward, the doctor had the usual nausea from the treatment. Soon the nausea kicked in beforehand, for each time he went down the corridor for his chemo appointment—at this one corner and not before—he would have to veer into the john and vomit. The power of the mind under stress.

So when Dr. Ronald Hamm strolled into Pete's room that afternoon, you might say that he brought with him a been-there, done-that attitude toward the human medical condition and the trials of the fighting man. He should have brought with him, as a counterweight, Pete's idiopathic medical history.

Pete Timmons had been admitted that morning, May 15, 1997, after traveling at dawn from his home in the Southwest. He had his blood drawn, his urine sampled and an electrocardiogram. He was assigned to a room with another sick veteran, Darren Moreau, who had arrived the day before.

Pete stretched out upon the bed, still wearing his street clothes. He lay quietly, a tanned young man with close-cropped hair, his hands clasped behind his head. His body ached, but in the rush of his departure he had forgotten his pain medication. He hadn't eaten all day, but he had no money to buy a snack in the canteen. Pete described his state in an account written later: *At this time I was in extreme pain, fatigued, and very weak, and confused.*

I didn't see that he was uncomfortable, only that he seemed to rest lightly on his bed, not settled in. I wasn't paying attention to Pete. He listened as I interviewed the other veteran in the room, Darren, and his girlfriend, Jackie, sitting together on Darren's bed. Darren was tall and pale and sat stiffly, while Jackie did most of the talking.

Dr. Hamm, clipboard in hand, came in and joined the conversation.

The four of us (with Pete harking, masking the tension he felt) talked about the impact of the wartime exposures.

"I don't question that veterans are ill," the doctor said. "I say, Let's just make them better."

"No," said Jackie, who is a strong-minded person. "Let's find out what happened to them, what it is, and let's neutralize it."

"We could care less about what happened," Hamm said, bridling a little, then catching himself. "Well, I have a prurient desire to know what went on, but it won't help us to help them." Rather than get into it with Jackie, who already had lodged two complaints about Darren's care, he turned to the new patient. Washing his hands in the basin between the beds, he introduced himself to Pete.

"I doubt we'll cure you while you're here," Hamm said after the formalities. "Our job is to diagnose you. But our track record at that is pretty good."

Pete began to speak. He had been sick for a long time. He was already 60 percent service-connected, he said, and was getting Social Security payments too. I inferred from this that he wanted answers for his illness much more than he wanted compensation. "You don't know how much hope I've been through," he said. "I've been to so many doctors I don't know if I have an ounce of hope left." Out of desperation, he said, he had twice tried to commit suicide.

Hamm had nothing to say to that. When Pete, continuing, said that he had hepatitis C, a chronic liver infection, Hamm broke in with a chatty lecture about the risk factors for this strain of the viral disease. "In your case it was probably contracted from sex," he suggested. That is where he started to lose Pete. The doctor was trying to establish a rapport, a dialogue with a patient about a case, but Pete thought Hamm was disputing him. Pete knew perfectly well what the risk factors for hepatitis C were (besides sexual contacts, they were needle sharing among drug users and blood transfusions), and he bitterly resented what the first two implied about his behavior. None explained his infection, in any event, nor did the infection explain his symptoms. It had to be something in the war, Pete thought.

"I've been through the 'let's blame it all on the liver problem,'" he said to Hamm. "Understand, all my symptoms started at the same time in the Gulf before I came home."

He moved to the subject of his pain. "I've been laying in bed for two and a half years. I'm a *father*, and it's hard for me to get up in the morning. I'm in pain right now. One doctor told me to go home and pray, but instead I'm going to school, trying to get my degree in social work. It's very hard. I get bad grades, because with so much pain it's hard to concentrate."

Pete had very good teeth, I noticed. The fact that he didn't look sick, while he lay there talking about being sick, meant nothing. In every facet of this illness the views were conflicting. Seven of his teeth were false, he told me later, replaced when he was in the military.

Pete's journal continued: *Dr. Hamm asked what do I think happened to me in the war. I replied by asking if he was serious. (Approx. 10 min prior I heard him telling the spouse of the other patient, it doesn't matter how we were contaminated). I told Dr. Hamm that I believe it was the PB pills. He replied that would be impossible, it would take a very high dose. I told him I was forced to take one every four hours for almost three weeks.*

"Why do you think you're ill?" Hamm asked Pete.

"Seriously? I think I'm ill because of the pills. Every four hours the staff sergeant would wake us up and make us take them."

"Pyridostigmine," said Hamm. "Did you know that myasthenia gravis patients take it at four times the dose you did?" Again the chatty tone, as if making conversation, not debating him.

Dr. Hamm and Jeff Wheelwright continued a conversation about PGW [Persian Gulf War] *and Vietnam. Dr. Hamm turned again to me and asked if I saw any celebrities during the war. I felt this was a very obnoxious question, and I replied I worked during the war, and I couldn't see my own hand in front of my face.*

I'm afraid I encouraged Hamm to expatiate, as a way to enhance my own standing with the people in the room. From discussing Ron's Vietnam injuries we turned to the smoky skies over Kuwait and then to the famous people who had visited the troops. Hamm told a funny story about administering shots to Brooke Shields and her mother before they left for Saudi Arabia. In the rear end, the both of them, and then he got their autographs. His trick, as he related it, was to give the shot *during* the warning about the forthcoming stick, kind of like the quick pitch in baseball. It was over before they knew it.

"You don't have to be brutal to be a doctor," he concluded.

Pete laughed. "Well, I wasn't being entertained. We were mopping up. There was no bottled water for us."

Dr. Hamm then told me my diagnosis for Hep-C seemed to be inaccurate. At this time I mentioned I had a liver biopsy at the Military Hospital Camp Pend. California. He then questioned that there was even a hospital on Camp Pendleton.

"I've had a liver biopsy, and I really don't want another one," said Pete.

"I'll be riding herd over this. I don't see the value at this juncture for invasive procedures," said Hamm.

"I never look jaundiced, that's the thing," said Pete.

"Yes," said Hamm, bending closer, "nice white eyes. . . . You *could* have a gallbladder disease, totally unrelated to something infectious or chemical. My hope is that you'll walk out of here with a hard diagnosis." Hamm had hoped for a hard diagnosis for John Cabrillo's tremors too, against the odds of his experience. But John got a soft diagnosis, somatoform disorder, and Carol too, fibromyalgia.

Further conversation proceeded with Dr. Hamm and Mr. Wheelwright. At this Dr. Hamm turned again to me and stated, "The Gulf War Syndrome does not exist." This confused me to say the least.

The veteran asked Hamm what he thought about Garth Nicolson's treatment for the "syndrome." Nicolson, an independent biochemist, claimed that infectious microorganisms called mycoplasma were driving the symptoms and could be knocked out by a stiff course of antibiotics.

"There's no such thing as gulf war syndrome," said Hamm. "It's a semantic term. There *are* illnesses, though. Nicolson has a treatment plan. He uses antibiotics in pulses, but it's indiscriminate. You know, death can result. I wouldn't do it unless it's been proven that an infectious agent was responsible. I wouldn't want to take any heavy regimen for six weeks except for food and water."

"How many Persian Gulf veterans have you seen?" Pete wanted to know.

"Four dozen in the referral program," Hamm said, "and about three hundred and fifty more through the registry exam. I've also done about one hundred and fifty compensation exams."

"You know, it's taken me five years to get here, and I don't want to be another statistic."

"We are not likely to satisfy you completely," allowed Hamm.

Pete became emphatic. "No one has done anything. I have had three colonoscopies and a liver biopsy, and they still don't know. I don't want to sit here and be tortured and picked at—"

"Three colonoscopies?" Hamm's eyes widened. He was used to veterans pursuing their symptoms, but three fruitless probes through the rectum were a lot.

I then proceeded to request something for the pain, he asked "What kind of pain"? I replied my entire body has pain. He asked if I can take Motrin, I said whatever, I have taken up to 20 aspirin for this pain in a day. He laughed and said I wouldn't recommend anybody to take that much aspirin, I said I do what I have to do.

Pete asked for pain relievers, adding that he sometimes took twenty aspirin a day at home, though he'd had none today since being admitted. Hamm's response, which I did not write down, displeased Pete, for he said, "Oh, you think that's funny?"

The doctor said he'd order some medication, and then began his final remarks, which were about the schedule of tests that the medical center would be conducting over the next two weeks. "I am making no promises, but at least you won't leave here and say they didn't do anything."

At this point I was experiencing a build up of mania. . . .

"You're not getting it! I've *had* every test. It always comes up negative and I go home and lay in bed."

Hamm, startled, took a small step back. "I do want to hear your frustrations," he said carefully.

"What I expect is some answers. I rearranged my life and I come here on only seventeen hours' notice and now I'm asking myself, Am I going through this for me? Or for the VA?"

The veteran paused. "I'm getting a little manic," he said apologetically.

. . . and I then stated "I am feeling some mania" . . .

"Are you speaking loosely? Are you bipolar?" Hamm looked down at the papers on his clipboard. "Is that in your chart?"

Dr. Hamm smiled and said, "You say that lightly", this confused me. I responded by stating "there is nothing in my record that I suffer from symptoms of Bipolar illness"???

"It should be—or I'm out of here. I'm a grown man with responsibilities, and I don't have to—" Pete's face was flushed, the tips of his ears were bright red. He popped off the bed and in the same motion reached down for his satchel.

Hamm fumbled with his papers. Pete brushed by him and headed for the door. The doctor followed Pete into the hall, trying to dissuade him from leaving. Pete, unswerving, went to the elevator and pushed the button. Finally Hamm turned away, palms up, looking angry too. "I can't keep him here," he said.

Aghast—guilty—for I had a part in this, I took the next elevator down. I found the veteran outside by the curb smoking a cigarette. He'd called a taxi and was going to the airport, bus station, somewhere away from here.

"He was still talking about Vietnam, man," said Pete. "He wasn't listening to me."

Pete would not change his mind about leaving. He admitted that his expectations had been dashed. "Yeah," he said, "I guess I was hoping to be cured—but they won't give me a goddamn aspirin."

Now he decided to go to a relative's house in a suburb of Los Angeles. When I offered to drive him there, he looked at me in disbelief. "I won't get in the car with you. I don't know you."

He was right, of course. I smiled ruefully. What a disaster.

"Yeah," he croaked. "Laugh."

I had nothing to lose. "It's incredibly lonely—isn't it, Pete—this illness. You're out there and you're all alone with it. You've made a *commitment* to it because your illness is your only friend after all these years."

"Yes," he said, surprised I knew. But he brought up another friend, who was holding his soul together: "My wife, she knows more about this than any doctor."

When the taxi had taken him away, I turned back to the hospital, and who would be coming out the glass doors but Carol, slow on her cane. I blurted the whole story to her.

"Oh, you can't learn anything that way," she said mildly. "Maybe the next test would show something." She proceeded on her walk.

Back in the room, Jackie and Darren were indignant.

"He [Hamm] let Pete down extremely," declared Jackie. "Not that he should have a cure for him, but he should be prepared."

"That's why I have Jackie speak for me," said Darren. "Because I get agitated like Pete did."

"After you live with a gulf war veteran, you learn to recognize the warning signs," she said.

Ron, when I caught up with him the next day, was contrite. "We were starting on a road to a connection, I thought. He was miffed that I missed his bipolar depression. I forgot he had a valid diagnosis. I came over there without his packet, and I was caught with my pants down. He had hopes that we'd be different, and when I showed I didn't know . . . I'm not going to hear the end of this. I e-mailed my boss and told him, 'I lost one today.' "

A week later, Darren Moreau also left in a huff. He and Jackie thought the testing plan was repetitive and wasn't leading anywhere. They were dismayed by the staff's "incompetence," as Jackie described it in letters to their congresswoman and various senators. "We have found that the medical and nursing staff is not properly informed or instructed in how to deal with the PGW veterans." The day before the pair departed, Hamm offered them mea culpas on behalf of the VA and himself. What a disaster.

5

Pete at Sea

Pete Timmons was on the deck of the warship, and something was stuck in his throat. Bad enough that the battle was about to start, a battle he'd never banked on when he joined the marines. Bad enough that his wife, half a world away, was about to bear his second child, and he not there to look after them, and they not knowing whether he'd ever come back. Something painful was stuck in his throat. Rather it was lower down than that—he concentrated on it now—a lump he located between his throat and his chest.

It felt like a roll, a piece of food that wouldn't go down. Maybe he should drink some water. . . . The water! That was it, he thought. The last few days, while the warships maneuvered on the Persian Gulf, feinting attack on the shoreline of Kuwait, Pete had taken more water than usual. The water tasted like diesel fuel or jet fuel—all the troops talked about it. The taste was in the powdered eggs, in the punch, in the tepid ejaculations of the drinking fountains. A petrochemical smell hung in the showers and laced even the laundered fatigues.

Pete's ship wasn't unique. Bad-tasting water was a source of disgruntlement throughout the invasion fleet. Since the onboard distilling plants operated in close proximity to the vessels' engines, diesel pollution from one sometimes got into the other. Harmless, the navy maintained.

"I was drinking a lot because I was dehydrated," Pete said to me on the phone. "I had a lump in my chest after this. I never told anyone about it." Some days he was convinced that the clog in his throat and his cascade of symptoms afterward were due to the ingestion of jet fuel.

I wrote "globus hystericus" in the margin of my notepad. "Did anyone else," I asked, "get sick from the water?" Dr. Jeff the friendly inquisitor.

Not that he could say. "You're worried about getting into battle. Everything's a big laugh, you know. You don't go complaining about your health. If you're sick, you keep your mouth shut for as long as you can stand it. They get mad at you. You're considered a slacker, basically."

I drew lines underneath my provisional diagnosis. Globus hystericus is the sensation of a mass or lump in the throat when no anatomical abnormality is evident. The condition has been around under other names for at least two thousand years. Because the Hippocratic physicians believed that the uterus could migrate within a woman's body, causing trouble wherever it landed, they attributed the mysterious discomfort in the throat to the wandering womb.

The words "uterus" and "hysteria" have the same root. The diagnosis globus hystericus dates from the time of Freud, when psychoanalysts were appropriating hysteria, still considered a bodily ailment, but no longer an exclusively uterine or female one, into the newly opened cave of the mind.

The "lump" you get in your throat during grief or anxiety: That's a run-of-the-mill form of globus. It's a transient physical response to an emotional state, akin to the headache or stomachache generated by tension, or the dizziness and palpitations following a violent argument. Nobody objects to this kind of reaction being typed as psychosomatic or psychogenic. Gastroenterologists, whose purview is the region where the globus sensation occurs, will permit such mild symptoms to be called hystericus. But when the sensation persists and interferes with swallowing, or makes the person feel as if he's choking or can't eat, or causes a high, clipped cough, such as I heard from Pete occasionally, trying to clear the constriction, the gastroenterologist will look beyond stress for an organic disorder.

The source of the sensation, if not in the anatomy of the throat, might be in the function, an impairment in gastroesophageal function. The esophagus muscles may not be contracting normally, or the tube may be disturbed by acid backing up from the stomach. Labeling the condition "globus pharyngeus" (in pointed rejection of Freud), the gastroenterologist will start treatment with a course of acid blockers.

A third possibility, neither hystericus nor pharyngeus: Was Pete having a toxic reaction to contaminated water, as he asserted? It could have been so in part. The exposure was mild and unless every marine aboard was concealing the same symptom, Pete's throat had to be much more sensitive than the others'. He would have experienced what doctors on either side of the mind-body fence call an idiopathic reaction.

It's been said that "idiopathic" means that the doctors are idiots and the patients are pathetic. Sore truth of the quip aside, idiopathic refers to a medical condition of unknown cause, arising of itself, peculiar to the individual. I grant that Pete had an idiopathic physical change in his esophagus on the ship because of the bad water or the fraught moment or some other factor. The standpoint of this chapter will be that Pete's reaction to the change was excessive.

It is the reaction to the reaction that is significant. Long before gulf war syndrome became a public issue, here was a pure case of a man heading toward a disabling illness from a state of good health. A soldier on a ship feels a twinge, and from there his symptoms grow like pearls, monstrous black pearls, accreting around the grains of irritation within his body. In the months and years hence, Pete responding to his idiopathies would make globus hystericus look like child's play.

By the numbers, almost 700,000 people went away to war, about 115,000 had special health exams in years afterward, roughly 20,000 posed symptoms that puzzled the doctors, and a smaller group, Pete Timmons among them, undertook repeated and elaborate testing to try to elucidate their conditions. But the answers to the hardest problems did not fall out. Similar syndromes, as I described in the last chapter, could encircle Pete's problem but would not capture it. Another approach is called for, the individual or idiopathic approach.

"I'm as much proof as one hundred thousand people, if you ask me," Pete said.

I did ask. I spent many hours over several years laboring with him on the telephone and by e-mail because since that one time in Los Angeles he never again would meet me face-to-face. He never provided me with any documentation to verify his military and medical history, and he forbade me to talk to his doctors about his case. In that regard he gave me less to work with than John or Carol, but still I have no reason to doubt him. I think each of us saw the other as an honest person, even though we were bound to disagree, like oil and water, on the meaning of his story. We disagreed because he believed in a disease and I believed only in his sickness.

Eric Cassell, the physician and author, has written of the "fallacy of the idea that different people with the same disease all have the same sickness." Likewise, Foucault complained that modern medicine had turned the sick person into an "endlessly reproducible pathological fact to be found in all patients suffering in a similar way." The distinction they draw is between a generalizable medical condition, a disease, and an individual's private experience of it, an illness or sickness. In Pete's case a further distinction must be made because he was privately ill with something that was broadly irreproducible: two huge barriers for me to cross in order to attain the core of his sickness.

Nevertheless, I pursued it. Fending me off, he boxed my ears again and again; my incessant interest made his symptoms worse. "I'm not going to like your book," he warned me, "no matter how many of my words you use." He was vituperative, wounded, brave, fascinating. I never knew a man who had actually examined his own entrails for the clues to his future.

HE WAS BORN in southern California, the youngest in a large family. His father divorced his mother when Pete was young. He isn't close to his father today and doesn't have much good to say about him. "I'm more into my mother's side of the family," he said. "My mother works in administration at a hospital. She's educated."

Pete was close to his stepfather too, after his mother remarried, but his stepfather died. He had a long illness, Pete said, following an exposure to carbon monoxide.

Pete doesn't remember having any problems with his health as a child. He mentioned being treated for low blood sugar, no doubt meaning hypoglycemia. The hypoglycemia diagnosis has gone out of fashion today, for the symptoms of shakiness or lightheadedness usually can be blunted by snacks between meals.

Health was not a topic that the family members explored. "If you had diarrhea, you didn't talk about it. It was all hush-hush," he said. This attitude made it difficult for his relatives to deal with his present illness because initially they were perplexed and put off when he tried to explain it. His mother, who was the most sympathetic, boning up on the gulf war illnesses, tried to understand. Even she would say, after one of his run-ins with the VA doctors, "What was it this time, Pete?"

Tanned and wiry, the teenage Pete was a skateboarder and a surfer on Huntington Beach. He was good enough at these sports, he told me, that he could have made money at them as a professional. But what he really wanted to do after high school was to become a cop. The local police department had a ride-along program, and he enjoyed catching glimpses of police work from the back of the squad car.

Life as a little brother in a big family wasn't easy. "Growing up, I got no respect," he recalled with a laugh, taking the sting out of it. "I used to be quiet. I didn't open my mouth." He believes that his reticence cost him his opportunity to become a cop. "I couldn't get through the exams for the police academy. On the oral part I'd choke up. I couldn't communicate the way I do now. One of the reasons why I went in [to the military] was to get help with this intimidation."

"You wanted to be toughened up?"

He thought for a second. "Yes, I wanted to be toughened up. I wanted to be strong verbally and physically. I still ask myself, Am I well enough to be a cop?" Then he made one of his characteristic shifts, changing gears without the clutch: "Hey, I'd be racked with ribbons if I were a cop now."

Pete had married his high school sweetheart, Alma, soon after graduation. He worked with his brothers in a family welding business, and it was great for a while, as he made good money and could call his own shots. Then there was a falling-out within the fold, and Pete quit. Early in 1990, with Alma pregnant and the young man feeling the pressure, the military beckoned him.

On the one hand, his wife and his mother were against his enlisting. On the other hand, he had relatives who had served honorably. Besides a steady income for four years, housing, and amenities, he would have a stepping-stone to police work when he got out, and maybe more, for Pete could see himself as an FBI or CIA agent down the line. He really didn't see how he could lose. If he decided to stay in the service and make a career of it, he planned on "picking up rank" fast. He knew he was smart enough.

Pete selected the toughest branch, the Marines. "I admired the Marines. I thought, These people are awesome. I didn't expect a war. I thought, Nothing's gonna go wrong. It'll work out, and they'll protect me.

"I was going to be a lifer," he told me another time, mocking himself. "I took all that abuse, I went through that prison camp, and for what? To hear, when I got sick, You're lying. Which they don't say to you in so many words, but that's what they mean. They throw you away like a piece of trash."

Pete had come to the point in his narrative where recall bias, to borrow an epidemiological term, had darkened his memory of boot camp. He was a good marine, he made clear in other talks, "flawless" even, before he got sick. An "expert gunner," he was trained to fire the eighty-one-millimeter mortar, which demands both mathematical calculation and manual dexterity. He was as tough as the others physically, having scored 295 out of a possible 300 on the fitness test he took on the eve of the war.

As for the hazing—"People are spitting on me, and you can't say stuff back to them"—of course it was mean, I suggested, but didn't every recruit have to endure it?

He was not every recruit, he protested. Whether dealing with me or other people, Pete insisted on being treated as an individual, not as a case study or an example or a moving part of any institution. Gradually I learned that regimentation and homogenization were anathema to him. In camp he put himself a notch above the other "grunts" partly because he was two or three years older and supported a wife and child but mainly because he prized his own mind. "They hire 'em out of high school and mold 'em to conform," he said. "Lots of these people get abused. They're from the trailer park. They're used to eating possum.

"I was way too intelligent to be in the military. I made a devastating choice, to go from earning twenty-nine thousand a year to thirteen thousand while having the same expenses. If I would have listened to my wife, I'd be making a hundred thousand a year now, I bet. But I go in and then I'm off to war, firing weapons."

Not that he had hesitated to answer the call to combat: "It was my duty to go, my turn to go, and I would have hated myself if I hadn't."

Pete coughed. "The military really whacked me out. I used to be quiet before I went in. Now look at me."

"You're a talker supreme, all right."

"I was never a stand-up guy before. I guess I have that to thank the military for. Jeff, it's no accident that I'm usually right. When the proof is out in front of me, I *fight*."

IN THE FALL of 1990 Private Timmons said good-bye to his pregnant wife and shipped out with the 3d Battalion, 5th Marines, aboard the USS *Mount Vernon*. The expeditionary fleet, massing in Subic Bay, the Philippines, departed for the Arabian Gulf in early January. In deference to the Saudi allies, U.S. forces used the Arabs' name for the Gulf instead of the Iranians'.

During late January, with the air campaign against Iraq under way, the marines practiced amphibious landings on the beaches of Oman. They trained with live fire in the desert for a week, then steamed through the Strait of Hormuz and drew close to the action in the northern Gulf. Everyone assumed that they would lead the invasion of Kuwait.

I wrote earlier that for the combat troops the most stressful period of the war, according to surveys by field psychiatrists, was the anticipation. In the cramped camps and ships the tension built over the coming fight. If a soldier juggled worries from home as well, the load could become precarious. Army researchers reported that "many of the problems surfacing in this deployed force seemed to be family-related. Chaplains, as well as other soldiers, believed those most at risk were young, recently married soldiers either with young pregnant wives or those married just before the deployment, and soldiers in relationships that were troubled prior to deployment."

The mental health counselors were able to nip most such problems in the bud—before they sapped a soldier's effectiveness, at least—by assuring him or her that feelings of distress were normal under the circumstances. A couple of talk sessions were usually enough; at most a soldier might need three or four days' rest in the mental health infirmary (optimistically dubbed the return-to-duty tent) before rejoining his unit.

I shall leave Pete on the deck of his ship for a minute. He is concerned about the mass in his throat. Ashore in Saudi Arabia, an army psychiatrist named David McDuff kept a record of the stress reactions that he and his colleagues were treating between late December and early February, before the invasion. Aggression, depression, and anxiety were the three most common expressions of prebattle stress, but the fourth was somatization. I called Dr. McDuff and asked him to tell me about the last one.

McDuff's definition of "somatization" was a "reaction out of proportion to a symptom and its severity." He said that the soldiers in this category had passed through one round of doctoring without result. He remembered a man who said he was paralyzed, another with persistent numbness, a third with a nagging gastrointestinal complaint. "You can't conclusively say there was no biomedical explanation," McDuff said, "but since there wasn't a biomedical treatment to offer them, the next best response was to make a psychosocial intervention"—i.e., give emotional counseling.

By this logic, if a soldier complained of a lump in his throat from drinking fuel-tainted water, the doctor, having ruled out tissue damage to the area, might reassure the patient of the body's capacity to detoxify low concentrations of hydrocarbons. That is why we have livers, he might say. Besides, nothing medical can be done for an exposure to jet fuel once it's past. If the strange lump in the throat didn't clear up, the doctor would inquire about stressors other than the water—the soldier's fears about combat, say, or his family situation.

"I look at all domains, I try not to think dichotomously," McDuff continued. "Anyway, we doctors make too much of the need for a diagnosis. What is the patient really asking us? The individual may be crystallizing a broad complaint into a specific symptom."

I asked whether the somatization that showed up in his caseload could have marked the start of the gulf war illnesses.

McDuff rephrased the question, dodging the loaded words. "How does combat," he said, "fundamentally change an individual's view of his general health?" He gave an unexpected answer: "Personally, my health changed, and I'd say it's changed for the worse."

Like Pete's, McDuff's summons to war came as a jolt. Having only recently stepped down to the army reserves from active duty, the doctor learned "to his astonishment" that two-thirds of the standby medical units were being called up. Because of his prior experience, McDuff was named commander of the Psychiatric Detachment for the 7th Corps. He visited every unit of the corps, traveling across the front in Saudi Arabia.

"I think the deployment was long enough and severe enough to be very stressful," he said. "If you were a reservist being treated for hypertension, as I was, and at home you got the best care and medications, and in the Persian Gulf the care was not available, then what do you feel? I ran out of medicine at three months. It made me pay more attention to my health and to the environment.

"I was *cold* in January. There was frost in the tent, after all those lectures about heat stroke in the desert. I had so much sand in me—in every orifice. You couldn't see the roof of the tent with your flashlight because of the sand in the air. Because of the blowing sand, I got *eight* infections of my tear ducts. I never thought about my tear ducts before.

"If there was an exposure to be had, I probably had it. I think of exposures in a very broad sense, chemical, environmental, being in a foreign culture. If I wonder about anything [causing the gulf war illnesses], it's whether there was something in the dust and sand, something microbial, an allergic reaction perhaps, as people moved into an area where they had never lived before.

"It gave me an insight into the veterans' mentality. There is a constant monitoring of your bodily functions. A shift in thinking can take place: I was a healthy man before, now I'm an unhealthy man.

"Today when there's any change in my health status, a part of me attributes it to the war. For example, I think I developed gastrointestinal problems from eating MREs [meals ready to eat], which are very constipating. I went three or four days without a bowel movement. Now I have alternating diarrhea and constipation. Also, I think my chronic headaches are worse. I know it's related to job stress, but still. . . .

"Then again," he said ruefully, "I'm six years older."

This happened to a man whose "intensive training in psychosomatic medicine" had well prepared him for tricks that the mind could play on the body. My evaluation of Dr. McDuff on hearing his story: idiopathic physical reactions during war. Patient's understanding of somatization prevented symptoms from spiraling. Symptoms declined during actual combat, when his mind was preoccupied with greater threat.

Was there anything else?

"I hated the Persian Gulf War, but now I'm pleased that I went," McDuff said. "It may be that personal growth is a more common outcome than illness." The experience had made his marriage better too; he didn't say how. The people like him who benefited from the war will be discussed in the last chapter. They don't include Pete.

ON THE AFTERNOON of February 24 Marine Battalion Landing Team 3/5 came ashore unopposed at a place called Al-Mishab, twenty-five miles south of the Kuwait border. Terns wheeled across the barren landscape. The next day the battalion rolled forty miles west through the reddish dunes. Turning north, the convoy arrived at its assembly area on the southwestern border of Kuwait on February 26.

Other marine and army divisions, having preceded the 3d Battalion into the smoke-blasted country, were pursuing the enemy at Kuwait City and points north. The mission that Pete took part in was to guard the supply routes, clear the mines, and mop up any resistance that had been bypassed in the blitzkrieg. Ironically, his battalion did not meet any hostile action until after the cease-fire was declared, on February 28.

"We were chasing people in the desert," Pete said. "Nine, ten guys at a time. They had Toyota trucks with fifty-millimeter machine guns, some of them rusted out. They were rebel soldiers." According to an intelligence report I obtained, they were probably commandos of the Iraqi Republican Guard who refused to give up.

"Were you trying to capture them?"

"We didn't capture anybody. They'd run into a compound and we'd blow 'em up. Initially we held our fire. They'd shoot at us and run, shoot at us and run."

"Were you scared?"

"It was pretty freaky," he said.

"You killed people?"

"Nobody goes through life trying to hurt someone" was his answer. "It would have been better for me at eighteen. The others were hard-core jocks—you're not afraid of death then. I had *kids*, man."

On March 2 Pete's eighty-one-millimeter mortar platoon was probing some abandoned buildings and bunkers in the Al-Wafrah oil field complex, close to the Saudi border. "We were setting up our gun line, and a guy was shooting at us from a distance. Boom—I saw the rounds as they sprayed in the sand, but we were right out of range. I guess I was the only one who noticed. So I went on to the radio and sent a warning, and I was punished for it. I got my ass chewed. They said I was jumping the chain of command. The attitude is, you're a private and you're not smart. So then the sergeant, he put me out there on the perimeter closest to the fire. I think it may have been deliberate."

The next day the marines used their heavy firepower to destroy an enemy-held building in the oil field. This was the lethal engagement that Pete mentioned, leaving five Iraqis dead. Immediately afterward, mission accomplished, the units were ordered to exit Kuwait. By March 4 they were boarding the ships with no casualties sustained in a week of action.

"My unit was the most decorated," Pete recalled. "We were stacked. I came out of there with seven medals, I think." The citations were awarded at the group level, not to him individually. One praised "your exceptional initiative, keen knowledge and unfailing ability to manipulate the 81 mm mortar with accuracy." Another observed that "your increasing optimism and Esprit de Corps spurred your squad to great heights across the desert from Saudi Arabia to Kuwait and back." Pete e-mailed the tributes to me in a rare wistful mood. "It takes a certain kind of person to serve as a marine," he reflected. "Those were the good ol' days."

He was sick when he got back on the ship. Figuring he had the flu, he didn't do anything about it. Then a rash broke out on his arms, which he covered for a while with long-sleeved shirts. He remembers the color of the rash as yellowish and even bluish. He wrote me:

> I was in fear of what to do, we were sitting on the flight deck in gun teams, sergeant Carter asked, "What the fuck is wrong with you Timmons, you have a rash on your arms, what have you been into?"
>
> "I feel like I have the flu, sergeant, I don't know what it is," I stated this in a way to make clear I did not sound like I was trying to get out of exercise. Nobody ever wanted to PT [do physical training] around the USS Mt. Vernon, it seemed useless, but however, you didn't want to be found in your rack down in the berthing area. . . . I didn't mind the exercise, just not today, I felt like my nerve-endings were exposed on the surface of my skin, I was either going to pass out, just sitting there, or vomit, but if I was to vomit of course I would have to clean it up.
>
> "Go to [the] corpsman, tell him to look at it."
>
> "Aye aye sergeant Carter."

The corpsman didn't know what to make of the rash. He took Pete's temperature and said, "You're fine. Suck it up, marine."

Pete went back to sick bay a number of times to have his temperature checked. "Six years later I still have the same feeling—achy," he said. "It never went away." Because he wasn't well, he was assigned to mess duty, the first snub of many to come.

On the ship he was informed that his wife had given birth to a daughter a few weeks prematurely. The news put him at the top of the list for demobilization, but it was not until late April that Pete rejoined his family.

In the interim, bivouacked on a beach in Saudi Arabia, he tried to relax. The flu, or whatever it was, didn't go away. "Nobody knew I was sick. There was a corpsman in camp, but what did he know? I thought, If I get really sick, I'll pass out and they'll help me." Gastroenteritis, an inflammation of the digestive tract, was diagnosed just as he left. "When I got home, I was very sick. I shit my pants, I was urinating on myself."

Home was Camp Pendleton, on the coast of California, north of San Diego. "I was in a new platoon, with no gulf war vets, and they thought I'd teach them about the mortars, but it wasn't working out. I was going to the doctors three times a week and getting no support at home." He had fever, chills, weight loss. Baffled doctors sent him for consultations off the base.

Pete was put on limited duty, and at first no stigma was attached to him, "because I'd seen the shit and done my job well. I wasn't considered a slacker. The 'boots' were hazed instead."

He kept up his physical conditioning, even tried to increase it as a bulwark against his symptoms. "I was still in for the long haul. I tried to run. I tried everything. PT was my way out of it, but finally I gave up. Now I can barely make it back home when I go on a hike."

All the physical problems afflicting him today started in the Gulf, he insisted. There was no delayed outbreak, no eruption of a postwar syndrome for him. Nor for many other veterans, I suspect. At this time hundreds or perhaps thousands of idiopathies were separately converging. But Pete was farther along than others on the continuum to debility. His illness developed so rapidly, especially in the condensed frame of his telling, that if you didn't know the stages of the illness process, you would miss them.

I WANT TO back up and dissect the process. As a starting point, remember the research showing that military personnel who were *not* sent to the Gulf also exhibited gulf war symptoms, but at lower rates and in milder forms. This finding can be extended to civilian populations—to you and me when we don't feel well.

When people go to the doctor with a new symptom or symptoms that are bothering them, their complaints often are familiar to the doctor, but whether they will get a hard diagnosis is by no means assured. Dr. Kurt Kroenke, an expert on medically unexplained symptoms, has written: "Symptoms account for over half of all outpatient encounters or, in the United States alone, nearly 400 million clinic visits annually. About half of these are pain complaints (headache, chest pain, abdominal pain, joint pains, etc.), a quarter are upper respiratory (e.g., cough, sore throat, ear or nasal symptoms), and the remainder are nonpain, non-upper-respiratory symptoms, such as fatigue, dizziness, dyspnea [shortness of breath], palpitations, and others." Analyzing the outcomes of the visits, Kroenke found that "one-third of the symptoms seen in primary care are medically unexplained."

The *Washington Post* medical reporter David Brown, who is also a physician, picked up on Kroenke's work in an article on the gulf war ailments in 1998. He wrote:

> The problem of chronic, poorly explained symptoms is a huge one in medicine. In this age of high-tech miracle cures, it may be the profession's best-kept dirty little secret. . . .
>
> In a study published in 1994, researchers [Kroenke et al.] recorded the frequency with which doctors couldn't come up with causes of 15 common symptoms reported by patients. Fainting was unexplained 33 percent of the time, headache 30 percent, dizziness 27 percent, abdominal pain 23 percent, breathlessness 19 percent, joint pain 17 percent. Other studies have found even higher rates.

The Pentagon got in hot water in 1995 for citing Kroenke, who at that time worked for the army, because three of his studies that were used for comparison to the vets' symptoms involved older patients and a greater number of females. When I asked Kroenke about this, he argued that, taking his research as a whole, "None of the studies show a large age effect. Symptoms are not that much more common in older than younger people. Symptoms are more common in women, but they remain common in men." Still: "Trying to say one is going to get an adequate comparison group [to the veterans] anywhere would be fooling the critics. We can't."

If comparisons between groups are inexact, there's no disputing that medically unexplained symptoms are ubiquitous. The positive news is that most people with symptoms manage to feel better soon. Again to cite Kroenke: "About 75% of outpatients presenting with physical complaints will experience improvement within 2 weeks. Of patients not improved at 2 weeks, 60% improve within 3 months."

They get better even if they don't go to the doctor. According to Arthur Barsky, a Boston psychiatrist who studies somatization: "Surveys of healthy persons who are not patients show that fatigue, headache joint aches and stiffness, upper respiratory symptoms, and diarrhea are common and generally resolve spontaneously, usually within 1 month."

Pete was one whose symptoms were going the other way. I've called his condition idiopathic, but another term that a physician may use is functional. A functional illness is one that can't be identified by physical signs. It depends on the patient's own report of it.

If a functional illness becomes chronic, it may be classed as a functional somatic syndrome. "Somatic," by the way, doesn't mean "psychosomatic." According to a recent paper by Barsky, functional somatic syndromes "are characterized more by symptoms, suffering, and disability than by consistently demonstrable tissue abnormality." The examples he gives are chronic fatigue syndrome, fibromyalgia, multiple chemical sensitivity, irritable bowel syndrome, temporomandibular joint dysfunction (a jaw disorder), and the conditions stemming from silicone breast implants and whiplash injuries.

The lead symptom of each condition tends to mask the syndromes' similarities. Observes the British researcher Simon Wessely: "[T]he differentiation of specific functional syndromes reflects the tendency of specialists to focus on only those symptoms pertinent to their specialty, rather than any real differences between patients." Barsky and Wessely put the gulf war illnesses firmly in the company of the functional somatic syndromes, although this syndrome is yet too new and amorphous to have been adopted by any one discipline or specialty.

From the patient's perspective, to have a functional illness implies that the organic evidence, the biomarkers for it, probably exist but aren't detectable with today's diagnostic tools. A functional diagnosis keeps the patient engaged. Somatization, which is the psychological creation or amplification of bodily (somatic) symptoms, need not come up as an issue to divide the patient and doctor. Even a manifestly psychological malady like depression can be considered functional. As the CFS researcher Benjamin Natelson points out, the mechanics of depression, a "biological disorder of neurotransmitter physiology," surely will be known in better detail in the future.

From the doctor's perspective, a functional illness is like a holding pattern to which the patient can be assigned while various approaches to treatment are tried. The bad news is that the longer such patients do *not* improve, the less likely they *will* improve. An unfortunate minority slip into the whorl of an interminable, though rarely terminal, sickness, as Pete began to do in the months after the war. There is no way at present to predict who these people will be. "Chronicity breeds chronicity," says Daniel Clauw, a rheumatologist at the Georgetown Medical Center.

Most physicians, especially in the managed care regime, don't have the time or insight for patients with unresolved functional conditions. Because of the way that medicine is organized, favoring disease over symptoms, "objective" evidence over "subjective" presentations, these patients tend to sink from sight unless they have an organizing proposition of their own to cling to, such as the immunological deficiencies claimed by chronic fatigue syndrome patients, or the silicone in the systems of women with breast implants, or the toxic exposures itemized by the gulf war vets.

I wish that the Pentagon and VA doctors had been less strict about epidemiology and had acknowledged gulf war syndrome as a functional illness. After the first year or so, when the mystery had not yielded to medical science, the goal should have been to agree with the patients on a nebulous identity, if not a precise name, for the symptoms, and then to shift the focus to treatment options. Maybe John Cabrillo could have been soothed, or Carol Best pointed in a new direction. But instead, when confronted with the difficult cases, most of the doctors within the military system fell into the mind-body, either-or trap: They either referred the sick vets to psychiatrists and PTSD clinics or, just as often, launched exhaustive and fruitless biomedical investigations.

For the person on the brink of an inveterate sickness, neither approach is likely to succeed. Either the patient, stung by the implication that it's all in his head, spurns the psychological intervention, or else the biomedical hunt, which he welcomes initially, turns into a wild-goose chase. A more intense, more reductive probe may well uncover scattered abnormalities, perhaps justifying the effort to the patient and doctor, yet never reveal what is wrong overall.

"This is the crux of the gulf war health issue," warns Charles Engel, an epidemiologist and psychiatrist at Walter Reed Army Medical Center and Uniformed Services University of the Health Sciences. "Continued diagnostic testing into unusual or unlikely illnesses or research into unlikely hypotheses that yield 'positive' results are highly likely to be false positives. To continue diagnostic testing into an illness when extensive research has already proved negative wastes society's money and leads to erroneous findings that can cause serious psychological and even medical harm to those individuals."

IN THE SPRING of 1992 the medical staffers at Camp Pendleton thought they thad found it—the key to Pete's illness. Evidently he had hepatitis C, a liver infection. His blood tested positive for antibodies to the virus.

Hepatitis C is an elusive condition. It was not isolated and named until 1989, after years in the shadows as "non-A, non-B" hepatitis. Blood screening for it became available only in 1992. Since that was the year Pete tested positive, it appears that he was a forerunner for both hepatitis C and the gulf war illnesses.

The two wouldn't be confused today. Surprisingly widespread, the hepatitis C virus is harbored by an estimated four million Americans, most having contracted it from long-ago exposures to tainted blood. Because an infection progresses to symptoms in only a minority of cases, hepatitis C is a silent epidemic. Usually it takes two decades before the slow scarring of the liver initiates the nausea, fever, fatigue, and wasting of chronic hepatitis. Patients may not learn of the disease until they're at a dangerous stage of cirrhosis.

In hindsight, however, the diagnosis was a good bet. Although not jaundiced, Pete had symptoms matching those of hepatitis, more or less, and it was not impossible that a young man could have rapidly developed an advanced case. The only way to assess the disease accurately is through a liver biopsy. In May 1992, more than a year since the onset of his symptoms, Pete submitted to the stilettolike thrust of the trocar, a tool penetrating his abdomen and plucking a sample of his liver cells.

The results were ambiguous. The microscope disclosed signs of chronic inflammation, but the signs were not severe. It was only a "probable" hepatitis, according to the pathologist's report. Pete read the highlights to me on the phone. Later tests of his blood for type C antibodies were not consistently positive, Pete added, and his liver enzymes, another indicator of hepatitis, were normal the last time they were checked. If he carried the disease, it was not active, nor had it been in 1992.

Pete dismissed hepatitis as the cause of his symptoms long before his doctors did. When a VA physician urged him, a few years into his illness, to start treatment for hepatitis C, he declined. He'd learned that interferon, the only drug available and far from a surefire cure, had harsh side effects. "My liver wasn't my problem," he said. "Why would I magnify my pain? Why risk losing my hair and my marriage—'cause few spouses can take it when you're on the interferon?"

He never thought of the hepatitis finding as a false positive, only that it had falsely led doctors away from the real issue of the toxic insults of the war. The implication of the diagnosis was that "my liver problem is my own fault." It was maddening to Pete that he had to say to people, "I'm not a heroin addict." The American Liver Foundation, which he contacted, assured him "it's not only from sex and drugs."

He did glean one useful thing from the episode: the opinion of the pathologist who did the biopsy that his liver was chronically inflamed. When he learned that agents other than viruses, such as bacterial pathogens, alcohol, and toxic chemicals, can cause inflammation, he began to fashion his own diagnosis for his problems. He had an image of a toxic chemical raking through his body, a one-time hit, no trace of which could be found today, and the agent had left his liver scarred and his intestines as well. It could have been the fuel in the ship's water, or the PB pills he had to take, or some "stuff in the sand," such as chemicals left over from the Iran-Iraq War in the 1980s and stirred up again by the U.S. bombing.

"I could have lain in something, I could have inhaled something," he maintained. "But I did become a little bit psycho too."

HAVING A BODY in distress will reveal the mind in distress as well. The more symptoms a patient has and the longer they go unanswered, the greater the probability that he or she will be psychologically disturbed. That's "be" disturbed, not "become," for the correlation between the two is not necessarily a consequence. The correlation has been charted by chronic fatigue and fibromyalgia researchers and by doctors who work at the mind-body interface—namely Kurt Kroenke, today an internist at the Regenstrief Institute for Health Care in Indianapolis, and Wayne Katon, a psychiatrist at the University of Washington. "People with high numbers of medically unexplained symptoms," says Katon, "almost by definition have had high numbers of lifetime anxiety and depressive diagnoses."

A corollary, if you will, of the correlation is that people who doggedly look for help for their chronic symptoms—starting with their family physicians and moving to the advice of specialists—are more likely to be clinically depressed, anxious, panicky, etc. than those who don't go for medical help. I have referred to this tendency among those who seek relief for irritable bowel syndrome. Katon says the connection applies to chronic fatigue too. "If you study chronic fatigue in the community," he says, by "community" meaning a random, non-medical sample, "about twenty percent of respondents will have chronic fatigue. About half of them go to doctors with it; the other half don't. When you look at who goes to the doctor, it tends to be the people with psychiatric illness and psychological distress. So distress plus symptoms tends to lead to health-care utilization."

I have an uneasy feeling conveying this information to you because it fits almost too neatly the gulf war veterans I met, John and Carol and now Pete. Moreover, my subjects illustrate, as if they were selected by me deliberately, statistics showing that the more symptoms a patient brought forward, the more psych diagnoses the VA and Pentagon doctors gave out. The vets who persisted in plumbing their health, they are the crazy ones—Is that what I'm arguing? Or were the psychiatrists just plugging diagnoses into the holes left open by the internists? These are the kinds of questions that are debated on either side of the mind-body interface.

AFTER COMPLETING the hepatitis investigation, the doctors at Camp Pendleton did not know where to turn. They sent their charge, who had become alienated and implacable, to the base psychiatrists. "I was worried they were going to lock me up," Pete said. "They gave me tests, asked lots of questions. 'Are you depressed?' 'Yes, because I'm sick.' "

Sometimes he was so enraged by his treatment that he felt he could kill somebody. "I was the shitbird of the platoon. They were treating me like a guy who couldn't pull his weight, like I couldn't make the hump. I was weed eating [doing grounds work], I was cleaning the head. 'We don't want you to contaminate anyone else'—that was the impression I got. Their attitude was, 'What the fuck's wrong with you?' Not 'Hey, buddy, how're you feeling?' But I needed that job. I needed that paycheck."

The psychiatrists came up with a diagnosis of bipolar disorder to explain his "manic" behavior. Pete spoke of this condition (and perhaps displayed it) during his short stay at the hospital in Los Angeles. Bipolar implies a cyclic pattern, whereby the down moods alternate with the ups, but the condition doesn't require episodes of depression. Agitation, talkativeness, irritability, and pronouncements of self-esteem—all these are elements of the case definition applicable to Pete. Still, the mania of a true bipolar illness has a feverish point to it, a goal that the person is driving toward, heedless of cost. If anything, Pete was backing away. He was not so much manic as exceedingly defensive, trying to keep his health together while meeting the military's expectations.

In January 1993, the most bitter moment of all, the Marine Corps discharged him. Pete was "boarded out" (medically retired) on the ground of hepatitis C. In the weeks before the move, he said, intelligence officers were following him around. "Finally they asked, 'How do you feel about being boarded out?' I gave up. I didn't have a choice.

"I didn't cry in combat," he added, his voice cracking, "but I'm crying now, because of the way they treated me. They destroyed my life and they are still lying about it."

Pete moved his family to Arizona and tried to pick up where he had left off, as a welder. On call for jobs, physically he couldn't do it. Appointments were being missed; work was backing up. He had to stop.

He applied to the VA for health care and disability benefits. More tests, more doctors scratching their heads, and inevitably there was friction over the nature of his ailment.

According to a checklist he sent me later, Pete suffered from twenty-two of the thirty-one symptoms most frequently entered by gulf war veterans. Of the leading complaints, he was spared only the headaches. He had aching joints, chronic fatigue, memory loss, sleep difficulties, skin rashes, concentration loss, depression, muscle spasms, nervousness, diarrhea, anxiety, breathing problems, chest pain, dizziness, nausea, stomach pain, loss of balance, sex problems, chemical sensitivities, frequent coughing, eye redness, and excess tearing. He could have added urinary trouble: "I either couldn't pee or couldn't control it. Is that incontinence? I used to leak all day long."

He was sliding into hell. His wife took the two infant girls and left. "Alma got tired of me laying around and saying I was dying, and I had problems with her believing me. I think she thought I had AIDS or something. I was going to a shrink then, and I asked, 'How come they don't understand?' "

He made a suicide attempt with a handful of tranquilizers but "forgot to take a lot of alcohol with it." Alma and the kids came back. When Pete threatened to do the job right, Alma got him admitted to the VA psych ward until he calmed down. "PTSD" went into his bulging medical file.

The most consuming of his physical symptoms were the stomach pain and diarrhea. Curled on the living room floor, Pete would moan and cry out, "It's not going away, Alma!' and he would hear his two children, in cruelly innocent mockery, making the same noises. He couldn't worry about what the girls were feeling. He was wondering, Is it a parasite wrapping itself around my insides? Are my intestines going through my hernia? My appendix? Every few weeks, it seemed, he would roust the family, and they would race to the emergency room, Alma at the wheel and the kids in back, because there was nowhere to leave them.

Between bouts of pain Pete read up on the organic features of gastrointestinal ailments: "*If a loop of bowel is trapped in a hernia, the bowel may be obstructed, resulting in abdominal distension, cramps, nausea and vomiting.*" He became familiar with the symptoms and signs of colon cancer: "*Polyps are abnormal growths on the inside lining of the intestine; they vary in size and shape and, while most polyps are not cancerous, some may turn into cancer.*" Growths or obstructions in the intestine could be detected: "*The colonoscope is a long, thin, flexible tube with a tiny video camera and a light on the end. The gastroenterologist carefully guides the instrument to look at the inside of the colon. The picture is shown on a TV monitor . . . .*"

"I've seen the inside of my body," he told me. "On the screen, during the colonoscopy. They make you look."

"Come on," I chided him. "They don't make you look."

"Well, it's true they don't. I'm kind of drugged up, but I'm looking to see if they are going toward something."

"How do you know what you're looking at?"

"Well, if they see any inflammation, I want to know what's causing it. Actually, I'm waiting for them to find something and to tell me about it. They biopsied in the inflammation, and one time they *did* find polyps, well, small ones, or they claimed to. . . ."

I gathered, however, that the first two colonoscopies were negative. The gastroenterologist told Pete that a third colonoscopy would be useful only if conducted while the pain was occurring. He should come for testing "while he was cramping up." Not long afterward Pete was back in the ER, demanding the procedure, but the VA physician who was on duty that evening either couldn't or wouldn't perform it.

The VA doctor was rude besides. "What do you want from us?" he said to Pete. "You come back here only if it's a matter of life and death." So the sick man stopped going to the emergency room and withdrew further into the shell of his pain.

The way I piece his story together, Pete by 1995 had completed his descent. From his idiopathic reaction to the water on the ship, to the persistent aches, diarrhea, and rash following the war, to the development of a full-blown functional syndrome, with its biomedical blind alleys and psychological swamps—poor Pete had bottomed out. He was disabled and nearly alone. It seems cold to say about a person in such multifarious disarray that his condition might also be distilled to a single word, one that you've heard before, "somatoform."

A SOMATOFORM ILLNESS, the condition that John Cabrillo was labeled with, is of course a psychiatric illness. It represents an extreme instance of the mind's tryst with bodily sensations. Many milder versions occur, since everyone somatizes to one degree or another. I have told about the army psychiatrist McDuff, who treated somatizing soldiers during the run-up to the war and at the same time fretted perhaps too much over his own health. Just before I began writing this chapter, to give another example, my father died, after two crises of illness. A change in my balance—I had noticed unsteadiness when putting on my trousers, etc.—became worse during the period my father was sick, and I was convinced, even as I researched the ins and outs of somatization, that I was headed for an appointment with a neurologist. Two months after the funeral my equilibrium abruptly improved. Relieved and a little embarrassed, I marveled at the metaphor. My father's passing had caused me to "lose my balance" temporarily.

That was an instance of acute somatization, and though it sounds more serious than chronic somatization, it is not, because it is short-lived. Chronic somatization can ramify and harden into a somatoform illness. In a new textbook Kurt Kroenke has contributed a chapter, "Unexplained Physical Symptoms and Somatoform Disorders," that offers tips to physicians on identifying such conditions. There are factors to look for, in addition to a high number of physical complaints.

One clue, which I've mentioned before, is a troubled childhood; a patient's past trauma may be repackaged. "Childhood family problems," writes Kroenke, "particularly physical or sexual abuse, but also alcoholic parents and family dysfunction are risk factors for adult somatization."

Another clue is that the patient relies on a battery of medications yet changes them frequently. He either can't tolerate the side effects or fails to find relief in any of the pills. Pete over the course of our talks commented that he disliked the effects of the pain medications, antidepressants and tranquilizers that had been prescribed for him. At the same time he wolfed aspirin and was forever switching his stomach medications. "In a nonsomatizing patient," observes Kroenke, "one drug from a particular class is typically as effective as another; in the somatizing patient, all drugs from the class are equally ineffective."

Third, though the reasoning seems circular, somatization is suspected when the patient absolutely denies that he might be somatizing. If the doctor says that the mind is at least *contributing* to the symptoms and the patient jumps up and objects, "You're saying that it's all in my head?" then he's protesting too much.

"The way it would work in your case," I suggested to Pete one day, going very cautiously, "is that you got exposed to something, your body overreacted, and your head learned a bad lesson."

"Yes, that has happened," he replied to my surprise. "My body's talking to itself—'Oh, shit, what's going on?' But also I have scar tissue on my colon and my liver."

A more typical response from him, which arrived by letter, dispatched the notion: "Just what kind of illness do you think this contamination could induce? The mind can not cause scar tissue on the liver, or colon, or inflammation throughout someone's intestines, I mean come-on. . . . It is clearly obvious you will hear what you want to hear and interpret things to make money not truth. You can come up with your own conclusions but we are talking about a cover-up, not a medical fallacy of the victims of this syndrome. This is exactly the problem victimizing the victim over and over."

Finally, says Kroenke, somatization is a diagnosis best made over time, not after one or two consultations. The workups must continue to be negative, yet the sick person must continue to strive for answers, even as his symptoms evolve, one failing part of the body crowing for attention over the others.

By the time I got to know Pete, in 1997, he had been on a health quest for six years and had become a student of his body's vicissitudes. Partial compensation by the VA hadn't made it feel better. He still had the dry heaves daily, but he noticed that his night sweats had eased, pretty much gone away. He used to have the rash constantly, but now it occurred only twice a year. Each time it came back, though, it was a harbinger of his other symptoms worsening, principally the diarrhea. He knew he would be sitting on the toilet for hours at a stretch.

A troubling new development was that his kidneys were pounding. Also, his esophagus had started to bother him again. "It feels inflamed. I want to have it checked out. I'm going to request that an upper GI scope be done— to go down the other way."

Most days, his outlook bleak, he had to fight to keep going. "Who knows what's going to shut down next?" he said. "My kidneys? My heart? Who's going to take care of my family if I die of a heart attack in ten years? How can I take control of my *life* back?"

At the center of the galaxy of his symptoms was an ineffable pain. The pain was a black hole, gobbling him up, invisible to the world, yet emitting a tremendous energy. Absorbing it all day wore him down. "I don't understand my kind of pain," he said. "I hurt up and down my body, not just in my joints. I don't want to know what cancer pain is like, but this—I'm admitting I don't know how to explain it to anybody."

He resented the VA's referring to it, in his medical files, as "aches and pains," as if the thing he felt were ordinary. "It's an extreme humming in my body," he insisted, "my nerves running up and down under my skin. You know after you've had the flu for three days, how you're hot and feverish and you can't bear to be touched? It's *that* kind of feeling. It's a *humming. . . .* That's the only way I can describe it."

But he was explicit about the effects: "I can't live with this pain until I die."

The philosopher Elaine Scarry argues that pain is the absolute definer of reality. For the person in pain there is no reality besides pain; if it hurts, it must be real. Simultaneously no one outside the person can be sure of the pain he feels. Those looking in, the doctors and relatives and the writer, must at some level harbor doubts.

"It puts you through a wall," said Pete tiredly. "The family doesn't understand. You *can't* be the same person that you were before. . . . If only you knew how I felt."

Since I do not know his pain, I cannot say that he had a somatoform disorder. As far as I know, none of Pete's doctors ever told him he was somatizing. A patient who would accede to that label is rare in any medical setting. If a person could grasp the wisdom of the somatoform diagnosis, probably he or she would not have got caught up in the thicket of symptoms in the first place. When an individual is proud but not worldly-wise, the idea of somatization is unavoidably going to be taken as an insult.

"Somatization too often is used to discredit the patient's experience," cautions Walter Reed's Engel. "The label alone minimizes the reality of the pain, the diarrhea, or whatever a patient is suffering. And it presumes to know what may be unknowable." Therefore I shall retreat to the safer ground of the functional somatic syndrome and continue my portrait of Pete from there.

THE GROUND IS still rather squishy. "Functional somatic syndrome" is an ungainly phrase, as is "chronic multisystem illness," another attempt that has been made to encompass the family of disorders to which the gulf war illnesses belong. Someday a crisper term will be offered, reflecting, no doubt, a clearer perception of the mechanisms of illness.

Whatever the mechanisms turn out to be, one doctor, the George-town University rheumatologist Daniel Clauw, has in my judgment done more than any other to illuminate the conditions. Introduced to the gulf war ailments in 1995, later than most physicians, Clauw tied the nosological strands together before the strands were even recognized by others. In talks at scientific meetings he would put up a slide of what he called the chronic pain and fatigue syndromes. His diagram, which looked something like a bruised eye, consisted of four concentric shapes: fibromyalgia, chronic fatigue syndrome, the "exposure" syndromes (multiple chemical sensitivity, the gulf war ills and others), and the somato-form disorders.

That Clauw subordinated the veterans' health problem to a broad spectrum of modern illness accounts for why you did not hear about him during news coverage of the controversy. But if anyone could have understood the impregnable sickness that Pete Timmons fell into following the war—I mean Pete struggling alone in the dark, before the politics took hold—it was Dan Clauw.

At the time of the war Clauw was five years out of medical school. He was working toward his board certification in rheumatology at the George-town University Medical Center in Washington. A series of events brought him together with four seemingly different groups of patients. These encounters were "serendipitous," he said, for his career and for his under-standing of the gulf war cohort on the horizon.

First he became familiar with fibromyalgia patients. Their pain was not a psychological creation, he decided. "When you see that many people with FM," he says, "you realize there's a physiological basis to it. Yes, you see stress issues and illness behavior in some, but you don't see it in others. Some people are just like you and me except they're in chronic pain."

Next Clauw treated a group of patients recovering from an incontrovert-ibly toxic exposure. L-tryptophan, a nutritional supplement meant to enhance moods and sleep, was sold in health food stores in the late eighties. A bad batch of the stuff produced in 1989 caused a miniepidemic of severe muscle pain and fever. Several thousand people were ill, and there was no uncertainty about the physical basis of their reactions. Yet even after their blood work and other signs had returned to normal, some patients still complained of diffuse pain and tiredness. Clauw suspected that they must have had fibromyalgia or chronic fatigue beforehand, but undiagnosed. That was why they were taking the supplement in the first place. If so, the toxic incident aggravated their conditions.

The L-tryptophan episode, which led to litigation over the health dam-ages, taught Clauw something else. "I learned what happens to a group of people when they're told they've been poisoned—the way they start to focus on it, the victim mentality."

Soon he met another set of victims, women who believed their health had been harmed by silicone breast implants. The epidemiological proof that silicone had caused their symptoms was never established. But as part of a settlement with the manufacturer of the implants, claimants had to be examined by a rheumatologist, and Clauw saw a number of the women. He concluded that their pain and fatigue and distress were due not to a chemi-cal exposure but rather to an exposure to the frightening publicity. In the medical literature he came across a term for this, "environmental somatiza-tion." "If you tell people they're exposed to a toxin," he said, "you *will* make some of them worse."

Lastly, when he started up his clinical practice at Georgetown, Clauw acquired a group of patients with low-back pain. They were referred to him by an orthopedic surgeon who couldn't find anything mechanically wrong with their spines. Chronic back pain, which accounts for the most frequent source of workers' compensation claims, has become an occupational epidemic in the United States, notwithstanding that the number of jobs demanding bending and heavy lifting is at an all-time low. For most of Clauw's patients, evidence of injury or abnormality didn't register on X-ray or MRI scans. The pain seemed out of proportion to the diagnostic findings.

Here were four groups of people in pain. Their backgrounds and their medical evaluations were unlike, and their own attributions for their health troubles varied. But their complaints were more the same than different. Since he had no objective test to tell such patients apart—no strict measures of disease or injury, that is—Dan Clauw tried to understand them collectively. He included in his thinking people with chronic fatigue syndrome and the less serious somatoform disorders, and later he added chemical intolerance.

As for the ostensible causes of these conditions—whether the ailment started with an injury, infection, emotional pressure, or chemical exposure—they worked as one, Clauw theorized. He lumped the causes together as stressors. From looking at epidemiological surveys, he realized that when subjected to a stressor, a certain minority of the American populace will come down with symptoms of chronic pain and fatigue and seek medical assistance. The majority do not, because they either aren't that ill or don't want help for their problems. "Everyone has a little FM/CFS," as Clauw put it, "and some people have a lot of it."

By framing the symptom complexes that way, he made the individual's susceptibility more important than any possible cause. If some people were predisposed to be ill, as he contended, what was different about them physiologically? Why did their systems get tripped up by the various stressors? Clauw thought the problem had to do with very subtle dysfunctions of the muscles, glands, and the immune and nervous systems. The dysfunctions he was talking about were not hypothetical, but neither were they conventional sources of pain or inflammation.

Patients like Pete, Clauw would say, have defects in their capacity to process pain. The stimulus causing the pain is real, but the nerves relaying the sensation make too much of it. "The volume control is set too high," he says. "The knob is turned way up." A specific muscular dysfunction he mentions is smooth-muscle dysmotility: If a person's esophagus and intestines do not contract properly, irritation and burning may result, leading to indigestion and diarrhea. All of Pete's physical symptoms, for that matter, might be related to small, idiopathic breakdowns in internal performance. The body's engine is running, but it needs a tune-up. It was very cutting edge, this theory of illness, but with his credentials he was able to stay in the mainstream.

When he presented his ideas to physicians who treated fibromyalgia and chronic fatigue syndrome, Clauw was well received. Patients' groups liked the message too because he seemed to favor the organic aspects of the etiology. He did not shy away from the role of psychological stress, but he was clear that the symptoms lay outside the patients' heads. "Psych stuff is OK with these people," he told me. "They just don't want to hear it's their primary problem."

Clauw's fact-filled lectures contained something for everyone. His low-key self-confidence and his steady gaze were disarming. "All the illnesses I've been involved with have been contentious," he said. "I know how not to put my foot my mouth."

At one program in 1995, General Blanck of Walter Reed was in the audience, about to give a talk himself on the gulf war illnesses. Clauw recalled that when Blanck got up to speak, he altered his text and repeatedly paid tribute to Clauw's analysis. Afterward Blanck invited Clauw to consult with the VA and Pentagon. A year later the rheumatologist and his Georgetown colleagues got the first of three large federal research grants. Their plan was to study the "dysregulation of the stress response," and the study subjects would be drawn from the spectrum of functional conditions, not just the sick veterans. It was late in the day, but the work might eventually shed some light on the illnesses of concern to the military.

Neatly Clauw sidestepped, or stepped over, the issues rankling the gulf war debate. "We have all been somewhat paralyzed," he said, "by the need to know what caused the illnesses." He had no trouble conceiving of a soldier getting a harsh whiff of nerve gas or a pesticide, or having a temporary reaction to a pill, or (another kind of stressor) being shocked by the sight of bodies on the battlefield, or feeling a disorienting disquiet on being returned to his or her old life a "hero" when he or she didn't feel very heroic. If the biomedical researcher had the right tools and was on the spot immediately, a measurement might be made of the stressor in action, the biochemical sting, the neuro-immuno-endocrino-, etc. structures trying to adjust and maybe misfiring. It would happen to one who was sensitive or predisposed.

In Clauw's paradigm of illness, though a lot is going on physiologically,

the emotions play a critical role. They can do more than just trigger symptoms. Once symptoms occur, emotions can create illness behavior. This is
the part of his presentation that appeals to psychiatrists. Also known as
maladaptive illness behavior and the sick role, it is a trap that some patients
fall into, reinforcing and perpetuating their conditions. Not that it happens
willfully, Clauw hastens to emphasize, but it can block the patient's recovery. In most cases the family goes along, "enabling" the behavior. The worst
of the patient's bad habits is the sense of being wronged, which focuses
attention backward to the circumstances surrounding the onset of the illness rather than forward to the actions and treatment he needs to get better.

An example Clauw uses for illness behavior is the victim of a motor vehicle accident. He has seen her often in his rheumatology practice. She is in
pain, sues for damages, develops fibromyalgia, becomes disabled and
depressed. (She sounds like Carol.) The other driver, the one at fault, who's
maybe injured also, does not become chronically ill. "I have never seen an
individual develop FM after they *caused* an accident," says Clauw. "When a
physical stressor has a fair amount of psychological stress accompanying it,
that person seems to be at higher risk of illnesses like FM, CFS or MCS.
And if you can't budge them from their belief system about what their illness is or what they need to do about it, you are not going to make them
better.

"I'm afraid we have a comparable kind of thing with the gulf war illnesses," Clauw concludes. "What has happened is that the veterans feel as
though their complaints were not or are not being taken seriously. It's a
negative prognosticative factor when they believe that the government did
it—that the government is lying and the government has to fix it. This
doesn't go away when they get their compensation."

PETE WAS HAVING one of his bad days. In the morning he lit the fire in
the fireplace as usual and got the kids ready for school, but he felt weak and
dizzy afterward and had to return to bed for several hours. Now that he was
up, the pain crackled through him. He was humiliated by an outbreak of
rash. The ringing phone got him started on the bureaucrats who refused to
acknowledge his gulf war condition and the doctors who had failed to treat
him.

"They're not doing anything for us," he said. "They're just following symptoms and making statistics for their studies. The anger I feel comes from not knowing, and from their betraying me, and for blatantly telling me there's nothing wrong."

"Anger and pride are not good for your health," I said.

"I know all that. But I'd be homeless if I gave up this pride and anger."

A curious comment. I think he meant that his anger could forestall the piteous collapse that he feared and that his pride was keeping his self-esteem and his family together.

"I was raised to always believe in the truth, to not back down and never conform. I won't go away. So the VA gave me what I wanted [service-connected disability payments]. But yet they won't call it Persian Gulf syndrome. I want to see Bush burn in hell and for Schwarzkopf to die of his colon cancer, which, by the way, I think must be connected to the Gulf."

Whoa now, Pete.

"I don't like what I see in myself," he admitted. "I can't control myself when the world starts spinning around my freaking body!"

A bad day, as I said. On good days he would say, "I don't want to be too mad at these people 'cause they're trying to help me," and he even could be humorous about himself. "I'm not your typical patient," he granted. "Most of the doctors at the VA are just holding down a job. They go home at night and say, 'Man, I'd have had a better day without *that* guy in my office.' "

When I laughed, however, he brought me up short. "They took away my health, and they haven't lived up to what they're paid to do. . . . They're paying me money to live, yeah, but they still have control of my life."

Pete had appealed his partial disability rating. He wanted the VA to find him 100 percent disabled and to increase his monthly compensation accordingly. One of his suspicions about me, initially, was that I was an agent sent by the government to test him, and he feared that if he failed the test by saying something wrong or putting something libelous on paper, not only might his appeal be denied, but he might lose his disability benefits altogether.

The issue of compensation is of course the stickiest wicket about the gulf war illnesses, what the epidemiologists call a confounder, and psychologists secondary gain, complicating the assessment. As Dan Clauw and others have noted, when a society establishes a disability and compensation plan for an illness or an injury and adopts lenient diagnostic criteria, the number of cases and claims increases rapidly. They decline when the criteria are tightened. The history of repetitive strain injuries in the workplace offers a good example of money's fertilizing influence on illness behavior.

To qualify for compensation from the VA for the murkier gulf war conditions was no piece of cake. Malingering by veterans cannot be ruled out, but the cases, I believe, must have been very few. I don't accept that thousands of men and women would have made themselves ill and falsely claimed disabilities, putting jobs and families at risk, for the purpose of obtaining government support. What happened was that people got sick, and then some of them surrendered to the sick role. According to the experts in this realm, it's not the desire for compensation per se that maintains the illness behavior, but the exercise of having to prove oneself impaired. The frequent medical exams and forms to fill out, the claims and appeal process, the angry pride and silent self-doubts act like padding on the trap of illness behavior.

Pete, whose wife worked, needed the money as much to prove he was not a useless husband as for the money itself. But he hated jumping through hoops for it: the mandatory appointments with the gastroenterologist and psychiatrist and the other doctors who had no cure to offer him, just as he had no recovery to show them that would allay their responsibility. Showered with diagnoses, he pressed his appeal on the basis that part of his health problem should be considered "undiagnosed." This was the VA category closest to gulf war syndrome, the thing the agency wouldn't admit. He was determined that it should.

"If my wife has to take time off work to take me to a doctor's appointment, she'll say to someone, 'He's ill from the gulf war, or, 'He has gulf war syndrome,' and I'll say, 'No, no, no. They haven't admitted it.'" An admission today might not satisfy him, he said, because "it would either mean they were lying then or lying now."

Nor did the emergence of the gulf war illnesses as a national issue make him feel vindicated. It just made him feel lost in the crowd. "They come up with a registry, and people come out of the closet to sign up. I thought, What about this little voice? What about me? I didn't wait to start crying about this—I was crying from the beginning." In the early years he had been involved with a Persian Gulf veterans' group in his community, but he dropped out, skeptical that others' symptoms could compare to his. When I asked him why he wasn't more sympathetic, he replied, "If they're sick, how's that going to help me?" That was on a bad day.

Although a chronically ill person has little leverage to exert in life, his neediness may give him control over immediate family members. Within his own house Pete seemed to be the commander. He did pay full credit to Alma, "my lovely wife," who since his illness had put herself through college and got a good job. Besides doing most of the housework, she made his VA appointments and ran interference for him, he being the only one permitted to blow his top. I once heard him in the background yelling, "No calls!" as his wife apologized that he couldn't come to the phone. His older daughter, who was eight, developed stomach pain of her own and had a gastrointestinal biopsy, which was negative. A bright student, she deserved accelerated instruction, or so her father maintained to her teachers. "I'm always at school arguing with them," he told me wryly, "as I'm sure you can imagine."

Pete's two children had never known him when he wasn't sick, I said. "Yes," he agreed. "I show them pictures of how I used to be. . . . I wanted my kids *not* to learn this stuff."

The family had no social life. "We don't go out to eat. It's all me, really. Because I'm like 'Don't pay attention to me, don't touch me, don't pay attention to how many times I go to the bathroom.' I can't keep the shit from coming out of my ass.

"A lot of people think I'm weird because of the way my symptoms make me act. If I tell them why, they say, 'You fought for our country and then they did *this* to you?' But they don't give a damn, really. I meet a friend who notices I'm in pain, and he asks what's wrong, you know, kind of an innocent question. So I get going and I won't shut up. That's the last time I see that person."

In his book *The Nature of Suffering* the physician Eric Cassell writes of the social isolation that occurs when "[p]atients with chronic pain discover they can no longer talk to others about their distress." Isolation is but one aspect of suffering, which Cassell defines as the conflict arising between the person's "simultaneous needs to respond to the demands and limitations of the body and to the forces of society and group life."

Thus Pete's first duty every day was to his body. He was constantly in negotiation with it. He had to wait to see what it would let him accomplish, since he could never outrun or outfox it. The painkillers, acid blockers, Kaopectate, anti-inflammatories were but lids upon symptoms that his body regularly blew off. Occasionally, though, the physical pressure dimin-

ished for a day. "When I feel good," he said, "I feel like I can do everything." In a buoyant, half-disbelieving mood he wrote letters, did chores,
got some of the week's reading done, maybe even exercised a bit, jogging a
couple of laps. He made plans. He was depressed when the pain flared
anew, usually because he had attempted too much.

Brought low again, he was reminded of his failure in his second duty,
which was to be a husband, father, and contributor to society. Contributor,
yes, because Pete thought he might still be of service to his country, if only
he could get better.

"Despite frequent anger and bitterness," continues Cassell, "occasional
expressions of unfairness, and attempts to hide, withdraw, or pretend indif-
ference, sick persons try to stick it out in the world . . . because the social
aspect of the person desires to keep trying, driven by the ineluctable forces
of human society."

Without relinquishing his sick role, Pete had issued a tenuous challenge
to his body. He set himself the goal of a college degree, and to get it, he
would have to leave the house and venture out into the world. Assisted by a
vets' service organization, the Disabled Veterans of America, he had
enrolled at a branch of the state university. He went to school part-time,
taking courses in psychology and sociology. The tuition was paid by the
government.

The classroom was a scary place. Pete was older than the others, as he
had been at Marine boot camp, but this time the competition was tougher.
Brash minds just out of high school adapted to the course material faster
than he could. The instructors didn't haze him, but they prodded him to
keep pace, wondered at his absences. Pete had a hard time being a follower
in the best of circumstances. "The professors have you see it their way
only," he complained. "They're brainwashing me. If you're not learning the
way they want you to learn, you're out of there."

Other disabled students, he noticed, ignored their impairments and
demanded no favors. Pete tried to do the same with an illness that wasn't
apparent. He took a pain pill before and after class. Sitting for an hour was
hard, standing up to deliver presentations an agony, because he feared being
disrespected. "If I would be totally disabled, in a wheelchair, I wouldn't
have to answer questions as much. If I don't feel well, you can see it in my
face. I don't look well, and I've got a horrible attitude."

Every day he asked himself how hard he should push in school. The choice was between "wanting a degree or wanting my health." Two courses per semester, three trips to the campus per week were all he could handle. He had to drop a psychology class when nausea kept him out for a while and he couldn't catch up. Social statistics, required for his major, was so difficult it was "a tumor in itself."

Still, by the middle of 1997 Pete had limped halfway to a bachelor's degree and had begun to imagine a career. He saw himself most often as a social worker and mediator, "helping people like me deal with the bureaucracy. . . . I've thought about working with the homeless," he said. "A sick person is the same thing. Once you're down, you're really down."

He wouldn't be Pete if he didn't dream big. Instead of a social worker he might become a lawyer, "because I'm very good at arguing." Or an anthropologist, since his studies had got him interested in travel. Or a politician, if you can believe it, a politician who would be very protective of his past. ("I might want to run for office someday, and if I give you my records, I'd be exposing the dark side of Pete Timmons.") The writer's life didn't sound bad either, working as your own boss and all. He asked me how he might go about publishing his Persian Gulf experiences; his angle would be the chemical threat of the new warfare technologies.

In my own unscientific study of the sick veterans, I found them to be smarter than their levels of education (mostly high school or a bit beyond) might suggest. Often I could hear their minds scraping against the ceilings of their experience—the mental gasping, as it were, as they strained to understand their collective health problem and the abstract and alien depictions of it by others. If the purpose of education is to open minds to new prospects, then education was beginning to have a salutary effect on Pete. The question was whether the rest of him, the suffering soma and the darker regions of his psyche, would go along. He summed up his quandary in an astutely paradoxical comment about his future. "I know I'm cut out for social work," he said, "but can I handle the people?"

MAKING A LAST-DITCH effort to get to the bottom of his symptoms, Pete traveled to the West Los Angeles VA Medical Center for a special evaluation. It was a fiasco, as I reported, on which he brooded for months. "The trip to L.A. convinced me that there is no plan for my health to get better," he said bitterly, "except for time, maybe."

During this period in 1997 Dan Clauw was voicing doubts that people like Pete could be helped. The Georgetown rheumatologist was concerned that the "undiagnosed" veterans had been through the medical wringer too often. They had seen too many doctors in the VA and Pentagon systems who did not know what was going on. The idiopathic symptoms of 1991 and 1992, which, though not simple to treat, might have been headed off, had become interlarded with psychological disorders and illness behavior. To correct such conditions now was extremely difficult, perhaps impossible.

"This is something that the military needs to recognize," Clauw said at an Institute of Medicine workshop in Washington. "We probably are too late in treating gulf war syndrome to have a major impact on what we do for these individuals. This is not to say we shouldn't try the same types of treatments that we use in fibromyalgia and chronic fatigue syndrome. But we would have been likely to be far more effective had this been addressed early."

Politically such a view was untenable, for Congress had been pressing the VA and Pentagon to demonstrate gains in treatment, even though the condition to be treated had not been defined. Later that year Clauw and other investigators were asked by the two agencies to come up with proposals. Clauw recommended trials of a program of cognitive-behavioral therapy and aerobic exercise—not magic bullets, as I've indicated before, but they have helped against chronic fatigue and fibromyalgia. Cognitive-behavioral therapy (CBT) has also been employed against depression, anxiety, phobias and somatoform disorders. CBT is not a cure for the patients but a tool to lessen their suffering.

"This stuff works," Clauw said to me, "but the subjects need to be involved, they need to be *open* to it." Participants must put cause and blame aside and commit to small, positive changes in attitude and activity. Their heads must be engaged as much as their bodies.

Nurse Jones had tried a light version of CBT with Carol. One of the techniques is to identify and dispute negative ideas, such as the idea that no physical relief can be achieved without a clear diagnosis of the problem. Relaxation exercises, another technique, can take the edge off pain, and you can be taught several ways to get a better night's sleep. Pacing yourself strictly, by working at a task no more than fifteen minutes at a stretch, for example, can promote a sense of accomplishment while avoiding the disheartening flare-ups. Moreover, if faithfully once a day you take time for something you like to do—make yourself enjoy your garden, or a movie, or dinner with a friend—you may end the day feeling a little brighter about yourself. Finally, keep a log of your progress to prove to yourself that you're not as helpless as you thought. Those are some of the items in the CBT bag of tricks. The goal is: You manage the illness; it doesn't manage you.

By the time the veterans' treatment trials were launched—late in 1999, as nothing moves quickly in this story—Clauw had softened his prognostication that vets were too hardened in the sick role to be helped. "The vocal representatives who have strong beliefs are a smaller portion than I thought," he said. "The vets I've seen don't feel well, but they may be amenable to therapy. Anyway, if they've signed up for a trial, they have to believe that behavioral interventions will have some benefit."

Pete lived about three hundred miles from the nearest participating medical center. It would have been impractical for him to join the trial, had he known of it, since the group sessions were held once each week for three months. I don't think he would have been tempted anyway, because I couldn't interest him in a somewhat similar program run by Walter Reed Medical Center in Washington.

Likewise, when I suggested that Pete might try meditation or yoga, he said, "It just might work, but I don't see myself doing it."

How about psychotherapy?

"I have had an outside psychologist," he said, "but I'm not seeing her now."

"Why not?" I asked.

"Bringing everything up and trying to get through the rest of the day was exhausting. The more I talk about it, the worse it is. Every doctor's appointment stirs it up again and I get manicky. But if I ignore it, it goes away, though not the pain. . . . Sometimes I think I should stay out of it and I'll have a healthy life."

IT WAS A strange and prickly relationship we had, conducted over long distance. We were like pen pals or a chatroom couple whose ardent correspondence doesn't lead up to a meeting but leads away from one. I was the prince repeatedly trying to put the slipper upon Cinderella, and Pete kept saying the shoe didn't fit.

The conversations went this way: I'd ask him how he was feeling, and he'd tell me at length, in the course of which he would relay new biographical details and much that was repetitious. Usually I'd ask him for copies of his medical records, and he would take the request as a sign I didn't believe what he'd been telling me.

He was only half right. The up-and-up aspect of my approach was that I believed him and needed his records to support my methodology, which was journalism. But the records also might support the emerging idea of my book, which I'd partly sensed in dealing with John and Carol, that the veterans' physiological reactions to the wartime events or exposures, whatever they may have been, had been superseded by distress and pain and the swollen predicaments of daily life. These were now driving the symptoms; to deal with these was a psychological, not biomedical, challenge.

Pete did send me a packet of materials, consisting of VA handouts and a cover letter. The letter contained useful information and colorful harangue, but there were no personal documents. The envelope bore no name or return address. The letter was unsigned. "You could be a spy for the VA," he explained when I called. "I'm afraid of the VA, I admit it."

I mailed him a copy of my first book as proof of my identity. Half jokingly, he said that still didn't prove it. He roved from cocky disregard— "No one is going to outsmart me"—to jackrabbit scared: "You could be a member of the CIA. You could wrap an explosive wire around my neck and make me carry your pack!"

I kept calling. He never hung up, but he blasted me for not respecting his privacy. "All this is more for your benefit than mine," he protested.

"I hear nothing from you that lies uniform with my research or [with] conversations with other vets," he wrote me. "Perhaps because I am involved involuntarily with this syndrome since 1991 to present and suffer each and every day I am closer to the truth than you can ever hope to decide. You can't change my past experiences with your words, no matter how it is interpreted by you."

His most stinging riposte: "When I was trying to kill myself, it was always because of people like *you* that I had to deal with in the VA."

"OK," I said finally. "If you won't show me any records and you think I'm out to get you, why are you talking to me at all?" On that day we'd been going for two hours.

"Everybody needs an outlet," Pete said.

My hope, or was it a self-justification, was that through me he might forge a passage back to health. Unable to do anything about the biological basis of his condition, and unable to change his views or break his sick role by *telling* him the facts, perhaps I could make him better by Socratic questioning. Let him rattle on and gradually reason his way out of the illness. I'd weather his storms and keep him on course, a steady current to his yawing.

No, I did not succeed, first because he would not be patronized and second because I could not get enough words in. Only at the very end of a telephone call would he allow me to suggest what he should do about his anger or pain or isolation. It was as if I were summing up a therapy session to a most grudging patient. "Talking adds to the stress the illness already has created," Pete said. "The only thing that is going to solve the problem is either a cure or a neutralizing medication." He blabbed mainly out of frustration in not being able to convince *me*.

Our relationship improved when the VA put through his complete disability rating, agreeing with the substance, if not each particular, of Pete's appeal. According to the VA readjudication that he read to me, his irritable bowel syndrome, hepatitis C, bipolar disorder, and "undiagnosed fatigue and body aches, consistent with fibromyalgia," all contributed to his disability, so that he would receive the maximum compensation.

"I'm satisfied with this decision," he said. "I've proved my case. I'm getting nothing that I don't deserve." Thereafter he stopped worrying that I was an agent provocateur or at least that I was government paid. Another thing that helped: I took to sending postcards announcing a date and time when I'd call, so as not to jar him.

I read him a passage from a Robertson Davies novel, *The Cunning Man.* The main character, a metaphysically oriented physician, offers "a lesson about being a doctor: you can't really form an opinion about somebody until you have seen the place where they live."

"Oh yeah, it's true," he said. "You have to know the context of the person. From social work I know that." Yet he refused to have me visit because, he said, the encounter would disrupt his health and domestic stability. "I don't have the fear of talking with you like in the past. But I can hide"—he added with a laugh—"if I talk to you on the phone."

For the first time he wished me luck on the writing. "I'm having a change in attitude. I'm developing a softer side. I'm gearing up for social work."

ONE DAY HE said, "Just last night I dreamed I ate something toxic—"

"Hey, that's interesting, Pete. So did I. Well, not that I ate something toxic, but definitely it was a toxic exposure."

I wrote up my dream and mailed it to him.

I was leading a group of journalists home. Five or six of us were inside a big hospital, and we wanted to get to the exit toward the west.

The hospital had many twisting corridors; I thought I knew a way through, a kind of shortcut. After a few turns and long passages we came to a door. When we opened it and went inside, I saw it was a dead end. The room was full of file cabinets and equipment: a cluttered but ordinary storeroom.

Then I felt a sensation of heat on my back, like a sunburn. We started milling around confusedly. Clearly something was wrong.

Suddenly a bunch of security guards came in behind us, all in an uproar. They moved us the hell out of there, but they weren't angry at us, more frightened. It turns out that we had stumbled into a dangerous place. The storeroom was full of live radiation, like an X-ray chamber. We were invisibly contaminated.

In the outer room there was panic. Hospital officials made it known that our group had absorbed a lethal dose of radiation. A few of my colleagues, who were looking ill, their backs leaning against the wall, now began to slump to the floor. I too felt nauseous (one of the symptoms of acute radiation poisoning). But I tried to fight against the feeling.

The hospital officials put out a press release. Instant news, complete with our names and thumbnail photographs. The gist of the story was that these hapless individuals had absorbed a lethal dose and would inevitably die.

I got angry at this. I knew about radiation, so I thought, and didn't believe we were dead men. I believed that if we could hold on during the short term, keep ourselves active and try to walk off the symptoms, like a person who is freezing to death is supposed to do, then we would survive. I stalked about the anteroom, scared but also convinced I could beat this.

Passing by a plate of glass, or mirror, I glimpsed my reflection. My hair had grown longer and turned gray, and all the tips of the hairs were scintillatingly white. Not a good sign, I realized.

I wanted to telephone my grieving family and tell them not to believe the news, that I would make it. But naturally I couldn't find a working telephone. I must have gone to three or four phones, and all the while the hospital officials followed me with their eyes, neither helping nor inhibiting me, this goner who wouldn't accept his fate.

Finally I got a call through. I reached one of my brothers, who is an upbeat and philosophical sort, but who may guard his share of anxiety below. My brother was wearing a black suit. I had reached him at my own wake. Although glad to hear from me, he was not moved or surprised, and I had the feeling as he chatted that he had missed the point of my ordeal.

There are items to gloss here, starting with my desire to lead the journalists "home" on the question of toxic exposures, but I shall spare you my interpretations as I did Pete. When we spoke next, he commented, "It's pretty close. It sounded so real for my problem." He remarked especially on the family not getting it. "I don't understand why my family blows me off. My mother still says, 'Oh, you'll be better.' " Much later it dawned on me that my brother's initials were the same as Pete's. All along it had been Pete and I on the phone line, in urgent and mutual incomprehension.

He never did relate his own toxic dream. On the verge of sending me medical documents—"I want you to see the dates. I could be a bullshitter, after all"—he hit a bad patch and decided against it. The memory of his trip to Los Angeles and the incident with Dr. Hamm got him riled up again. He talked about his cycle of pain and the "throwing up that never goes away.

"At least I know now I'm not going to need a doctor if I go into sudden pain. I'm trying to develop a new way of dealing with things, but then *you* remind me how angry I am."

"Still," I answered him, "you haven't told me to fuck off yet. You know you can whack me and I'll take it. I'll keep coming back to you until I get what I want, you know that."

"Yeah, I do." He laughed. "But maybe there's something else going on too. . . ." He coughed, his throat tightening. "Maybe you care about me."

PETE'S LATEST PHYSICIAN at the local VA hospital was Dr. Black. Pete liked him much better than others he'd had. Dr. Black hung in there with patients, full knowing that the ride would be rough. Having taken care of scores of Persian Gulf vets, he believed that gulf war syndrome was a legitimate entity, a real condition they were suffering, but he stayed neutral about its cause and did not promise any remedies. "If I can't cure them," Black said, "listening to them is at least second best." He was just the thing for a (somatizing) symptom-juggling patient.

Kurt Kroenke advises physicians to use "healing words" with such patients. Reassure them, Kroenke says, that their symptoms are as real and even as disabling as they say, but dissuade them from further consultations with specialists with the argument that their conditions are idiopathic and "poorly measured by current diagnostic tests." The patients should be told they are not getting worse, and why not. "If they have arthralgia [joint pain], affirm it is not a crippling type of arthritis (e.g., rheumatoid arthritis). Explain the reasons why their chest pain is not the type seen in heart disease, why their dizziness does not suggest a tumor or a stroke. Inform them that while their symptoms may wax and wane, many patients may have long periods of symptom reduction or remission, more good days than bad."

This is, in effect, cognitive therapy, and Black seems to have practiced it with Pete. "He'll talk about what he *doesn't* know," Pete said. "The honesty of the guy. There's nothing *he* can do. . . . I have to wait until this blows over or until they find something in Washington, D.C." But other times he'd grump, "Why should I go to the appointment? When he just listens to me and writes it all down again."

Kind, receptive, yet sparing with his help, Black was like a parent teaching an infant to walk. During 1998 Pete discovered he had less need of medical attention. He found himself able to stand back from his body, not battling it as much but observing it. He started to make a daily record of his symptoms, as if they were engrossing pieces of natural history. "If you are interested, let me know," he said. He almost let me have them.

"Not fighting the symptoms seems to help me move on with my life," he wrote in an e-mail. "Understanding that I have no choice but to except [sic] my chronic illness, I am not as angry day to day. I've recently regained hope for myself, knowing I can depend on myself, not so much on the VA. I can't rid the ignorance in the world, but use what I have. . . ."

At school he did better; the professors were supportive. Joining a college club, he took part in an Easter food drive for the community. He and Alma contemplated moving back to California after his graduation because he felt resilient enough to deal with his relatives.

His main physical complaint during this period was in the gastroesophageal area, the burning and the globus, his aboriginal symptom. In truth it had never gone away. "The pressure in my chest is a great concern," he wrote, "and seems to be getting worse. I can't swallow properly. It's obviously inflamed. I'm thinking of having an endoscopy. Then I say, Why bother? I'm not gonna get cured. I'd have to drop everything to go take the test."

Dr. Black, trying always to normalize Pete's complaints, remarked that "half the country has indigestion."

"What kind of a comment is that?" said the veteran, offended. He continued to ask for the test. He told the doctor he had nightmares about a tumor growing in his esophagus. Black acquiesced, but the procedure did not take place until six months after he had begun to request it.

Arriving at the GI clinic of the VA hospital, Pete was not pleased that the doctor performing the endoscopy would be a certain Dr. Bird, whom he'd seen five years earlier, when his health had been in crisis. The two had not got along. "Dr. Bird kept saying that hepatitis C could cause my GI symptoms and the rest, and I said 'No, I have inflammation throughout my entire body.' "

Today they were snippy to each other, the doctor recalling that Pete had skipped an appointment in 1993 and Pete reminding him "to treat me like a patient." After administering a mild sedative, Dr. Bird snaked the endoscope down Pete's throat, to see what might be there.

Kroenke and colleagues have studied the overlap between people with psychiatric disorders and people who undergo upper endoscopies for unexplained GI symptoms. The researchers conducted their study at a GI clinic at Walter Reed Army Medical Center in the early nineties, before the gulf war illnesses became important. One hundred and sixteen patients, including both genders and several races, agreed to participate. The subjects filled out psychiatric questionnaires before they went in for their endoscopies, and the results of the survey were compared with the outcomes of the diagnostic test.

The organic findings were inversely related to the psychiatric findings. That is, the people who came out having major GI abnormalities, such as tumors, ulcers or esophageal strictures, were less likely to have emotional problems. The people who came out of the procedure *without* something seriously wrong in their gastrointestinal tracts were three times more likely than the others to be suffering from anxiety, depression, or a somatoform disorder.

Therefore, the researchers suggested, it might be wise to make a psychiatric screen of GI patients requesting the upper endoscopy. According to their study, patients who were untroubled had a fifty-fifty chance of having something seriously wrong. At those odds the endoscopy certainly should go forward. But if patients had an emotional illness, especially if they scored high on the somatoform scale, the probability was very low that the scope would uncover anything major, and the money for the test would have been spent fruitlessly. By contrast, a ten-minute psych survey cost almost nothing.

I don't foresee the American medical establishment adopting this sort of measure, even under the most tyrannical of cost-cutting programs. It would presume an acceptance of mind-body interactions by both doctors and patients. More important, it would dismiss a large gray area of the study, which Kroenke and colleagues duly discussed.

Half their study subjects had signs of "minor" inflammation in their digestive tracts. The endoscope had detected something organic, in other words, though the doctors did not consider it serious enough to have caused the extensive pain, heartburn, or vomiting that had prompted demand for the procedure. But say you were the patient at the GI clinic. If the scope could show your esophagus to be inflamed even slightly, though a "minor" inflammation to Kroenke, would you ever agree that your mental state was the dominant factor in your condition? I hardly think so.

"Good news for me," e-mailed Pete a few days after his endoscopy test. "I believe we found the cause for the acidic problems, (vomiting, tight chest, serious indigestion, inability to digest) I've been having for the last 7 years. I will have to speak with Dr. Black and confirm what was found, but the good news is I was sent home with meds that should take care of it within a few months."

I telephoned immediately. "They got a picture of what it is," he said excitedly. "A cyst, something like that, and it can be dissolved with medication, I think he said. I need a follow-up to see the extent of damage from the acidity."

He felt vindicated to have hit the crux of his GI problems. "I'm getting somewhere because *I'm* suggesting what test to run. There are a few things still up in the air that I want to get to next. I get this acidic problem taken care of, and then I want to go to the pain problem. . . .

"I was told at the VA that nothing I had was life-threatening, and for the first time I believe it. It's been six or seven years, and this intestinal thing isn't going to kill me, the hepatitis C isn't going to kill me. . . . Now I know, it's my life, it's not my death."

What a sea change in attitude, all thanks to an anatomical abnormality in his esophagus. But what was it, exactly? When I followed up with a request to talk to the specialist, he wrote: "Do not attempt to speak with any doctors that are attempting to help me, past, present, future. I will no longer entertain this issue with you. Looking through documents I realize, speaking with you will get me nowhere."

ALL RIGHT, THIS time I left Pete alone for eight months. When we were back in touch, he named it: a hiatal hernia. The endoscope had revealed a hiatal hernia as well as esophagitis, inflamed tissue of the esophagus, caused presumably by stomach acid.

Oh, the ambiguity of diagnosis.

A hiatal hernia is a pooching out of the stomach into the lower esophagus. It breaches the sphincter that normally closes off the tube from the stomach and makes it easier for digestive acids to bubble through where they don't belong.

People with chronic heartburn and acid reflux commonly have hiatal hernias. However, stomach acid may get into and inflame the esophagus without there being a hiatal hernia to pave the way. The sphincter just relaxes at the wrong time, inappropriately, usually after a big meal.

Hiatal hernias also occur in people who have no gastroesophageal complaints whatsoever. Thus the two conditions should be considered correlates, not cause and effect. A hiatal hernia is a risk factor for a reflux disorder, as are obesity, alcohol consumption, cigarette smoking, and high use of aspirin or ibuprofen. Of the three risk factors that characterized Pete (hernia, smoking, and analgesics), only the first was anatomical.

Surgery is not usually an option for hiatal hernia. Although there are serious types of esophageal hernias that do require surgical correction, this one does not unless it becomes very large. Considering it "minor," Kroenke et al. ignored hiatal hernias in their study of the psychological correlates of endoscopy-seekers.

In short, the finding is not the holy grail that Pete made it out to be. He had put things backward, seizing upon the signs in his throat when they merely confirmed his reflux disorder, which could have been diagnosed without the endoscope.

Dr. Black did not exaggerate by much in saying to Pete that "half the country" had indigestion. According to surveys, 20 percent of Americans experience heartburn or acid regurgitation at least once per week, and 40 percent once per month. Some of these people will see a doctor about their conditions, and if they go more than once, they are likely to be diagnosed with reflux disorder, or, formally, gastroesophageal reflux disease (GERD). A minority of GERD patients will in turn have difficulty swallowing, will cough or vomit, will have chronic inflammation of the esophagus. They will be taken into the care of specialists. Diagnostic probes may or may not reveal structural abnormalities.

Whatever their symptoms, most GERD patients can be managed within a three-step progression of medication. Start with simple antacids. If they don't help, move up to the so-called histamine antagonists, the Zantac, Pepcid, and Tagamet class of medications. The third echelon, the most expensive but also the most effective in preventing acid flow, is represented by the proton pump inhibitors, lansoprazole and omeprazole. The upshot in Pete's case: He had been taking cimetidine, the generic Tagamet, and after the endoscopy he was assigned lansoprazole.

Placing his stomach disorder in this context normalizes Pete, and I could do it for each element of his symptom complex, I suppose, except that a man having so many "normal" disorders is decidedly abnormal. Still, the context of the symptoms is familiar, broad, close to home—it *is* home. Instead of a discrete illness known as gulf war syndrome, which seemed to tramp out of the desert in the early nineties, what happened to the vets was a group of native symptoms grimly reorganizing themselves. Pete and the others who were vulnerable came together on the far tail of the bell curve of American health. Why it happened that way, why the war should have catalyzed this thing in these people, I do not know. Savvy doctors insist it does not matter. If the patients were ever going to recover, they would have to stop seeing themselves as victim-veterans.

It was happening that way for Pete. Stubbornly hewing to his private biomedical path, he was moving away from his gulf war identity. "I'm just a guy trying to solve my own medical problems," he said. "I'm interested in *me* and in what I'm gonna do." As he slowly improved, he noticed, at the GI clinic, that not only Persian Gulf but also Vietnam veterans had stomach symptoms similar to his. "These are pretty typical problems," he concluded.

The last time we spoke, he said, "I try very hard not to get upset any more." Then: "They [the Marines] kicked me out!" Uh-oh, I'd done it again. But the jag of temper didn't last, and with his anger spent he had nothing further to say to me.

OUR FINAL E-MAIL exchange:

"When you tell me you are not including me in your Book, it makes me very suspicious of your intentions from the beginning, as I had said before. Since your first contact with me, you seem to want me to believe what you want me to believe, not what I know. This certainly is not respectable & furthermore fears me of an attempt to slander, not to mention the lack of respect for my privacy & health (mental & physical)."

"Pete, when I wrote, <<It's kind of a hopeless task, me writing about you>>, I didn't mean I am not including you in the book, just that you probably won't like it. I am writing about four veterans from the WLAVAMC referral program, and except for Darren, all the subjects are suspicious of my intentions and probably won't like the results. Darren is giving me the benefit of the doubt, but who knows whether he'll like his portrait. Maybe a different writer or a kinder writer would withdraw, but it's too late for that. I am too far along."

6

Darren Is Dying

Warfare gas has become almost a fetich [*sic*]. To what extent it should be held respon-sible for a great train of symptoms of which so many ex-soldiers complain, is an open question, and one that requires a solution. The blame for every conceivable sort of ailment has been placed on gas. There is scarcely a functioning organ of the body whose disturbed action at some period during or since the war has escaped the blame for its erratic performance being laid at the door of poison gas.

> *H. L. Gilchrist,* A Comparative Study of Warfare
> Gases, *U.S. Army Medical Corps, 1925*

During the past several years the world, in general, has been undergoing critical social, moral, and economic changes; and, in the present state of upheaval, an ever-increasing number of patients are observed who present a symptom-complex which is intimately associated with the individual's struggle for security, for independence, or for whatever state is presumed to assure the spiritual and material happiness of the individual. This symptom-complex is essentially a representation of the interaction between emotional and physiological factors. . . . Patients presenting the well-known pattern of symptoms haunt the offices of physicians and specialists in every field of medical practice. They are often shunted from one physician to another, and the sins of commission inflicted upon them fill many black pages in our book of achieve-ment.

> *William J. Kerr, James W. Dalton, and Paul A. Gliebe,*
> *"Some Physical Phenomena Associated with the Anxiety States and*
> *Their Relation to Hyperventilation,"* Annals of Internal Medicine, *1937*

After twelve years in the military, Darren Moreau returned to the Palouse country of Washington and Idaho, where he was raised, with the expectation that he would die.

The Palouse joins the wheat fields of eastern Washington to the high forests of northern Idaho. The agrarian terrain, as you pass through it from the west, rolls and dips sharply, seeming to accelerate as it nears the mountains. As you wind upward, the bottom drops out into huge evergreen-lined gorges, the rivers so far down you cannot see them.

Darren was the third of five children. Until Darren was six, his father worked on the family farm in Washington and after that in the lumber mills in Idaho. Strict and rough, Phil Moreau was not mourned by Darren's older siblings after his death at fifty-five, of a heart attack, but Darren loved and missed the old man, knowing his strictness and roughness better than anyone. In the air force at the time, Darren came home for the funeral. He overheard someone at the graveside remark, of his mother, "She's better off without him." Darren bridled at that but held his tongue; he always tried to think the best of people, even when he had reason to be angry with them.

Since he was young, Darren had loved old cars. One of the paradoxical aspects and perhaps the only benefit of being terminally ill was that he was free to indulge his hobby. His duty to his country behind him, his future foreclosed, Darren's dream was to restore a 1957 Bel Air Chevrolet to glossy running order. Though the '57 Bel Air was his favorite car, he was partial to many other makes and models. The vehicles he acquired—a dozen, two dozen, three dozen, in the years following the onset of his illness—were antiquated both in vintage and in appearance. In short, Darren's cars were junkers. Stowed in a borrowed pasture, on a bench of land above the river gorge, they were all beauties to him.

"When Jackie and I get to where we want to be, in our house," he said, "the cars will be in their stalls side by side. They will be *drivers,* and they'll be safe. Just turn the key and go."

"Kind of like your children," I said.

Darren nodded. He could not, would not have children himself, but he used the word discipline in regard to managing his family of cars. "They all can't be treated like trailer queens," he explained. "They have to be able to take a ding or two."

It was an end-of-summer evening, crickets sounding in the grass. A cool breeze fell off the prairie and filtered through the pine and fir trees on the way to the river.

"I've got records for each car, what parts they need, what's been done. If I do die and we have to sell a car, the owner will have all the paperwork, with the hours I've spent working on them."

I had asked Darren to give me a tour of the stock. We strolled past several cows and came to the first one, a '68 Charger, which struck me as too streamlined to belong to Darren. "It's Jackie's car," he said. It was only a few parts shy of being ready to go. He sketched its qualities: "A performance-minded car. Six miles per gallon if you're lucky." I remembered Jackie's hard-charging performance at the VA hospital in Los Angeles a few months earlier.

We came to a '42 Plymouth, sunk in the weeds, and beyond that a '51 Belvedere, which seemed to be trying to return its metal to the earth. Yet Darren said he had the parts in hand to make the Belvedere run. He had paid $350 for it, he and Jackie hauling it all the way from Albuquerque.

Why would he do that, I asked, when he had so many others at home to be restored? He talked about the Belvedere's rarity and potential value and the like, but I began to sense that Darren was a soft touch for any august auto that had been beaten down and abandoned.

In the summer of 1997 Darren was about to turn forty years old. A tall man, over six feet four, he was what you would call a sharp dresser, without being flashy. Tonight, in casual clothes, he wore a green shirt, black pants and a western-style belt buckle. His dark lace-up work boots, unscuffed, sported a fringe upon the tongue.

Good grooming was important to Darren. Every three weeks he had his hair razor cut. He wore a thin handlebar mustache that gave him a slightly rakish look; but he lacked the rake's cockiness, or maybe he had lost it, and he was too pale besides. Darren was less bulky than when he had been a weight-lifting, distance-running military policeman, a guy who would bolt forward in emergencies while other men stood paralyzed. Briefing me on his cars, he crossed his arms and put his hands into his armpits, I suspect to stop them from trembling.

"When we hit the rod runs [car shows]," said Darren, still on the subject of the Belvedere, "they'll have to take a look at it." The wheels on the car were chocked, but it wasn't going anywhere. In a few months it would be peeking from the snow.

A smallish buck stepped out of the trees, fuzz still on its antlers, tense as a spring. The deer walked through the upper rank of the cars. Past the '57 Ford coupe, the '53 Bel Air, the '53 Chevy coupe—which was "the business coupe," Darren noted. His two prize '57 Chevy Bel Air hard-tops rested nose to nose, one set to donate its organs to the other.

A moon appeared on the lavender sky. I was overloaded with impressions of the lovely landscape, the rusting specimens and their tender owner, who was rolling now himself with his plans for the winter, telling me what he would accomplish in the shop. The tension was out of his body.

"Everything I have is going to be automatic 'cause I can't stop and start in a procession that long. . . ."

"Why not?"

"The pain from working the clutch."

"The cars give you a reason to be positive about your health," I suggested.

"This pickup," he said, standing before a '52 Chevrolet truck, "is going to have a nineties flair. The grille will be different. I'll change those wing windows. The back lights will be different too."

We arrived at a fence, and he threw over some hay for Jackie's horse, Stormy. A warm dark enveloped us. Already I felt closer to Darren than to my other subjects. I can feel his eyes on this page right now.

"I'm the doctor of cars. I can make 'em healthy, I can shine 'em up," he said, as if to answer me.

By his own account, Darren's life was going to be cut short by "terminal arthritis" and "brainstem inflammation due to neurotoxin," which had been diagnosed in 1992 and 1996, respectively, and attributed to the war.

Staff Sergeant Darren Moreau was deployed to Oman from Charleston (South Carolina) Air Force Base in August 1990. Oman, the country guarding the entrance to the Gulf, was well back from the front. Darren's squadron supported the 1702 Air Refueling Wing. He lived in a tent city that was sprayed with pesticides, he said, and was ordered to take pills and shots whose purpose was never explained. He remembers the continual landing and taking off of aircraft and the flares in the sky from the navy ships.

He was assigned to food services and mortuary affairs. In the latter job he readied body bags and registration papers for the American corpses that would be airlifted to the base prior to their transport home. "They were expecting thirty thousand dead," Darren said. "Fortunately that didn't happen." He never did handle any bodies because there were too few casualties to be processed through Oman. He was redeployed to Charleston in April 1991.

Those are the details of his wartime service as furnished to the Presidential Advisory Committee, the Senate Veterans' Affairs Committee, and individual politicians. For after Jackie had begun to campaign on his behalf, Darren became a relatively prominent veteran. Invited to testify about his illness, he—or more often she, since he pleaded he was unable to read his statement because of his condition—described how a rash had covered his legs when he was in Oman. No one was able to diagnose it. He had mysterious abdominal pains. Back home, six months later, he had an acute episode of dissociation, a "dream-state feeling," he called it, lasting fifteen or twenty minutes, during which he experienced lightheadedness, loss of feeling, blurred vision, and weakness. Since that day a flood of symptoms had engulfed him.

When asked by a senator if he had had any major health problems before the war, Darren said no. Just the seasonal ailments and childhood illnesses "that anybody could experience." He acknowledged one surgical procedure, a correction of a toe deformity called mallet toes, a condition acquired after he entered the air force.

I checked Darren's statements against the medical records he supplied me. In histories taken during and following the war and in a VA claims adjudication, which drew upon his full military record, I found references to at least one prewar incident of pain in the areas tormenting him afterward: pain in his head, neck, lower back, knees, and abdomen.

But if there was a precedent, what of it? His complaints in the years before the war were conventional, such "that anybody could experience," and the pain afterward so dominant as to be of a different species. The war was the watershed event, the wellspring of his illness, either because he encountered harmful chemicals there or because other factors, individual factors, were triggered there. Or both.

Darren's prewar records revealed that he was twice divorced, and that he'd had a bout of genital herpes and subsequently a vasectomy. Ashamed by the viral contamination of his body, he had the vasectomy so as not to infect any child he might produce in a future relationship. This radical step was medically unnecessary. But later he considered the decision to forswear children, and marriage, for that matter, all the more justified, for he believed his gulf war symptoms were communicable.

In the fall of 1991, though, Darren Moreau was just a man with escalating pain and no inkling of gulf war syndrome. In the wake of his scary "dream-state" episode, he went to the doctor at Charleston AFB. Darren presented with symptoms of what seemed to be arthritis in his neck, back, shoulder, and knees, but he didn't show the redness, tenderness, or audibly cracking joints of arthritis. After running some basic tests and not getting anywhere, the base doctor sent Darren to an army rheumatologist, the expert in this specialty for the Defense Department in the Southeast. The rheumatologist met with Darren five times over the next six months, examining him closely, and Darren learned from this doctor that he was dying.

A major theme of this chapter is the doctor-patient relationship. My previous subject, Pete Timmons, distrusted authority figures, including physicians. Quite the opposite, Darren was polite and cooperative with whoever was treating him. At the early stage of his illness he gave no grounds for skepticism or quarrel. He was searching for answers to his health problem with an open heart, desperate for direction, but at the same time, I think, he had an instinct for where he wanted to go.

Charles Rosenberg, a historian of medicine, has written of the "negotiation" that takes place between patient and doctor. It happens at the margins of medical certitude, where the patient's malady is less than explicit. "Some ills have a well-understood biological basis," observes Rosenberg, "others none that can be demonstrated. Meaning is not necessary, but negotiated, the argument follows; disease is constructed, not discovered."

Functional illnesses especially lend themselves to a negotiated interpretation, one that can satisfy both parties and keep them working together toward a solution. If a medical solution is achieved, the patient gets better, and the relationship ends. If not, the patient has no choice but to carry out the part of being chronically ill, and he may do that with a doctor's help as well. Paradoxically, until Darren found the right doctor, he could not fully express his sick role, his chronic illness behavior. He couldn't do it solo like Pete. He needed partners.

The army rheumatologist, whose name shall be Dr. Smith, became Darren's first partner. Smith established a good relationship with the patient, though the negotiation between them was incomplete because during the time Darren was seeing the doctor he was also preparing to leave the military.

At the beginning of 1992 the air force offered an incentive to certain personnel to quit with cash settlements. The catch was that if not enough people accepted the offer by the deadline, involuntary separations, or RIFs (reductions in force), would follow, and no bonuses given. "My rank was targeted," Darren recalled. "If I didn't take the voluntary separation and was riffed, I'd only get one-third the settlement." His health made the decision for him. Darren would take the thirty thousand dollars and get out, but he always felt that he had been pushed, like an old car that is left to rust.

After his initial evaluation of Darren, Dr. Smith wrote at the top of the consultation report: "Impression—diffuse polyarthralgias [joint pains]; I am unable to identify unifying theme or diagnosis that clearly explains the various symptoms. Therefore will address them individually."

Smith filled two pages full of speculations on various disorders, endocrine and hereditary, plus cancer and several arthritic conditions, as he chased the pain from the back of Darren's head to the temple, radiating into the neck; to the throbbing left shoulder and subsequently to the right; to the hip feeling as if it were going out of its socket; to the lower back, which burned in cold weather; to the knees, constantly aching, especially when climbing stairs. Only the pain in Darren's feet could be comprehended by the doctor, as a consequence of the aforementioned mallet toes.

Many scans and tests later Dr. Smith threw out the obscure possibilities and tried to choose between basic types of arthritis. Rheumatoid arthritis (RA) is a systemic disease, an autoimmune attack on multiple joints, in the worst cases making subjects profusely ill. Darren would have fitted RA if there had been signs of inflammation and the proper blood markers, but there were not. As for osteoarthritis, it usually starts in people older than forty and strikes a joint or two at a time, the weight-bearing structures and not usually the shoulders. In short, it is a degenerative process, painful but rarely producing inflammation. Darren was just thirty-four and rather too sweepingly afflicted for osteoarthritis, but it appeared to Dr. Smith, scrutinizing the X rays again, that a process of degeneration was under way.

Still without an exact diagnosis, the doctor delivered his prognosis to the patient at their final meeting, a week before Darren's separation from the service. Smith said that Darren was not a candidate for surgery, for the degeneration of his hips, knees, and back was still mild. But he would need considerable physical therapy just to stay even. The neck pain was "most worrisome," and improvement in that region couldn't be expected. Darren was cautioned against "running or jumping or exercise." From the record it's evident that Dr. Smith was discouraged by Darren's illness and also by his failure to have identified the cause.

Next—I have switched from the doctor's notes to Darren's account—the rheumatologist took the patient aside. Saying that he was under orders to soften his findings and that he would deny telling Darren this, in order to protect his career and family, Dr. Smith came out with the truth. Darren should know he was dying, that there was a "road map of arthritis" in his body, that this particular form was one of five types of terminal arthritis.

I located Dr. Smith in Hawaii, where he'd been transferred. There was a strangled pause at the end of the line. "Dying? That's what he says?" the doctor said. "I can honestly say that I wouldn't say that to a patient. I can't imagine, for the life of me, that I'd say his condition was life-threatening. I know of very few types of terminal arthritis, if I'd even call them that"— Smith named a bone cancer, and a severe infectious joint disease, and described an advanced rheumatoid arthritis of the neck—"which does cause patients to die fifteen or twenty years sooner than they might. But why would I be discussing this with Darren?"

Dr. Smith still retained a copy of Darren's record, and he looked it over.

"On the other hand," he reflected, "there's a grain of truth in what he says. The tone was pessimistic, I admit. There was evidence of degenerative arthritis in his neck and hip. I was looking at a steady progression. I could possibly have said to him that surgical replacement of his hips might be necessary in the future. But I'm at a loss to explain this. Especially the part about protecting my family."

He cited "the conspiracy theories" that some gulf war vets were prey to. Darren had become politicized in the intervening years, especially after meeting Jackie, but that didn't explain the opposing accounts.

"What about fibromyalgia?" I asked Smith. "In your first evaluation you didn't consider that."

"I didn't think of FM because he wasn't female. Seven years later it sounds FM-like, the burning sensation in his back, but he was talking more about his joints than the pain in his muscles."

Dr. Smith recalled that he had treated gulf war veterans before Darren, men who had ready diagnoses, mainly rheumatoid conditions. After Darren, "those I saw mostly had chronic pain amplification syndrome, and they were easier to figure out because they were more dysfunctional. They had a paucity of objective findings and a plethora of subjective complaints. But Darren didn't fit into any entity in rheumatology. He simply had a lot of pain at those sites."

Smith rang off saying he had learned something valuable about patients. If Darren had misread him, he had misread Darren. Idiopathic, apolitical, hurting, worried, searching Darren. A pure case. In a few years Darren would find a better accomplice, a physician to articulate his dire illness fully. He would find the right confidant too, a mate who believed.

DARREN WAS RELEASED by the U.S. Air Force into the care of the Department of Veterans Affairs in June of 1992. Returning to the Palouse region of the Northwest, he took a job in the distribution center of a news-paper plant. In September he went to the VA hospital for the compensation and pension exam in order to establish a service-connected disability.

The VA's assessment of Darren was not as gloomy as Dr. Smith's. X rays indicated nothing seriously wrong with his knees or vertebrae. Still, the VA examiner noted, "His complaints regarding joint pain are no doubt real and an inflammatory disease, early, could well be developing." Darren was awarded a 30 percent disability. He learned he would receive no money until he had paid back his separation bonus; at the monthly rate of his dis-ability compensation, that would take him ten years. Rather than appeal the decision, he washed his hands of it, for at heart Darren was not a battler of the system like John, Carol, and Pete.

Too proud to give in to the sick role, Darren kept up his appearance and went to work every day, although he changed jobs a number of times. After the stint in the newspaper plant he worked for a snowmobile dealership, as a clerk in an auto parts store, as a car salesman—aching and on his feet nine hours a day—and lastly in a state employment office, helping other veter-ans find jobs. Jackie said to me later, with considerable pride, "Darren has never *not* worked," to which Darren added, "Even if it's going to kill me, I'm going to continue on working."

Darren kept using the VA for health care, but unhappily. His medical records for 1993 and 1994 were lost. Passed from doctor to unknowing doctor, he soon became frustrated. In the fall of 1994 he switched to another facility, hoping that the treatment would be better at the Spokane VAMC.

Darren's new doctor at Spokane VAMC was Dr. Long, a rheumatologist, like Dr. Smith. "My first visit he was very interested," Darren said of Dr. Long. "I liked him. But the next visit, when the lab tests came back, he just changed. He was a whole different doctor. 'You're healthy,' he said. 'There's nothing there.' He said it over and over. He quit being a doctor to me."

Brusque but not insensitive, Dr. Long never said to Darren that the illness was all in his head. Rather, at each appointment, he seems to have tried to buck up the veteran by insisting on the positive. "How's this healthy-looking specimen doing today?" he would greet Darren.

"I'd go up there, bent over like an old man," Darren said, "and he'd move my knees around a bit. 'You're a fit young man,' he'd say. Abrupt. He ends everything so quick, and he doesn't do anything for you."

The collaboration between Darren and Dr. Long over the shape of his illness never got off the ground. Dr. Smith at least had agreed with Darren that his health was deteriorating, but Long by contrast would make no prognosis without a diagnosis. Absent a diagnosis, the prognosis so far as he was concerned was good.

Dr. Long was a practitioner of scientific medicine, and in scientific medicine the doctor-patient relationship was not a negotiation but a quid pro quo. The patient provided information in the form of test results (if symptoms alone were insufficient), and the doctor proffered a disease to fit the malady. Then the doctor gave treatment, and the patient reciprocated by getting better. In Dr. Long's model there was no middle ground, no chronic limbo to fall into. The downside of strictly scientific medicine is that if tests are negative and the doctor cannot arrive at a diagnosis, he may think he has failed the patient, an unsavory thought, which he subdues in favor of believing that the patient has not cooperated and at some level must not be sick.

"Doctors don't like patients who aren't easy to treat," said an administrator at Spokane VAMC. "It's scary for them." He spoke of Dr. Long as "an accuracy freak . . . compassionate, but his personal delivery isn't the best when he doesn't have support for a diagnosis."

Dr. Long was not used to being questioned, not by a patient, not by a writer. The very notion of negotiating or collaborating was too touchy-feely for him. "The doctor is not there to please the patient," he told me tartly. "You like him because he does the right thing, not because he kowtows to you."

Not unexpectedly, the rheumatologist did not recognize the gulf war syndrome, dismissing it as a "diagnosis of emotion." Therefore I asked for his views on fibromyalgia, the closest alternative label for Darren's condition.

Long believed in FM if only because "physicians have seen it so many times and the patients all tell it the same way. So, OK, it must be something—we'll call it something. But everyone has their thoughts on the side about how disabling it is. I'm on the side that it's not too disabling. It's possible to be perfectly healthy and to have fibromyalgia too. FM is just aches and pains."

Without Darren's permission, he was reluctant to address Darren's case specifically. "When you see this kind of patient," he generalized, "you say, look out, I'm dealing with a guy with a lot of symptoms, and I'm not going to find much." He called up Darren's records on his computer. "Hmm, an awful lot of normal test results there. . . . A hundred tests he's had done, and most of them are normal."

Finally, to shake me off, Dr. Long urged that I read *From Paralysis to Fatigue*, by a historian of medicine named Edward Shorter. I already knew the book, which is subtitled *A History of Psychosomatic Illness in the Modern Era*.

"There seems to be a considerable exaggeration with him [Darren]," said Long. "If he's not in Shorter's ballpark, then I'm all wet."

BEFORE THE ERA of scientific medicine patient and doctor *had* to collaborate, there being no alternative. In most cases the patient's symptoms were the only testimony of the disease. Listening to the patient, the doctor tried to classify the disease, following a somewhat arbitrary if no less scholarly path than today's differential diagnosis.

The doctor asked the patient about aspects of himself beyond his physical sensations. Foucault has likened the inquiry to botanical prospecting. The person's humors and his daily habits, the influence of the local atmosphere and the season all contributed to the species of ailment in question. Both doctor and patient believed that a man's body interacted continuously with his environment; likewise his mind with his body, his morals with his health. Everything was bound together, and occasionally one of the elements slipped out of whack. To locate the problem and restore order demanded a thorough exposition, during which trust was built between the two parties.

From roughly 1800 onward, as the patient stood to the side, scientific physicians broke down the elements of his disease, put them in compartments, and ranked them in importance. Out went the boxes with the person's morals and the atmospheric conditions; in came the boxes of clinical anatomy and physiology. New boxes, containing pathogenic microbes, were opened, along with the tools for manipulating them, such as antisepsis and vaccines. Also, the physicians put the mind into a separate box from the body, a heavy black box, and moved it to the back room.

If the atomization of the disease process improved the patient's chances of recovery, he had less to offer the investigation than before. Provided with biological signs, the doctor often did not need the patient's symptoms in order to diagnose or cure him. But as disease was being excised, so to speak, from the patient's individuality and his place in the world, the holistic modes of caretaking, the alternatives that used to be the originals, kept up-to-date too. Illnesses that did not yield to scientific medicine were attended to by mountebanks and patent remedies (science's biased terms) or by practitioners of the mental control of disease, such as the mesmerists and Christian Science healers, who were the mid-nineteenth-century placeholders for psychiatry.

Nineteenth-century scientific medicine had difficulty with the ailments of the spine, brain, and nerve fibers. Spinal irritation was a common diagnosis for vague and disturbing symptoms, and in more pronounced cases the diagnosis was hysteria, particularly if the patient was a woman. Hysteria and its counterpart in the male, hypochondria, both were considered organic disorders. The terms have since been debased, but to physicians of the day, you may be sure, the outbursts of hysterical patients were not signs of emotional weakness.

Hysterics were prone to fits, paralyses, convulsions, numbness, heightened sensitivity to pain: extreme expressions of bodily distress. The Frenchman Paul Briquet made the first hardheaded study of hysteria in 1859. It was not seated in the uterus, Briquet declared, but in the brain, and one in twenty sufferers was male. According to his mechanism of the disease, the "affective part" of the brain, in predisposed people, became disturbed and injured by long periods of stress, such as could befall "maltreated children, unhappily married women, or subjects tormented by profound grief." From the altered brain the disorder extended to other organs and induced uncontrolled bodily manifestations.

In the 1870s and 1880s the neurologist Jean-Martin Charcot, whose research base was the Salpêtrière infirmary in Paris, split off the epileptics and other neurologically damaged patients from the hysterics. Subdividing hysteria further, he tried to distinguish cases caused by brain injury from those stemming from frightening events and accidents. While Charcot the neuroanatomist failed to find brain lesions—the concrete signs of hysteria that he expected—Charcot the clinician grew famous for his weekly demonstrations of hysterical symptoms in his infirmary patients. Charcot epitomized the doctor-collaborator. His patients swooned or writhed or fell entranced when he probed their "fixed painful points."

The powerful idea of Shorter's book *From Paralysis to Fatigue* is that in every era of medicine certain disorders are deemed "legitimate" by society and others are not. People with psychosomatic illness, says Shorter, unconsciously pick and choose their physical complaints from a "pool" of acceptable symptoms, a pool managed by true-believing physicians. Thus Charcot's medical exhibitions gave persuasive, even pleasing proof of hysteria's authenticity.

The neurologist Sigmund Freud, who studied at Salpêtrière in the 1880s, concluded there was nothing neurological about hysteria. Freud thought that repressed memories of traumatic experiences, including memories of childhood sexual abuse, instigated the hysterical symptoms. The person's pains, fits, and contractures represented a "conversion disorder." As Freud developed his theory of the unconscious, he made a fateful turn away from the role of sexual traumatization in childhood, deciding that the memories being repressed were but fantasies and projections, although the psychological conflict was nonetheless real. He maintained that neurosis was just as capable of producing physical symptoms as actual trauma, and so he decided to treat the neurosis.

Because of Freud and other informed critics of neurology, hysteria lost its legitimacy as a disease. The next generation of doctors put Charcot down as an entertainer, his patients as unwitting performers. Hysteria was defined as any symptom that could be "induced by suggestion and abolished by persuasion." The upshot was that hysteria began to disappear—to be precise, the diagnosis of hysteria disappeared. Patients with chronic, unexplained maladies had to go back to the symptom pool, as Shorter would say, and reformulate their conditions.

After 1900 psychiatry acted as a sort of vacuum cleaner for physical disorders that fell out of favor. Along with hysteria it scooped up something known as railway spine, in which the victims of railway accidents developed peculiar symptoms, seemingly out of proportion to their injuries. It was noticed that railway spine was often attached to litigation for compensation. The term compensation neurosis, the successor to railway spine, is still in mental health manuals.

Also, neurasthenia, after a prolonged debate, was stripped of its organic status. Neurasthenia was first classified by the American neurologist George Beard, who produced several books about it in the latter half of the nineteenth century. Beard listed scores of symptoms. Chronic fatigue was the hallmark indicator, and various other manifestations were itching, palpitations, salivation, incontinence, and "vague pains and flying neuralgias." Beard believed the disease resulted from an injury to the nervous system, which became drained of propulsive force. More men contracted it than women, more upper-class people than lower-class. Although overwork and the buffeting of modern life were the prime agents of neurasthenia, Beard insisted that it was a physical, not a mental, state.

Neurasthenia was a victim of its own success, for in the early years of the twentieth century it was broadly diagnosed, reaching into the working classes in both the United States and Europe, until it lost its meaning and physicians pulled back from it. When the mind doctors sought to put the neurasathenics on the couch, soon there were no more neurasthenics wanting treatment.

Neurasthenia's immediate offspring, which went by the names of neurocirculatory asthenia and neuromyasthenia, did not survive long either, being without biomedical support. In the realm of fatigue they were succeeded, as the decades of the last century passed, by chronic brucellosis, postviral syndrome, myalgic encephalitis, and chronic fatigue syndrome.

Always psychiatry put predatory pressure on the paradigms of unexplained illness; always it stayed one step behind, as the conditions were reformulated by contemporary attitudes about illness and by advances in the diagnostic technology of scientific medicine. Although psychotherapists earnestly desired to collaborate, negotiate, etc. with the patients who might need them, most patients disbelieved and turned elsewhere for medical partners. The stigma attached to emotional illness seems constant in society.

IF OPPOSITES ATTRACT, Darren and Jackie were made for each other. "She was fun and had a lot of energy for life," Darren recalled, which sells her short. Jackie was a red-haired, brassy-voiced live wire, ten years younger than he, as outgoing and clear as Darren was drawn in and cloudy. She was an ex–rodeo rider and an ex-wife, no stranger to hard knocks. She loved to drive trucks, the bigger the rig the better, but was employed at present operating a school bus on the back roads of Idaho.

They started to date late in 1995, during a period when his symptoms were on an even keel. They enjoyed snowmobiling and dancing together. With his expressive eyes and soft-spoken charm, Darren was quite a catch, Jackie thought. She owned a home in the trailer park by the river, and he moved in in June 1996.

Darren professed not to want a sexual partner or anything more than a friend. Although he had had several physical relationships since the war, there was an air of abstemiousness gathering about him. During sex with his last girlfriend he had felt a "tightness" in his testicles, a "burning" in his semen, and he wondered if he might have infected her. From herpes and the gulf war contamination, he felt doubly defiled.

Jackie professed not to mind. When she learned about his gulf war condition, she promised to take care of him. "Who else would go into a relationship knowing I'm a dying man?" he said gratefully.

Her first intervention was in the spring. For two weeks Darren had been bothered by a tightness in his chest and a tingling in his arms. It seemed to him that his heart was beating irregularly. He didn't want to go the hospital, though. What good would it do? he said. The VA never found anything. Jackie became alarmed, pointing out the ashen color in his face when his chest was hurting. The change in his color was news to Darren. She insisted they go to the emergency room at Spokane VAMC.

But when Darren's heart was found to be normal, and the problem dismissed as a passing inflammation in his chest, Jackie was skeptical. She was angered by the response. On the drive home she cried over the cold way the VA had treated him.

In August Jackie brought Darren to his regularly scheduled appointment with Dr. Long. The doctor reviewed Darren's complaints, some old and some new, summarizing them in his notes as "aches and pains." Dr. Long then asked Darren about his smoking and drinking habits (none and minimal) and also whether he was homosexual or heterosexual. There are grounds to ask this of a patient with persistent symptoms, but Darren was astounded and hurt by the question. Jackie, when she heard about it, hit the roof. After that they agreed that he would not meet with any doctor without her being present.

Through the fall Darren got worse, jumpy and snapping at Jackie in the evenings, and in the mornings so painfully stiff he couldn't get out of bed unless she pulled him out. Now that she was there to support him, his spartan, half-scornful attitude toward his body, his sorry, decaying body, as he regarded it, began to crumble. He was tired of suppressing this illness. He needed help! But without medical guidance Jackie was floundering. "I'd go meet the devil himself if it would help Darren," she said. What should she do?

One night in early December of 1996 she and Darren were watching a documentary on the gulf war illnesses produced by a Spokane television station. The only doctors who were shown to help the veterans were those who worked outside the mainstream. Featured were Garth Nicolson, Edward Hyman, Katherine Murray Leisure, and William Baumzweiger, all national names in the veterans' community, each having a different theory of the illnesses. Jackie was struck by the interview with Dr. Baumzweiger. His idea was that there had been neurological and immunological damage to veterans from low-level chemical exposures during the war. Three veterans in the Spokane area had improved under his care, notwithstanding that one of the patients, according to Baumzweiger, had a terminal illness.

Here was the specialist Darren must see, Jackie decided. Besides, things were so frayed at home a dramatic move was needed. "It was our last chance to make it as a couple and maybe get him some help," she recalled.

The next day she made contact with the doctor, and three days later they were on their way to Los Angeles, where Baumzweiger was based. Without the push Darren never would have gone. "I was going to beat this on my own," he said, smiling weakly, "though of course I wasn't."

BILL BAUMZWEIGER WAS a neurologist. In late 1996 he still worked for the Department of Veterans Affairs, but under increasingly hostile superintendence. He told Jackie and Darren they had better come down to his clinic at once because he might not be there if they waited until January. He already would have been fired, he believed, but for a U.S. congressman, who was blasting the agency for trying to muzzle him.

A psychiatrist by training, Baumzweiger had returned to medical school late in his career in order to take up another specialty. When the gulf war illnesses broke out, he was doing his residency in neurology at the West Los Angeles VAMC. The patients he saw intrigued him. Following his hunches, Baumzweiger ordered extra lab tests for them and performed detailed neurological exams.

The vets had all kinds of deficits that the other doctors weren't picking up, he determined. Sorting the test results of ten patients, Baumzweiger found abnormalities in heart rate, body temperature, blood pressure, lymphocyte (white blood cell) count, spinal fluid, brain waves, and diverse other measurements. Even more abnormal were the symptoms that the doctor recorded in his extensive interviews. The veterans suffered from "olfactory hallucinations"—strange tastes in their mouths and strange smells having no external source. They had blurry vision, sensitivity to sunlight and noises, lack of coordination, loss of direction, seizures, lassitude, and phobias.

Baumzweiger acknowledged there were psychiatric symptoms in the mix but argued they were a consequence of brain damage. The phobias, for instance, might have occurred when neurons, knocked out by environmental toxins, grew back and reconnected in novel ways.

Indeed Baumzweiger's theory of the gulf war illnesses managed to encompass every region of the body—and every rival theory too—because he ran everything through the brain. An inflammation of the brainstem caused an immunological breakdown, permitting the arousal of latent viruses and lurking bacteria, from which, or along with which, resulted a cascade of cellular, hormonal, and cardiovascular irregularities, plus the neurological damage from the original insult.

I don't have the background to critique Baumzweiger's theory, but then he has not provided data defining the disease process so that his peers might critique it. You might object that I have put stock in Daniel Clauw's model of illness, which also contains esoteric physiologic connections. Clauw, however, met many scientific tests, as required by his peers, while Baumzweiger was just out there propounding.

"I may be an outsider," he told me. "But I have proof that their [the vets'] heartbeats increase twenty-two beats per minute when they stand up, and then you give them the medicine and it's reduced."

OK, about the patients with surging hearts, Darren being one. The formal name for their condition is postural orthostatic tachycardia syndrome, POTS. The fact that doctors have made it a syndrome with its own acronym suggests that it did not arise with the Persian Gulf War. POTS is another in the constellation of functional disorders that appear in the background when you focus upon the gulf war illnesses. POTS has an objective core, tachycardia, which distinguishes it from the other functional syndromes, but it's like them in having satellite symptoms of dizziness, fatigue, breathing difficulties, and gastrointestinal discomfort.

Addressing the POTS patient, first the doctor rules out cardiovascular disease. So why then does a healthy heart race upon the simple exertion of standing? There is divided opinion in medicine on what to make of POTS. Some physicians, the minimalists, advise patients to drink more fluids, increase the salt in their diets and try not to worry about it, for the pounding sensation and dizziness are not dangerous and may well go away in the coming weeks or months. Other doctors, making a stronger response, will prescribe beta-blocking medication to slow down the heart rate. The third echelon—to which Dr. Baumzweiger belonged, minus the technical apparatus—plunges into an analysis of the autonomic nervous system, which regulates the involuntary ("automatic") muscles of the body, including the heart. In this approach, special tables to tilt the person up and down and special tests of his blood pressure and respiration rate attempt to fill biomedical data into the blank areas of POTS. Some of the data may point to subtle abnormalities in the function of the brainstem.

This triage doesn't take into account the patient's wishes. The more distressing or disabling the POTS symptoms, the more likely that he or she will end up lying on the specialist's tilt table. The unspoken compact between this type of patient and this type of physician is the desire to generate test data for the worst case, just in case. Who knows if POTS could turn into something major?

Baumzweiger, a specialist of the gulf war illnesses, ordered many tests to flesh out his interpretation of the disorder, of which a racing heart was but one of the signs. At the same time he spurned the opinions of other specialists. "I don't care what they think of me scientifically or personally," he told me. He likened the VA administration to "the emperor's new clothes" and "a satrapy." "I feel they don't handle this thing medically, but politically," he said.

You'll agree he does not sound like a physician who will get ahead in a government bureaucracy. Baumzweiger was moved to an outpatient clinic in downtown Los Angeles, away from the big medical center and the referral program for Persian Gulf vets. He was not on the VA staff but was paid under a short-term neurology fellowship until mid-1997. Yet by word of mouth Dr. Baumzweiger still attracted patients, many from other states. The VA cracked down on him for ordering too many costly tests and then brought him before a disciplinary committee for conducting unauthorized and unproved treatments. As a result, his story was publicized, his cause championed. John Cabrillo heard about him, and so did Jackie.

"The complaint was that I was treating people I was not supposed to be treating," Baumzweiger said, "though the vast majority got better. People were coming to see me in this tiny clinic in L.A. A lot of the VA's problem is jealousy."

"The official position is that you're not qualified," I said.

"Oh yeah," he said sarcastically. "I'm only a neurologist and a toxicologist and have studied neurotoxicology. And I'm not qualified."

He pulled down a medical text from his bookshelf and began to quote from a section on organophosphate poisoning. Organophosphate chemicals, the OP agents, include insecticides and nerve gases. The Pentagon's critics, led by James Tuite, charged that nerve gases were released by the bombing of Iraqi munitions factories during the war.

"'Well-known delayed neurotoxicity,'" the doctor read. "'One to three weeks after ingestion . . . progressive muscle weakness. . . .'

"It says 'diminishing after three weeks,'" Baumzweiger continued, "but I have seen abnormal electromyograms [a gauge of nerve damage] as long as four years out. This looks to be a delayed neuropathy."

"You're adapting a text on acute poisonings to the veterans in the Gulf," I said.

"I am refining, yes, what I read, based on my experience."

We were off Baumzweiger's area of expertise, if not exactly onto mine. The debate over neurotoxic exposures hung on whether the amount of OP agent—from the bombing, from the pesticide spraying, from wherever—could possibly have been great enough to be harmful.

"Tuite has NOAA [weather satellite] photos of gas going into the air," he said.

"Actually, Tuite says the photo shows a thermal plume occurring at the time of the bombing, but even that's far from certain."

"Well, OK. . . . But I know from soldiers there that they had severe olfactory reactions. We have no idea how dangerous the OP agents are. There were people hiding in tents, people turning around and stabbing their best friends. Sexual acting out. Nymphomania even. That comes from a disinhibition of the brain, the lower brain centers being released from higher control. And that's consistent with neurotoxic exposure. Subsequently the people have the other symptoms. They start seeing double, they lose sensation."

"Isn't that all anecdotal? Will you publish this in a journal?"

"Oh, I can't publish this," he said disdainfully. "The VA will not allow me. They will have my head."

"Is this a terminal illness? Do you think Darren has a terminal illness?"

"I do think his life's been shortened. All these guys. They gotta be."

In William Baumzweiger Darren finally had a doctor who showed him how to be sick. Darren already *was* sick, you understand, but since he did not know why, he didn't exactly know how. Baumzweiger, in a three-hour session with Darren and Jackie that was part examination, part elicitation, demonstrated how the illness worked.

First the doctor recorded the standard information: height, weight, blood pressure, etc., adding a few twists. Darren's heartbeat accelerated from seventy-six to ninety-two beats per minute after he stood up. Though not an insignificant increase, it was about half of what most physicians require for a diagnosis of POTS.

The doctor asked Darren about his exposures during the war. "Had I been exposed to the oil fires, chemical explosions, et cetera," remembered Darren, in a written account. They went through each possibility, Baumzweiger nodding and taking notes. By this exercise they assembled the rationale for his illness.

Next Baumzweiger wrote down all of Darren's symptoms during the past five years: not just the major complaints of pain and diarrhea but also his individual quirks, such as drooling, "whiteness" in his field of vision, prickly hot skin on occasion, compulsions about salty foods, metallic taste in his mouth, claustrophobia, and others. That there should be so many strange and disconnected symptoms was no impediment to diagnosis. When he explained it, Darren and Jackie grasped that a brainstem inflammation could be responsible for everything.

Then came the neurological exam. Baumzweiger's battery of tests was an eye-opener for Darren. His reflexes were judged abnormal; "in some instances no reflex at all," Darren recalled. "The knees and arms didn't respond, but my whole body did." The two played the schoolboy's game of hand quickness. Shakily Darren tried to slap the doctor's hands resting on his. He missed badly.

"He then had me close my eyes, and he would snap his fingers and ask me to point where I thought I heard the snap. Most often I was several inches off." When Baumzweiger had Jackie try, "she was generally within one inch or less of where the sound had occurred."

Asked to balance himself on his tiptoes, Darren couldn't do it. Dr. Baumzweiger had to grab him by the forehead to keep him from tipping over.

Puffy-faced, wide-eyed, Darren looked awful during the exam. I saw a tape of part of it, for the patient was put through his neurological paces a second time, when the Spokane TV reporter who had put them in touch with Baumzweiger arrived with a film crew.

The doctor clapped his hands at Darren's ear to provoke a reaction. Eyes closed, Darren jerked his head away, even though he knew the noise was coming. "That's it," said Baumzweiger. "A very exaggerated startle reflex. That shows you the brainstem is extremely irritated and cannot inhibit it."

I was reminded of Charcot's medical salon in Paris, where the neurologist had put patients with hysteria onstage. The sick people would not have participated had they not trusted their doctor completely, and they must have believed the presentations would further the understanding of their illness. Likewise Darren went on television, he said, for the sake of other sick veterans. He was literally in Baumzweiger's hands, being manipulated and jumping in pain, until the doctor, with the insight of a psychiatrist, said, "Darren's had enough."

His performance on the neurological tests devastated Darren. "I felt anger, hurt, and pain," he told me. "That was the first time Jackie realized why I was agitated. And when Baumzweiger said it's killing me, like Dr. Smith did, that's when I understood the severity of it." He testified later, "On two different occasions while in L.A. I threatened to walk out of the motel room not to be seen from or heard from again. This was brought on by having to face just how sick I have really become."

Driving on the freeway after the exam, Darren "froze up" at the wheel, narrowly escaping an accident. Sent by Baumzweiger to the hospital for an MRI scan, he became terrified by the thought that Jackie had abandoned him there. "When Jackie was finally able to return, she found me in a hospital gown rocking back and forth, unable to speak to anyone, and tears running down my face."

Meanwhile his blood had been sent for analysis to a private lab. A neces-

sary cost, said Baumzweiger, which the VA wouldn't cover. Jackie paid the
eight-hundred-dollar bill. (She also paid the travel expenses for their
eleven-day stay.) The blood screening indicated that Darren was infected
with the Epstein-Barr and herpes viruses, a common pair of findings, but it
was conveyed in Baumzweiger's report as part of the evidence of his special
condition.

The veteran was told that he might prolong his life only by limiting his
activities; by avoiding contact with pesticides, sunlight, and stress; and by
embarking on a lifelong regimen of strong medication. Yet Jackie and Darren, once they got over the shock, were vindicated and even bolstered by
the consultation.

"I came home with an understanding of the neurological damage that
the Gulf veterans are trying to live with," said Jackie. "This has allowed
Darren and me to build a stronger relationship." Darren talked about making a will. When he showed Baumzweiger's report to his mother and
brother, they had to accept that though he had always been the strong one
of the family, this time he might not bounce back.

Not having to protest his condition any longer, Darren relinquished to
Jackie all the medical details. She took over his files and appointments
and medication. While he concentrated, as it were, on being sick, she
expressed his sickness to the world. She wrote letters about his care, or
lack of it, to senators and representatives. She collected hundreds of pages
of information on gulf war syndrome, which was back in the news
because of the Khamisiyah incident. Through the network she learned of
vets in the same boat as Darren and called attention to their cases too. "I
may be a little peon from a small state," she said, "but I am going to be
heard."

Soon Jackie knew more about the issue than he did and was able to brief
him. Darren referred to her in public as "my brain and my speaker" because
it was "a known fact that Persian Gulf War veterans experience short-term
memory loss and lack of concentration." Spunky and direct, big teeth flashing, Jackie announced herself as "Darren's spouse, wife, girlfriend, fiancée,
whatever." And now he said "we" when asked about his health.

I am confident in describing their mutual roles because I knew other
couples who made similar arrangements. In one instance it was a brother
and sister. The sick veteran was always the more genial one, the less political, while she spit fire and cleared away bureaucratic obstacles for him. At

the same time she made it known that he could explode unpredictably ("If you think I'm bad . . ."), and so part of her responsibility was to keep him calm and controlled. In their symbiotic, intense exchange the woman often contracted a milder version of the man's symptoms. Jackie did, or worried that she had.

All this composed Darren's way of being sick, his illness behavior, as opposed to Darren's unexplained illness, the private hell beyond my ken. Illness behavior is augmented when there is support from a spouse or family member, sanction from a doctor, and, not least in importance, a cultural explanation of the illness, which the sick person plugs into because it gives a coherence to his experience. Darren embraced the idea that he got sick because of toxic chemical exposures.

But that wasn't the worst part for him. "My being sick is OK," he said to me. "I served my country, I got sick because of it, OK. It's the aftermath that strips you of your pride."

A CHANGED PATIENT, and not for the better, presented himself to Dr. Long at the Spokane VAMC, just a week after the pair returned from Los Angeles. Darren's resting pulse was rapid; his weight had ballooned to 240 pounds. With Jackie sitting in, he complained to Long of stiffened joints, diarrhea, headache, chills, tightness in his chest, rash, pain radiating to his groin and abdomen, and a brand-new symptom, swelling in his lower legs and ankles.

Dr. Long affirmed the swelling as "edema" and labeled the rash on his legs "mild eczema." The doctor said he would order a new round of blood and urine assays and X rays. "Jackie asked what he was going to do about the swelling in my legs and ankles," Darren recounted. "He stated that there was not anything to worry about or uncommon about the swelling. When Dr. Long finished writing, Jackie attempted to address a couple of issues with him. He informed her that, 'This appointment is over. There will be no further information admitted.' "

Jackie followed the doctor into the hall, demanding to know if he had any "compassion and respect" for his patients. She held a copy of the blood results from Baumzweiger's lab and angrily pressed it into his hand, saying it should be entered into Darren's records.

Long's version of the incident ignores Jackie: "He pulled out some old

tests at the end, as I'm leaving the room. Some people call it door-knob-
bing. Others call it sandbagging. He was laying in wait for me. We had run
twenty minutes over, but I sat back down. I didn't say, 'We don't have time.'
I said, 'Let's get the labs—I'll reorder these tests.' "

That was on December 23. On January 4 Jackie brought Darren back to
the hospital. For two weeks he had been completely constipated and vomiting in the bathroom most mornings, yet he was still getting in his car and
going off to work. It was the blood in the toilet that spurred Jackie to call
Dr. Baumzweiger in Los Angeles. He advised her to hurry Darren to the
nearest gastroenterologist. She picked Darren up at his office, and they
went to the emergency room in Spokane.

A barium enema was performed, the barium highlighting his colon so
that X rays could detect any obstructions. "I was so backed up," said Darren, "I lost ten pounds of stuff when they flushed me."

According to the radiology report, his bowel contained pockets of gas
and undigested pills. Under the Baumzweiger regimen Darren had been
taking seven types of medication. They were not placebos, far from it. I will
list them in order of their potency: a sulfa drug normally used to combat
stomach inflammation; a calcium channel blocker normally taken by people with high blood pressure; an antidepressant; a tranquilizer for sleeping;
Motrin; Tylenol with codeine; and Metamucil for constipation.

The doses Baumzweiger prescribed were not extraordinary, but the
potential side effects of the accumulated pills were considerable. I learned
that swelling of the legs and feet, constipation, and nausea could result—
and maybe had in Darren's case, sending him to the hospital. When I
found out that the two strongest medications made patients sensitive to
sunburn, I grimaced, recalling Baumzweiger's warning to veterans to avoid
the sunlight. It appears he was speaking to the perils of his own treatment
plan rather than to the condition he claimed to have diagnosed. Even the
modest Motrin was implicated in Darren's emergency, because the medication may cause bleeding in the stomach, and he had seen blood when he
threw up.

Darren and Jackie, however, would not hear that the pills might be at
fault. After a weekend in the hospital Darren asked the nurses for his medication. It would not be forthcoming, he was told, for Dr. Long had
ordered it stopped. Moreover, no further testing was planned.

The patient rebelled, demanded to be let out of the hospital, almost ripped the IV out of his arm. "If that's the case," Darren said, "I'm going home to die where I have family and friends around me." As he dressed and packed, he placed phone calls to Jackie and to the Spokane TV station.

In short order the hospital administrators came around to placate him. There was a lengthy meeting, which Darren stalked in and out of while Jackie argued his position. The result was that Dr. Long was removed from his care. Assigned a new doctor, the more sympathetic Dr. Short, Darren agreed to remain in the hospital a few more days. Additional tests were scheduled for him, and his medication was restored except for the Motrin.

On January 8, 1997, still an inpatient, Darren appealed his VA disability rating, citing Baumzweiger's assessment of "brain stem inflammation secondary to neurotoxins."

DR. SHORT WAS the fourth doctor to grapple with Darren's illness. For better or worse the other three had taken their shots, leaving the illness, if anything, more entrenched. Had he known the full story, Dr. Short might have been forgiven for ducking this patient, but he was an inquisitive, dogged, and upbeat physician, as well as something of an eccentric, just the traits needed to care for the sick gulf war veterans. Lately the Spokane hospital had been sending difficult cases his way.

"If somebody comes to me and says, 'I've got these symptoms,' I'm not going to say, 'No, you don't,' " Short told me. "I may say, 'I don't know why or what caused them,' but you don't dump over someone because you don't know the answer. You don't go pick a fight with a patient because you have a hole in your knowledge."

He was fifty-five years old and in ordinary times tended veterans with geriatric ailments and skin diseases. Having been with the agency during its last environmental health crisis, over Agent Orange, he saw an identical conflict unfolding, the push for an explanation clashing with the push for a settlement with the veterans. "Persian Gulf syndrome will go on for another decade," he predicted, "while they fight about it and get data. Then they will establish service connection. It's a political problem and a scientific problem. The political problem will be resolved, and the scientific problem is of less interest to those who would resolve it. I approve of it getting fixed. I want to give the vets the benefit of the doubt. But if they get taken care of [compensated], they are not going to be interested in the science either."

Short, who *was* interested in the research, knew about the similarity between the gulf war illnesses and other functional syndromes. It showed in his initial evaluation of Darren: "History and physical compatible with so called Persian Gulf Syndrome, specifically fibromyalgia, chronic fatigue, possible migraine, and irritable bowel symptomatology."

But Dr. Short was not content to toss around labels. One of the syndromes was not academic to him since his wife suffered from fibromyalgia. A registered nurse, she had collected articles from the scientific literature on FM and CFS for years. "I live with fibromyalgia," Short said. "You can't measure it, tests are negative, but patients are hurting all over." When he probed the veterans, they showed the same trigger points on their bodies as his wife.

As a child growing up on a farm his wife had nibbled "seed wheat." The wheat seed in those days was coated with a "pink pesticide." Mulling over her history in light of the research he and she had collected, he came around to the toxic hypothesis. "My wife probably has it—chronic pesticide poisoning," he said. "The gulf war stuff smells that way to me. I bet you, when they do the work, that's what will turn up."

Short's opinion of the illness and his openness to patients enabled him to form a good relationship with Darren and Jackie right off the bat. "He goes the extra mile," said Darren. "He is interested." Darren was pleased besides that Dr. Short took Baumzweiger's workup seriously. "He says, 'I don't agree with everything that Baumzweiger is doing, but he's on the right track.' "

"What's the difference between the two?" I asked.

"Baumzweiger says to attack and use higher levels of medication. 'Hit it hard, and then back off,' he says, while Dr. Short likes to start off slow."

The latter withheld from Darren his full reservations. "Baumzweiger may be right," Short told me, "but he's a little bit crazy. I wouldn't start patients on six or seven drugs at a time. These things are toxic. Cardiac drugs have side effects. If he is going to go out on a limb, he should have a protocol behind him."

That spring Darren and Jackie appeared before the Presidential Advisory Committee investigating the illnesses. He, another veteran, and James Tuite read statements. Darren told his story evenly but faltered halfway. He apologized to the committee, adding that in the service he had been known as a good speaker. Jackie finished the statement for him. "I could barely whisper and walk on my own accord," he said afterward.

When they got home, Dr. Short persuaded them that Darren should discontinue two of the medications. Coincidentally or not, the swelling in his legs eased. He felt somewhat better in April, good enough to go dancing a couple of times. The doctor also started Darren on a regimen of twelve vitamins, the same that his wife used for her fibromyalgia.

All told, Darren swallowed thirty-five pills a day: fifteen in the morning, four at lunch, nine at dinner, seven before bed. A welter of sizes and colors, the medications and vitamins were doled out to him by Jackie from a clear plastic dispenser. The dispenser, like a three-dimensional checkerboard, sat on a coffee table in the middle of their trailer.

"He doesn't even know what he takes," Jackie said half-proudly.

"She counts 'em out, I take 'em" Darren shrugged, knees up, sitting on the couch, playing with the cats.

"What have they done for you?" I asked.

"The drugs have helped my energy level and my standing-sitting pulse level, and they control my temperature at night and intestinal problems. But they are no help for the joint pain, eye problems, central nervous system—where I shake. Baumzweiger didn't have time to address that. Anyway, there's no cure for neurological damage. When you become brain-dead, everything shuts down."

Dr. Short put Darren on the list to go to the West L.A. VAMC referral center, which had the expertise, he thought, to detect a neurological injury if there was one. "When you look at these people," he told me, "they're pretty normal, functionally, until you push them. Then you notice they're a little ataxic [uncoordinated], they're a little stupid [cognitive deficits], and they ache all over. You notice that. It's no one thing in particular. It's across-the-board neurological damage. But a whole lot of people, separate from each other, have these symptoms, and the VA hasn't been sophisticated enough to pick it apart."

Because he was not a neurologist, I pressed Dr. Short for his research citations, intending to compare his material with mine and see perhaps where we had diverged. He sent a smattering of papers having to do with pesticide exposures, and this permits me to give a short exegesis, which is somewhat delayed and I hope will be fair, of the neurotoxic framework. You will need to be familiar with it when you meet Jim Tuite.

ORGANOPHOSPHATE AGENTS, AS I noted, include nerve gases and insecticides. The insecticides that were used to control bugs around U.S. troop concentrations in the Gulf included malathion, diazinon, and chlorpyrifos (Dursban). Also used were carbamate pesticides, such as Sevin, which are similar in action but less toxic. For personal use, there were sticks of DEET and spray cans of permethrin. Some soldiers, not many, went so far as to wear flea collars containing chlorpyrifos.

Subsequently veterans got sick. Why? Scientific research can be like the drunk who looks for his lost keys around the lamppost because that's the only place where it's light. Of the chemicals under suspicion, the organophosphate pesticides were the most familiar. They had track records. They were better known, in terms of effects, than the nerve gases such as sarin. Other compounds, principally pyridostigmine bromide, the nerve gas prophylactic, were considered for their synergistic potential, the prospect that they could have interacted with the OP agents and caused a bigger bang within human nervous systems. But the best guidance to researchers came from studies of farm workers and pesticide applicators who had accidentally high contact with OP pesticides, either inhaling the vapor or spilling the penetrating liquid on their skins.

The literature was about poisonings and their aftermath. Almost no studies were available of aftermath pure and simple, which is to say, of chronic effects in the absence of at least some kind of acute or immediate reaction. There had been no call for such studies, for the pesticide poisonings—the escaped fatalities, you might say—were the driving issue. Researchers went back to see how the victims were doing.

Months or years later the subjects had got over the nausea, narrowed pupils, dizziness, runny noses, cramps, and shakes that they had suffered initially. But in bad cases there was some residual numbness. In severe cases, permanent damage to the nerve endings had occurred after a hiatus of a few weeks. A hard tingling in the hands and feet, which went away, was succeeded by paralysis. Limbs dragged; wrists flopped. "Organophosphate-induced delayed neuropathy" was the name of the condition. It was the worst thing known to happen to a poisoned person short of dying.

The "delay" was the part of the ailment that jumped out to gulf war researchers. Could a milder form of OP neuropathy have crept over the veterans—an infirmity not forecast by any symptoms at the time of exposure? Or if symptoms were noticed by soldiers, perhaps they were misattributed to the flu or the stress of war. Robert Haley, the leading scientific proponent of neurotoxic injury, thought so. The neurological syndromes that Haley labored to demonstrate sprang from the theory of silent delay. The theory had some support from toxicological experiments on animals.

Assume for the sake of argument that low OP exposures had left some of the veterans "a little stupid, a little ataxic," as Dr. Short put it. Even a trained observer had to have sophisticated tests to pin these changes down. The basic neurological exam wasn't sufficiently sensitive, to judge by the work of VA and Pentagon specialists, who, Baumzweiger excepted, did not detect neurotoxic damage in the health registry participants. Similarly, when Darren Moreau went to the West L.A. VAMC for his consultation, in May 1997, he did not impress the staff neurologist on first look as impaired. Darren pulled out of the program before further testing could be performed.

Elsewhere, advanced technology having been brought to bear, the sick veterans were shown to differ from healthy veterans in some minor respects. Haley's team, for example, found differences in sensory reflexes, as when the eyeballs moved in response to stimuli. By absolute measures and published norms of neurological performance, however, Haley's subjects were not impaired. The effect came out only in comparison with the other subjects in his sample.

Differences also glimmered on brain scans, but the scans that were employed, such as functional MRI and MRI spectroscopy, were so new that nobody could say what the differences meant, or what may have caused them, or whether they even qualified as anomalies. "You see differences in how the brain lights up," said Roberta White, a researcher at the Boston VAMC, "but I don't know what the explanation is." The older imaging systems, the X rays and basic MRI scans, did not illumine any such subtleties in the veterans. Findings in this field should be put aside until scientists have mastered the new hardware and verified its implications.

Other differences emerged through applications of medical software. Here I refer to neuropsychological testing. Neuropsychology is a relatively new specialty, springing up in the gap between two disciplines sharing an interest in the brain, neurology and psychology. When the brain becomes damaged, not only can there be a physical response—in reflexes and motor capacity, the traditional purview of neurologists—but also changes in mental and emotional states, of concern to psychologists. Neuropsychologists have put together low-tech methods to measure the brain's performance across the board.

A neuropsychological evaluation is lengthy. A battery of tests can take up to eight hours, as it ranges from personal questions (about health status, stress, nightmares, sad and happy moods, etc.) to tests of attention and memory (i.e., recalling the number of fingers that were shown to you a minute ago or identifying a sound that was played before); tapping effort (how many presses of a button you can make within a time period); and mental quickness (how long it takes you to push button A correctly when the dot on the computer screen appears *inside* the rectangle, versus button B if the dot is *outside* the rectangle). All the tests in the battery are standardized, meaning that an individual's overall score can be matched to the profile of known groups, be they healthy adults or patients with a particular type of brain damage.

Neuropsychological testing first proved itself on victims of industrial exposures, workers who were damaged by chemicals. The tests measured their loss of cognitive function. Although to the neurologist these people had recovered from their acute episodes, their normality was belied by small dips in memory, vision, and coordination, as calibrated by the neuropsychologist.

Such was the outcome in four or five studies of agricultural workers who had run afoul of OP pesticides. This work, from the late eighties and early nineties, became the foundation for the gulf war research. As one investigator told Congress in 1996:

> Taken in concert, the properly controlled studies indicate that humans who have experienced acute, high-level exposure to organophosphate pesticides may experience lasting deficits for as long as two to three years after the poisoning episode.
>
> What is not clear is whether a poisoning episode has to occur to cause these clinically significant persistent effects. . . . The most important question that needs to be considered in relation to the gulf war illnesses is whether repeated low-level exposure to organophosphates would also produce these effects.

To reiterate, there was little support in the literature for believing this, but then the question had hardly been addressed.

So the researchers addressed it in tests of Persian Gulf veterans, with the important caveat that actual exposures were unknown. By 2000 most of the results were in. Haley's neuropsychologist, who compared the scores of sick subjects with those of healthy subjects in the same unit, reported that the sick vets were brain-impaired. Researchers funded by the Department of Veterans Affairs came to more scattered and cautious conclusions. No effect, said one. Small decrements in motor skills, said another. Lapses in memory and concentration characterized a subgroup of the veterans sampled, reported a third team, but the strongest finding by this team was the high rate of psychological distress.

"We're dealing with very tiny effects," conceded Kent Anger, the psychologist contracted by the VA's Portland Environmental Health Research Center. "You have to go to heroic measures to find something, plus there's no baseline." Not only was the picture incoherent, but it didn't resemble the earlier profiles of OP-exposed workers, Anger added. If there were a "whopping" effect, he said, the case for a neurotoxic exposure would have been closed "within six months," instead of the six years and counting after the studies were begun.

"I can't tell you I am any closer to knowing the cause than before," conceded Roberta White, who is chief neuropsychologist at the Boston VAMC. "We still think something happened to the veterans. I haven't stopped looking."

Like Anger's, White's expertise was in neurotoxins in the workplace, where exposures, or at least specific hazards, were known and where worker health could be monitored prospectively. She commented, "We're not used to being told, 'They came back sick. Figure out what happened to them.' "

White's group, like Haley's, did find an association between a veteran's poor health, lower neuropsychological scores and his or her claims to have been exposed to harmful chemicals. But in the ideal scientific world, said White, her test battery would have been given to troops before they shipped out, so as to allow and correct for the role of IQ, learning disorders, substance abuse, and psychological conditions, not to mention disease and prewar exposure to toxics, all of which can alter the finer behaviors of the brain and nervous system.

The toughest nut to crack was the baseline personality. "How do you define," White asked, "a character tendency to express things physically?" How to identify, please, the ones who will be more likely to have symptoms, regardless of what happens to them during the deployment or what chemicals are in the air? How to know the sensitive few most at risk? No test battery, no statistical profile for them are available. You can only look back at damaged individuals, *into* individuals, as deeply as they will let you, and speculate as kindly as you can.

DARREN SAT ON the edge of his bed at the West L.A. VAMC. He wore pale yellow pajamas beneath a red bathrobe. The cardiologist had just left the room, and the rheumatologist was on his way—the fragmented consultations of the referral center process.

It was our first meeting, and Darren was relating to me the events leading up to his deployment to the war. He and some other airmen had lined up for their shots, not sure what the shots were for, and jokingly he asked the commanding officer what was the penalty for refusing to be vaccinated. This was the prewar Darren, who wasn't angry. His goal then was to break the tension, "to put the rest of the guys at ease."

"Darren's a leader," interjected Jackie. "He draws people to him." Having been chatting with Pete, who was on the next bed, now she came back to sit beside Darren. "Scoot over," she said, rubbing shoulders.

"It's been second nature to me," he continued. "People who were about to be discharged would be referred to me. I'd start counseling 'em, though they'd be unaware of it. Master sergeants who'd been there eighteen years would come to me and tell me their life stories."

I didn't know what to make of this man in chronic need of care who also would dispense it. Needy of help, yet needing to help, as I would learn. Darren broke up fistfights in the service. He pushed a little girl out of the way of a car that had slipped its breaks. At a party he saved a woman who was choking, administering the Heimlich maneuver while other guests hesitated. The motorist in the car wreck in Germany—stationed there, Darren was driving by—stabilized by his CPR. A fire put out in a building, possibly saving lives. All this told (not told all at once) with a quiet pride and no boasting. "I've been a hero in my own right," he said, "an unsung hero. I see a crisis, I rate it, I respond. It made me a good cop."

Today he didn't look like a heroic MP. Darren's face was as pale as his pajamas. Even his mustache was pale. In order to turn his head, he had to swivel his entire trunk, he was that stiff.

In Oman the first bad sign was the rash.

"When was the rash?" I asked.

"February," said Jackie.

"Jackie, please," Darren said, and continued his story.

The rheumatologist came in to examine the new patient. Jackie and I stepped back from the bed.

"I have shocks up and down my spine," said Darren, as the doctor flexed his limbs. "Can't bend."

"His whole body contorts," Jackie said.

"Anything else going on?" the doctor inquired.

"I have speech difficulty. . . . There's some stammering."

"See how he said that? It's a forced effort—"

Darren waved her off, frowning.

"Any headaches?"

"It's not how many headaches he has or when. It's when doesn't he."

"We'll have to take a look at that. . . ."

"He has dry eyes!"

Dr. Hamm entered, and the rheumatologist departed. We tripped down the path to Pete Timmons's blowup. After Pete fled in the taxi, I came back to the room and picked up the interview with Darren and Jackie. Each of us was shaken.

"They send them to war healthy," said Jackie, "then contaminate them, then bring them home and say, "We're through with you.""

"It's up to *us* to prove it was caused by the war," said Darren, incredulous. "They can infect us and not take responsibility for it?"

Head bowed, he let Jackie give the story of the crisis at Spokane VMAC and the switch from Dr. Long to Dr. Short. Now they had come to Wadsworth, where Dr. Baumzweiger wasn't allowed to visit them, just one of the complaints they had about the VA referral program—which was not what it was cut out to be, propelling Jackie to the phone and fax machine.

"The personnel aren't trained," Darren said. ""What's your problem?' they ask. I don't have one problem—I have ten."

Jackie was finishing his half-eaten lunch. "I'm expecting Darren won't survive this—the toxin in his body," she said. "I want to help him have a decent life for what time he has left—and to help other vets."

Darren was clutching his pajama legs with both hands, wadding the fabric at the knees.

"If I am terminal, I deserve one hundred percent service connection. So it's there when I need it. Any dying person shouldn't have to work."

This frankness alarmed me. "Are you sure that's the prognosis?" I asked.

Darren hedged a little. "Well, if they don't find something. . . . It's short-ening my life span. Baumzweiger said I was one of the worst he's dealt with. Even Dr. Short says, 'I don't like what I find. It's getting darker.' "

As the consultations at the hospital progressed, Darren was unhappier by the day. The food disagreed with him as much as the attitude of the staff. The neurologist took him on a "mind chase," said Darren, and "left us feel-ing he found everything to be normal." Another doctor scolded him for not knowing what pills he was taking and why. "That's what I've got her for," he said, irritated, "to do that for me. Anyway, it's in my records, look in my records if you want to know."

He went one morning to Pulmonology for a lung function test, in which he had to exhale hard into a tube. By the time he got back to his room, his chest was hurting, he was panting, he felt very chilled and weak. Jackie hit the call button for the nurses. Darren got under the covers fully dressed and, still cold, asked for extra blankets.

"I couldn't breathe. I couldn't get enough air," he remembered. "I was fading in and out. I didn't know whether I was dying or living. When all the doctors started showing up, that's when we started thinking heart attack."

Jackie was beside herself, because although Dr. Hamm and Dr. Fergu-son, the doctor on call, were paged, no physician arrived at his bedside for a half hour.

"I heard Jackie crying in the background," said Darren. "I was far away. It was a peaceful feeling. Then I heard Dr. Hamm say, 'Darren, don't leave us.' "

The nurses, and the doctors as they arrived, didn't think Darren was hav-ing a heart attack, but since his EKG was a bit suspicious, they decided to move him to the coronary care unit. The staff there gave him nitroglycerin under the tongue, just in case of angina, and heparin intravenously, against possible clots. However, the follow-up tests of his cardiac function were negative, and a day later he was returned to his room. "My EKG is normal for me but not normal for other people," Darren said. "But I know my heart has changed since I have been sick."

Hamm's summary of the incident was different: "Darren hyperventilated after the lung function test. The people attending him were not impressed with the gravity of the situation. His nails were pink, which told me that his circulation was OK."

Hamm's own prognosis to the couple: "I don't see dying vets. I see ill vets. Darren will get better, I hope—all the vets will get better—in a few years."

But after eight days Darren had had enough. When he and Jackie realized they could get the same tests at home under Dr. Short, who understood the illness and believed in it, they left Los Angeles in disgust. Ron had lost another one.

IT SHOULD HAVE been obvious that scientific medicine would never break the impasse between the stress hypothesis and the toxic hypothesis. Science would never resolve the dialectic over the cause, in Darren's case or any other. Too many ingredients were missing: a biological marker, epidemiological definition, exposure data, baseline information on the patients, follow-up information on the patients. The lacunae would never be filled so as to support a winning argument, whatever position you took on the mind and body etiologies.

Science must fail, and the kindest thing to be said about journalism, the other fact finder on the scene, was that it could do no better. What was left to make sense of the problem? What engine for insight? Well, history. Around the time that Khamisiyah was the big story journalistically, and Haley's neurotoxic findings were the big issue scientifically (journalism playing a double hand), a valuable piece of history appeared, although it did not get through the snarl of news to Darren and Jackie.

In September 1996 the *Annals of Internal Medicine* published a paper titled "War Syndromes and Their Evaluation: From the U.S. Civil War to the Persian Gulf War." The lead author was Kenneth C. Hyams, an infectious disease specialist and epidemiologist with the U.S. Naval Medical Research Institute. A Desert Storm doctor, Hyams had worked to minimize disease in the troop encampments during the war; drawn to the postwar mystery, he studied and wrote about it repeatedly. On this paper his coauthors were F. Stephen Wignall of the U.S. Navy and Robert Roswell of the VA.

From scouring the medical archives, Hyams and his colleagues came to three main conclusions. First, "Despite enormous progress in medical science, poorly understood war syndromes have recurred at least since the U.S. Civil War." Second, the symptoms of the war syndromes were more alike than different, with fatigue, shortness of breath, headache, disturbed sleep, and forgetfulness the core complaints, and diarrhea and pain also occurring. Third, in each war in which the syndromes cropped up, their interpretation by doctors cut along mind-body lines.

Finally, in syntax suggesting a desire to avoid controversy, the researchers stated that "no single recurring disease that is unrelated to psychological distress is apparent." As Hyams explained to me, there was a pattern. "Occult organic diseases are put forward," he said, "but they're never identified. Eventually they're ascribed to psychological factors."

It was the Hyams paper that alerted me to irritable heart. If Darren Moreau, who had symptoms in the region of his chest and heart, had served in the Civil War, he would have doubtless been diagnosed with this condition. Sharp or burning chest pain, accelerated heart rate, palpitations and shortness of breath, particularly upon exertion, were the hallmarks of an irritable heart. In hindsight it seems to have much in common with neurasthenia, which was about to be codified by George Beard under a sharply different social premise.

In the First World War again there were many of the "heart" cases, but new labels were given for the condition. The U.S. and British medical corps called it soldier's heart, disordered action of the heart, effort syndrome, or Da Costa syndrome (after the doctor who had studied it in the Civil War). Effort syndrome was the term that prevailed, while doubts grew about its cardiogenic basis. Sir Thomas Lewis, the British authority, wrote that effort syndrome existed "in the borderland between health and disease" because the same dizziness and palpitations and breathlessness could be induced in healthy people if they were worked hard enough. But the sick soldiers of World War I succumbed to strain and exercise rapidly. Their heart symptoms appeared premonitorily, in training and before battle, and also as a result of their effort during the action.

Separately World War I produced shell shock, a more notorious ailment than the irritable heart. The stark manifestations of shell shock were blindness, muteness, paralysis, amnesia, and muscle contractures, twisting its victims this way and that. At first the signs were attributed to neurological wounds, specifically a faint hemorrhaging in the brain caused by the concussion of exploding munitions. Then patients came in who had no proximity to the front. When doctors autopsied shell-shocked soldiers who died of infections, they failed to find brain damage, and the neurological model lost favor, just as it had with civilian hysteria. In fact, before the end of the war most physicians were decided that shell shock was the battlefield version of hysteria. In the new language of Freud, it represented the conversion of psychological distress to physical symptoms.

Shell shock was the founding lesson of military psychiatry, yet once recognized, the lesson was never repeated in as dramatic a fashion. You could say that like hysteria, shell shock had served its purpose. During the Great War the purely emotional reactions to battle, such as crying and panic, were viewed as either cowardice or malingering, and the penalties for such "weak" behavior were severe, including summary execution. Therefore, if soldiers unconsciously chose from among socially legitimate symptoms, as opposed to those that were frowned upon, to have a brain rattled by explosions and a contorted body ought to be above suspicion. If the shell-shocked soldier wept and trembled besides, he was assumed to have an organic reason for it.

The 1920s were not unlike the 1990s in that surprising numbers of war veterans struggled with ill-defined infirmities. Tens of thousands of compensation claims were filed in both the United States and United Kingdom. "[T]he majority of patients suffering from 'effort syndrome' remain in a state of imperfect health without developing serious disease," wrote Lewis. By another estimate, only one of six men had recovered. Moreover, irritable heart syndrome appeared to merge with shell shock syndrome, as in the case reports of "shellshock disordered heart" and "shell neurasthenia."

World War I had a third medical legacy. Poison gas had been used for the first time, and to horrible effect, leaving some men, the survivors of attacks, suffering from "gas neurosis." The symptoms of this condition were not in accord with the usual consequences of chlorine, phosgene, and mustard, the main agents deployed. Gas neurosis was instead a functional illness overlapping the effort syndrome and shell shock. Lewis estimated that only 5 percent of the cases of effort syndrome in Britain were due to poison gas, but in America gas seems to have been the greatest source of postwar illness.

Some seventy thousand American soldiers had been hospitalized during the war because of gas, the largest category of nonfatal casualties. In 1925 an army doctor named H. L. Gilchrist reviewed the compensation claims by all who had been wounded. The applications to the Veterans Bureau for ailments blamed on gas *exceeded* seventy thousand. In a passage that could have written in the present, Gilchrist observed that "the number of cases not gassed severely enough to require medical attention at the time was especially noticeable. A large number of applicants stated that the after effects did not become apparent for months, and in some cases years. There is no doubt that they honestly believed that this was so, but, from medical standpoint, it would be impossible." The soldiers would have to have been knocked down by the gas, Gilchrist maintained, in order for there to be long-term damage.

When World War II began, the British, who mobilized ahead of the Americans, discovered that effort syndrome (irritable heart) was once again sapping their troops. In 1940 Thomas Lewis published a second edition of his World War I monograph to guide military doctors on the illness. But the next year another researcher, Dr. Paul Wood, deconstructed the illness in the *British Medical Journal*. Reviewing two hundred cases, Wood declared effort syndrome to be a psychoneurosis, without cardiac or physiological basis. After that the syndrome faded out, because it either wasn't occurring or wasn't being diagnosed.

The coup de grace to the irritable heart may have been administered in the 1947 edition of *The Principles and Practice of Medicine*, the standard text for physicians of the day. The entry under "Effort Syndrome, Neurocirculatory Asthenia, Disordered Action of the Heart, Irritable Heart, Cardiac Neurosis" acknowledged that this functional condition, variously labeled, occurred in both the civilian and military populations, including women and children. As for the doctor's response to it, the editors sternly advised: "In treatment any suggestion of 'heart disease' should be avoided and every effort made to explain the condition. All too often a casual remark of the physician firmly fixes in the patient's mind that he has serious heart disease. . . . The whole method of life should be reviewed, and every effort made to improve the general health by proper exercise, bathing and good hygiene. Cardiac drugs are not needed and to advise them may undo all assurance that there is no 'heart disease.' "

World War II and the Korean War don't illuminate the mind-body argument as well as earlier and later conflicts do, because after the dismissal of effort syndrome there was no unexplained illness to report, no split in thinking between the etiologic camps. Doctors had much work to do on the battlefields, but the conditions they saw were all comprehensible to them. Soldiers had traumatic injuries or infectious disease or combat stress. That no mystery syndrome took shape I think is due to the power of the psychodynamic model, which by the mid-1940s had taken over military medicine completely.

When soldiers came down with stomach problems, rashes, headaches, or cardiac symptoms that did not seem to have an organic connection, the diagnosis was likely to be combat stress. "With normal acute emotional reactions, there are always somatic expressions," wrote Roy Grinker and John Spiegel, doctors with the army air forces, in 1945.

Psychosomatic symptoms were just one expression of battle stress, explained Grinker and Spiegel. Confident Freudians, they assigned the reactions to "passive-dependent states," guilt and depression, aggression and hostility, "psychotic-like states," or "psychosomatic states," pursuant to the soldier's nature. "All the disturbances are regressive in a psychological sense, in that the individual no longer has a mature and adult capacity to discriminate reality and adapt to his environment, but uses infantile reactions or 'lower level' visceral techniques, which bring him into new conflicts causing anxiety or produce crippling physical symptoms."

With the men in the field, the psychiatric pitfalls of combat were not addressed in this language, but rather with the euphemism "battle fatigue" or "operational fatigue." Physicians had learned that soft-pedaling the symptoms and keeping a victim out of the hospital, if possible, was the best way to speed his return to duty. A patient with a psychiatric diagnosis was not only stigmatized but also slower to recover. Of course Freudian enlightenment was not universal. This still was the army in which General George Patton slapped a terrorized and hospitalized soldier for being a "coward" and "yellow son of a bitch."

The Vietnam War did not produce a mystery illness either—during the time of the fighting. Acute stress reactions occurred, and infectious disease occurred, each managed for what they were. It might be said that during the war no unlimned pool of symptoms was available to soldiers trapped idiopathically in limbo. But as described in an earlier chapter, the delayed health consequences of the Vietnam War were novel and diametrical: posttraumatic stress disorder (PTSD) and the Agent Orange conditions. The Hyams paper noted that though the reputed mechanisms differed, both conditions were accompanied by the sorts of symptoms that had characterized other war-related syndromes. The vets exposed to Agent Orange and the vets diagnosed with PTSD voiced similar bodily complaints, and now they have been joined by the Persian Gulf group.

If you didn't stand too close, each generation of sick veterans looked alike. Such a broad perspective on the illnesses, offering many jumping-off places for thought, was a welcome change from the incremental, reduction-ist pieces of information that science and journalism had been putting out, pieces puffed up beyond their significance. If the past syndromes were anal-ogous, the probability grew that the experience of war in general had spawned the symptoms—not, in the current instance, sarin or OP pesti-cides, radioactive munitions, or pyridostigmine pills. And what was the abiding experience of all war but psychological? "We're not saying it's all psychological," said Hyams, "because there may be subsets of organic dis-ease. But it's the most unifying explanation."

"I WALK AND wobble all over the place like I'm a drunk," Darren said. "I shouldn't drive, but I do, and I have to make a living. If I got stopped, I'd never be able to walk in a straight line. They'd make me take a blood test."

It was June, the start of a jagged summer. He was weary from twelve-hour days, leaving home at 6:00 A.M. for the long drive to work and not getting back until evening. His job as a counselor at the state employment office was provisional. He had to take a written exam in a few months in order to become a permanent hire, and he was worried he wouldn't pass it.

Dr. Short so far had failed to stanch the decline in Darren's health, although Darren and Jackie believed the VA doctor was doing his best. "He's not exactly treating Darren," Jackie said. "He's helping Darren *exist*, with less pain and complications."

Darren said that Dr. Short had seemed "surprised" and "gave a lot of weird expressions" during his most recent evaluation, which was under-taken to upgrade his disability rating. When I called the doctor, he con-firmed the gloomy assessment, because "when I start seeing neurological stuff, when I see cognitive damage, how does it get put back together? The adult neurological system has very little repair mechanism."

The veteran continued to be bothered by chest pains and a feeling of constriction. On July 22 he was away at a training course in Boise when the symptoms flared anew. The pain started during the morning session. Dar-ren went outside with a coworker, tried to walk it off, but when his breath-ing became labored, the coworker took him to the hospital.

The Boise VAMC, which didn't know the patient, responded to the emergency with heart monitoring and nitroglycerin and a sedative. By the time Jackie arrived, several hours later, "They were already medicating him," she recalled. "I said, 'Stop what you're doing! This is like what happened in L.A. You aren't going to find anything on the tests.' "

Jackie wanted Dr. Short to be consulted, or, if not him, the VA cardiologist in Los Angeles. Neither doctor could be reached. She had harsh exchanges with the Boise staff. After a while it was smoothed over, and Darren was brought home, pale and silent.

Dr. Short's response to the episode was to schedule a thallium scan for Darren, a more intricate test of his heart function than previously had been done. "If you're telling me you're having chest pains, you don't screw around," Short insisted. "At his age you've got it check it out. I don't know about gulf war syndrome, but you can sure die of a heart attack." To be fair, there was a family history. Both Darren's father and grandfather had died of heart attacks in their fifties, and his two older siblings had high blood pressure.

But recall that Hamm and the Wadsworth doctors had diagnosed hyperventilation. It was a simpler explanation for the episodic symptoms in the area of Darren's chest. Hyperventilation, or overbreathing, causes the body to lose carbon dioxide at too high a rate. This shifts the biochemical balance and constricts the arteries, which cuts the blood flow to the brain and heart. A host of unpleasant sensations and reactions follow, in the worst cases mounting to locked muscles and loss of consciousness.

Hyperventilation is so familiar that you probably don't think of it as a medical disorder. A bad habit or tic, more likely. But not very long ago it was elevated to a syndrome, and before that it was a baffling collection of symptoms, energetically discussed in the literature. Perhaps I am overly fond of nosology, the history of medical labeling, but I think that the multiplicity of labels preceding "hyperventilation" nicely illustrates the mind-body imbroglio. In the period of the 1930s and 1940s the continuum of symptoms was variously known as: effort syndrome, autonomic imbalance, anxiety states, irritable heart, cardiovascular neurosis, clumsiness of the circulation, hyperventilation tetany, psychophysiologic respiratory reaction, neurocirculatory asthenia, pulmonary dystonia, and cardiorespiratory tetaniform symptom complex.

A half century later, though much winnowed, the terms have not been unified; they still mirror the outlook of the physician more than shed light on the ailment of the patient. You have hyperventilation syndrome, plain vanilla, which is flanked on the left by panic disorder, a purely psychological interpretation, and on the right by tachycardia syndrome (POTS) and neurocardiogenic syncope.

Dr. Short took the organic approach to Darren's chest symptoms, but was not so far to the right as to make a fancy organic diagnosis. He simply referred to Darren's attacks of pain and faintness as "heart." And ordered further tests.

THAT SUMMER DARREN and Jackie were roiled by another fear, involving his eyesight. After an eye exam at the VA hospital Darren was told he needed new glasses. "My eyes are having more of an effect on me every day," he said. "The ophthalmologist stated there is evidence that I have been exposed to toxins."

Darren stumbled over the name of the condition. Jackie got on the line. "Toxic optic atrophy," she pronounced. "The nerve is damaged by a toxin. Dr. Short says it fits with what he's been thinking.

"Darren's gonna go blind at some point," she continued. "Maybe we can slow it down, but we're moving toward acceptance of it. We're thinking of having him learn braille, but with his memory and concentration, that'll be difficult. . . .

"If he were blind, then he'd be unemployable. And then he'd need at-home care. It's kind of a glorified baby-sitter, but if push comes to shove, I'd get the training and I'd become Darren's certified caregiver.

"Then I think I'd give him what he's always dreamed of. The '57 Chevy. While he can still see, he'd be able to work on the car and paint it and the rest. I've got a loan out now, to buy it. And later I'll drive him in it, and he'll have the picture of it in his mind. He'll have his one goal. . . ."

Were those violins playing in the background? Oh, Jackie.

"At the street shows I can describe the cars to him. 'Here's a '42 coupe. It's chrome and red.' He can bring it to his mind 'cause he knows the cars already. . . ."

She got a little choky. "What I wish for is a normal life. We'll never be, quote, normal, like other people. Normal for us means not too many blowups, not too many medical emergencies, less of this running here and there, et cetera. I said to Darren, 'Has it really been worth it?' And he said, 'Yes, because of the other veterans.' Because of Darren's case, they're watching over the other veterans better."

The optic nerve, connecting the retina to the brain, consists of myriad fibers. Optic atrophy describes a loss or degeneration of the nerve fibers, which can be detected through the ophthalmoscope. Vision slowly deteriorates. The causes are various: eye disease, injury, a genetic flaw or, least commonly, poisoning. When there has been nerve damage from poisoning, it doesn't affect the eye alone, but hurts the entire body.

I would explore the condition further except that when I called Dr. Pearl, an ophthalmologist at Spokane VAMC, he said that although he had identified a few cases of optic atrophy in gulf war vets, Darren was not one of them.

"He thinks he has optic atrophy, but he doesn't," the doctor said.

What? Where did Darren get the idea then?

Dr. Pearl couldn't exactly say. He put part of the blame on Dr. Short, who he said had information that organophosphate chemicals could trigger this condition. Therefore Dr. Pearl's practice in examining the vets had been to tell them that he was *checking* for signs of atrophy. "I say it's a theory, and there's no proof. . . . I would *never* suggest a problem to a veteran who didn't have it," he said, sounding indignant.

But Dr. Short told me it was Dr. Pearl's opinion that Darren had optic atrophy. Short did have one medical article, though, by a doctor in Japan. The article reported cases of optic atrophy in children who had lived in areas that had been sprayed with the pesticide malathion in the 1960s.

"I made a little bit of a number over Darren's eyes," admitted Short. "You want to exaggerate a bit for the [VA claims] adjudicators. I don't think he's going to go blind, but I can't tell the future."

Though by this point in my reporting on the gulf war illnesses I'd heard just about everything, the eye episode made my blood boil. This was not a negotiation between a doctor and a patient over what to call an unknown condition. This was two doctors tossing out dangerous theories like crumbs to pigeons, which was medically outrageous.

Well, now that I have called Darren a pigeon, and Jackie too, I suppose I cannot take it back. It may get worse before it gets better, because I'm on my way to Spokane to meet with the couple and Dr. Short. For the hash-out session, you know. Jackie and the doctor are unsuspecting for the most part. Darren is fatalistic: "You can't say anything worse about me than what's already been said. I mean compared to the VA officials or senators who say it's all in our heads. I trust you to be caring and objective."

But I don't know how to balance being "caring" and "objective." So I am going to broach another possible label for Darren's health condition, the most bitter label of all: hypochondriasis.

A psychiatric disorder, one of the family of somatoform disorders, hypochondriasis involves more than being a hypochondriac in the popular sense. It is more serious than becoming preoccupied with a state of health or running to the doctor frequently. The true hypochondriac not only has frequent symptoms that resist tests and treatment, but also refuses to be reassured. He (hypochondriasis is the one somatoform disorder in which men match women in numbers) harbors the deep conviction that he has an irremediable disease. The patient's ideas of what *could* be wrong with him are not impossible or off the wall, but he won't give up the ideas in the face of contrary evidence. The symptoms, which are real, ratchet up rapidly, as if to vindicate his fears. If he is feeling anxious, he may hyperventilate; hyperventilating, he may induce a panic attack; in the panic state he may believe he is dying.

The criteria for diagnosis are strict in that the first doctor can't label a patient a hypochondriac. It has to be the second or third or fourth doctor, reviewing the latest test results in light of the failures of his or her predecessors. Still, the doctor may hesitate, because "hypochondriac" is terribly pejorative, and the patient almost certainly will disown the diagnosis. By ignoring or missing it, however, the doctor may invite complications from endless tests or treatments that are wrong. Together, an accommodating physician and a somatizing patient can do more damage than a reckless quack. In the end, though, it's only the patient who suffers.

DARREN SAT IN the waiting room of the Nuclear Medicine department at the Spokane VAMC. He wore clean jeans, sneakers, and a T-shirt depicting three "Chevy Classics," one of which was the '57 Bel Air, in red. He looked thinner and shakier than when I'd seen him last.

Thallium, a radioactive tracer, had been injected into his bloodstream, and the intravenous lock was still taped to Darren's forearm. When the tracer had fully circulated, he would lie under a scanner, which would record the illuminated blood flow within the walls of his heart. Any damage to the structure of the organ should be revealed. He would repeat the test on the treadmill, to make an image of his heart under effort.

While he waited for the tracer, Darren put his signature to the paperwork that Jackie had prepared for him. They were writing to U.S. senators and representatives about his recent unsatisfactory stay at the West Los Angeles VAMC. This was their second letter, challenging the hospital's reply to their initial complaint.

Jackie came into the waiting room with more letters, which they each proceeded to sign. "I'm in it till beyond Darren and till maybe I develop it myself," she said. Yet she was in a good mood. The week before, they had testified at a hearing of the Senate Veterans' Affairs Committee, and it had gone well.

"I can see Jeff writing in his book, 'There's Jackie licking envelopes and sending letters to the VA, causing trouble,' " she said with a grin.

Darren sat straight-backed in the plastic chair. I noticed that his hair was streaked with gray. "When you hear the word Persian Gulf War veteran now, you think of the illness, not the war," he said. "It makes you ashamed to say you're a Persian Gulf veteran. I know how the Vietnam vets feel. I was a proud American, and now I don't feel quite the same."

The next day I went to visit Darren at work. Everyone at the job placement office was dressed in jeans and casual shirts, except for Darren, who wore a necktie, a white shirt he had ironed himself, brown slacks, and brown tassel loafers. His illness was well buttoned down. He wished to look presentable for his clients, he said, who were military veterans and might appreciate it. Darren in his cubicle seemed attenuated and delicate, with long fingers that might have been manicured. I was reminded, I am not sure why, that he had an aversion to rushing water. He couldn't swim, because of having to put his head under, and when showering, he held his face out of the spray.

We went to lunch. What did he think had caused his illness? I asked.

It was the toll of organophosphate chemicals or, as he put it, "sarin-related type poisonings. We all have a little trace of it in us because of what we use on our fields as agriculture. It is also found inside a lot of the stuff we used to fight insects and as well in the bombs that they used over there. So you take a little bit of it, and then you add a lot of it, it's like having an apple and sticking a little worm in it, and it eats out the center of the apple."

How could he be sure this was the illness? "Because my central nervous system has been affected. You cannot have an infected nervous system and it not damage other vital organs in your body. It's not just Baumzweiger saying it. It's others noting the reflex problems, the toxic effects to my eyes."

I said there were no tests that could definitely tie his symptoms to toxic exposures. The chemicals themselves would long since have passed from his body. Darren thought there were "patterns that could be checked," though he conceded he wasn't as knowledgeable on that score as Dr. Short.

"Until DoD releases the information, there's not much we can do anyway," he said.

"What information?"

"They may have info on drugs they gave us, or the types of bombs, or stuff in the environment. Until it's all released, how can the research centers do the right toxic tests? Let the commander in chief step in and make them tell the doctors what they know."

"Doctors can work *without* that information," I said, deciding not to debate whether such information existed. "Scientists make assumptions about exposures—they assume they happened—and then do their studies. They still can't make connections to these symptoms." Except for Haley and a very few others, I should have added.

"OK, then, how about collecting info on the patients and what they're suffering, the types of diseases and all, and pass it on?"

This type of information had been collected, but Darren was right that it hadn't been packaged cogently. Also, the epidemiology was a snapshot, because most veterans were examined only once, when they had signed up for the registries. The ongoing health of the group was unknown. Recently a congressional agency had drawn blood from the VA and Pentagon with that charge. To Darren it was proof that the government was ignoring "the progressive nature of the illness."

A sneer drew down his face, accentuating the long-handled mustache. "If I had to go through it again—go to war and come back sick—I wouldn't go to doctors at all."

Arrestingly, he likened himself to a farm dog that'd been abused and beaten. "You know how dogs like that cringe? Well, people take care of them better than us, and we're allowed to die. I'm laying here, a sick, dying veteran, and people don't give a shit."

"If the illness is terminal," I said, "or as serious as you say, don't you think you'd benefit from psychological counseling for how to deal with it?"

"I don't think I need it." Darren paused, and then tried to illustrate his self-sufficiency. He told about a gunfire incident at the base in Germany in the eighties, a false alarm, as it turned out, but he felt he had responded to the crisis well. "I realized if I had to face death, I'd be comfortable with it. I had a sense of it in the hospital in Los Angeles, when it was black, and I was far away, like I might have been dying."

"The hyperventilation episode?" I ventured.

"Whatever it was," he said. "On earth we are here to help people. When I do go, I don't want to answer to hell but to heaven."

"Are you religious?"

"No, but my father raised me strictly, like the church would do."

I asked about his feelings of anger, or maybe he raised the topic, but in any event he replied with another anecdote. Early in his illness he'd wanted to bust a guy's neck when the guy crossed him at a gas station. He had wanted to strike out at other people in his path too but had controlled himself. "I decided not to go that way, to be hostile and not to care. Because of dealing with my marriages, the two that I had, I recognized the phases of anger. I've read books about anger. . . ."

His contempt for the cringing farm dog had subsided. He put on his best face. "I still like Darren," he said. "I'm comfortable in the illness, a little frustrated at the government, I guess." He smiled bravely. Oh, Darren, are you reading this?

WE TROOPED INTO Dr. Short's empty office and sat down. Jackie was in shorts and short sleeves, and Darren wore a white shirt and bolo tie, pressed slacks, and black tassel loafers. Through the window, we saw smoke on the horizon. A wildfire was burning on the outskirts of Spokane.

Flushed, Darren told Jackie to quit running her jaw and go and find Dr. Short. She went and did. The doctor was a friendly, grizzled, bug-eyed man with braces on his teeth. A yellow smiley-face button was pinned to his green scrubs.

The first order of business was Darren's heart. Short called up the results of the thallium scan on his computer and read them aloud. "Maybe a small area of ischemia [reduced blood flow] . . . an enlarged left ventricle . . . no evidence of a heart attack. . . . Nobody would do anything on this," he concluded, referring to treatment.

Jackie asked a number of questions. At the same time she was crocheting a border on a dish towel. Darren squinted and frowned, as if he might be smelling something unpleasant.

"Baumzweiger would say you have a pulse irregularity," said Short, leafing through a pile of Darren's records. "I *could* talk to the cardiologist in Seattle about this scan. . . . Do you want a B-twelve [vitamin] shot?"

"His headaches are worse," said Jackie.

Dr. Short got up and craned his head at the window, trying to follow the progress of the fire. It appeared to be closer, the smoke fuller, but there was a river between us and it.

"If you can go ten minutes on a treadmill with minimal change," the doctor said, "I'd probably rule out anything but lifestyle changes to treat a heart condition."

"I do have tightness in my upper chest," said Darren.

"During exercise?" asked Short. "Or at rest?"

"All the time," he said.

Jackie brought up Darren's "toxic optic atrophy," which led to a discussion of neurotoxic effects. There was a recent magazine article on the subject. Veterans' advocate Jim Tuite was quoted in the article.

"The article confirms what I picked up from the farm literature," Dr. Short said. "You take Tuite's arguments and the military's admissions—it adds up to some kind of a chemical/organic nerve disease."

Holding the floor with Darren and Jackie's tacit approval, Short gave an account of the hazards of OP pesticides and connected them to the downwind exposures to OP nerve gas, such as Tuite had proposed. Short pointed to a map of the Gulf on the wall behind his desk and said the prevailing winds were right. Fine, I thought, I wasn't here to debate that. Many winds and many hundreds of miles lay between the bombed Iraqi factories and Darren's post in Oman, and you couldn't even smell the smoke that was visible across the Spokane River.

When Dr. Short said that certain individuals were susceptible because their detoxifying enzymes could be overwhelmed, which was correct in principle, I said, "How's this going to help Darren?"

"Well, before you can treat, you have to know where you're at. I don't know which pills work. If you shoot at the brush, you might hit something, but—Baumzweiger, for instance, he's brush hunting. First we need to find out from DoD and Saddam Hussein what went on. I think we can get something out of them. Then let's look at the [pesticide-exposed] farm workers, to see if it's a multichemical process. You're going to have to do some subtle testing. . . ."

Still, there were no treatments for chronic pesticide exposure, he conceded. Dr. Short came around to where he began. Basically his attitude was, I'm just a poor clinician in the hinterland. Give me something at least half-valid that I can use to help my patients. But don't tell me they've got a stress disorder.

"What is Darren's diagnosis?" I asked. The smoke in the distance was really billowing now.

"Ordinarily I'd make a diagnosis of fibromyalgia," Short said, "plus optic atrophy and a few other things. I could do that. But if I say it's an *undiagnosed* illness, I think I can get him service connection. . . . We're playing a game, I admit. I condemn it, I don't like the system."

"What is the sick veteran supposed to do?" I said. "Try to get well? Try for service connection? Expose the errors and cover-ups of the government? Which? You can get a rush of endorphins when you show up the government. Is that the goal?"

Short liked the question, but before he could speak, Darren and Jackie jumped in. Darren was coldly furious.

"When our nation does something to us, it ought to be responsible," he said. "We're treated like abused farm dogs. Yeah, we do get satisfaction when we can show that."

Jackie was talking, and Short was talking, but now it was between Darren and me.

I said something about his anger, and he said, "If I went off my medication, *then* you'd see how I could get angry."

"You haven't seen Darren angry," echoed Jackie.

"I don't need to see it. I know he carries it."

"There's a missing piece of the puzzle," Darren said stoutly, "and until we have it, we can't know what to do."

"If you had the missing piece—if you saw the whole puzzle—it wouldn't matter. There's a big black hole between whatever the exposures were and the symptoms."

You could see smudges of flame on the hillside. "Your book is going nowhere," Darren sneered. "It's a dead-end book. 'These guys can't figure it out and we'll never know.' What good is that?"

Switching sides, Dr. Short said to Darren, "Don't let anger control you.

Think of Luke and the Dark Side. You may have fewer episodes of heart, or whatever, if you're not angry. It's not a helpful emotion."

"That's why I have Jackie, so I *don't* get angry."

"She does it for you," I shot back. "That's how it works."

"If you're on a marathon," Short said soothingly, "you can't sprint. You don't die of this very soon. Think of the serenity prayer. 'Give me the strength to accept that which I can't change. . . .'"

Jackie and the doctor kept things going a few minutes longer, but Darren and I had shut up, unable to look at each other.

"There are not many I can make well," Short was saying, "when they're chronically ill. But I try to be there for the patients. You cannot allow your anger to hurt you while we wait for answers."

"You're treating me like a kid," Darren protested. "I know all this! I'm thirty-nine years old!"

"Do we stop eating or do we stop spraying?" the doctor rattled on. "The tradeoffs we make for food. If they hadn't sprayed Agent Orange on the vegetation, we'd have had a lot more people shot. . . ."

Jackie broke in: "What about his nosebleeds?"

"It's probably the dry air," said Short.

After Darren had his vitamin shot, we went outside to our cars. The fire seemed to have been put under control. Darren came up to me and said, "Thanks for letting me vent."

"It's OK, Darren." Then he and I clasped each other tightly, to everyone's surprise but especially Jackie's. I never had anyone hug me before who had to stoop to do it. My briefcase, still in my right hand, flapped against his trembling back. "It's not dignified for a proud man to be angry, is it, Darren. But it's OK. Get it out."

OVER THE NEXT two years I spoke with Darren and Jackie fairly often. They seemed to be muddling through. Insomnia, bowel problems, and a racing heart continued to plague him, but he stopped worrying that he was going blind. He went to a specialist for neurological testing, in part to buttress his disability claim. Sarcastically he asked the neurologist, "What brain size do I have? Big? Small?" I gathered the tests were inconclusive.

He cut out the Baumzweiger medications cold turkey, having decided that the side effects were responsible for what he now called his anxiety attacks. To hell also with keeping out of the sun, as Baumzweiger advised, or avoiding the fumes of automobiles. He even swore off Dr. Short's milder regimen of vitamins and Tylenol. Then Darren reinstated some of the pills, even adding lithium for a while, but it didn't help.

"Live life!" Dr. Short urged Darren, his new tack. Then Short retired, and his VA successors, though sometimes veering off on organic tangents, gradually steered the veteran toward the psychological pole of his illness. He tried biofeedback, saw a psychiatrist for evaluation, went several times to the VA's PTSD clinic. It didn't help.

So he didn't die, but he continued to suffer. It was difficult for Darren to still like Darren, as he had put it, because Darren was disgusted that Darren could no longer hold a job. He failed the exam to be hired permanently at the job office and then failed the U.S. Postal Service entrance exam. He was surely bright enough to pass, but anxiety during the tests and his illness undid him.

"When I can't think clearly enough to leave the house," he said to me, "that'll be the end." But I objected when he referred to himself as "this disease-infested jerk" and "a brain-dead asshole."

"Thinking of yourself that way can't help," I said.

"You're not gonna *think* away bowel problems or bladder problems, just as I didn't think my way into them," he replied.

Out of work, Darren applied for Social Security disability payments, a move he had promised never to make. To qualify, he had to show the medical examiners that his reflexes were shot, that the pain in his joints was intractable. When his application was denied, he got an attorney and appealed. Meanwhile the VA upped his disability rating to 50 percent—not satisfactory, and he appealed. Mulling bankruptcy, Darren slipped from being unemployed to unemployable.

His state sounds bad, but like Pete during this period, Darren started to move away from his Desert Storm identity and its cantankerous medical appendage, which had faded from the headlines. He wrote me:

There is no secret medical condition. Any and all of the conditions have existed long before the gulf war came along. The label gulf war illness involves political sparring with no winners. Take the label away and the bullshit goes away with it, now I'm a regular patient with normal complaints. The doctor no longer needs the administrators to establish a medical profile. A headache is once again a headache, nerve damage is once again nerve damage, you get the idea. Diagnosis and treatment are now back in the doctor's hand, nothing new about this, just old-fashioned doctoring.

In the same vein he added, "More people are starting to believe I'm sick. My family is kinder. They'll let me go through the door first, the times I'm walking with a cane. It's kind of nice. Before they weren't really sure, because they were still waiting for Darren kick back and be strong again. To be the backbone guy again."

William Baumzweiger, now in private practice in Los Angeles, came up for a TV interview. Afterward he bought soft drinks for Darren and the other vets who were on the program. Darren said teasingly, "Is this the same doctor who told us we couldn't have caffeine? There's caffeine in this Pepsi."

"Oh, one won't hurt," the doctor said. "Anyway, the sugar's good for you."

Darren made a crack about his heartbeat racing up and down.

"Dammit, Darren," Baumzweiger said. "Don't joke about it. You're gonna die in five or ten years."

Darren said he'd shoot himself if he had to take his illness that seriously. He would live his life the way he wanted.

Probably the best thing to happen to Darren was that Jackie got a good job driving trucks and snowplows for the state. Her work stabilized their finances and took her away from home for days at a stretch. That seemed to relieve some of the pressure on him. As the two figured out how to live together, I don't believe that Darren bore the greater burden.

Jackie bought five acres out of town. They moved the trailer onto the property, along with her horse and his fleet of old cars. Darren said he would consolidate his unruly stock, but instead it kept growing. "I did get some work done on the '57 Chevy," he told me. "I'll fix one up and sell it and build the other one for me. The cars don't let me down at least."

"Trauma": a wound caused by an outside agent, an injury to the body or mind or both. "Traumatic neurosis": a hundred years ago, it was the diagnostic term for a trauma affecting the nervous system. Neurosis was not a pejorative then because it denoted an organic defect. In railway spine, a form of traumatic neurosis, the victim's bodily damage from an accident was overlaid by a nervous-mental injury. This was before litigation and compensation confused the issue.

I suspect Darren Moreau had a traumatic neurosis in the original sense, a wound to his mind-body apparatus. His was not a compensation neurosis; he wasn't a guy striving after money for getting sick, clearly. Did something genuinely traumatic happen to Darren? At the end of my reporting, in 1999, he provided me two possibilities, one having to do with the war and one not.

First, a brief review of the study of trauma. The battlefield was its twentieth-century laboratory because wars provided large numbers of subjects undergoing all sorts of wounds. World War I demonstrated that war produced traumatic neuroses (shell shock), as did World War II (battle fatigue). Vietnam's contribution was to show that an emotional injury managed by the individual at the time of onset might overcome him later. This phenomenon, PTSD, affecting people long removed from battle, opened the eyes of physicians and social scientists to the shadowy persistence of trauma in nonmilitary populations. As Harvard psychiatrist B. A. van der Kolk, an expert on PTSD, has noted, "Only in recent years has the correspondence between men's reactions to the trauma of war, children's responses to abuse, and women's responses to sexual and domestic violence been made explicit."

The Persian Gulf War, a short scrap with a long buildup, caused PTSD in a small minority of U.S. troops, and these were also the men and women who had the most nagging physical ailments afterward. The correlation between PTSD and physical symptoms is familiar to researchers, but PTSD, I'll say again, does not account for the gulf war illnesses. The government agencies did not claim that the larger medical problem was PTSD either, though the government was widely disbelieved because the two issues, psychological stress and PTSD, were conflated. Darren's Dr. Short, for instance, after attending a VA medical conference in California, said, "They want to call it PTSD. That's what they were peddling. There's no reason for PTSD. There are too many people, like Darren, who went over and sat at a desk, far from the front. They didn't see their buddies chopped up and hung like the Vietnam vets did."

No, they did not. But, interestingly, the rate of PTSD (and postwar health complaints) was highest in the reserve units whose job was to pick up human remains from the battlefield and match body parts to identities in the lab. In a sensitive person such an experience might be trauma enough. Darren was tasked for mortuary duty with the air force, but never had to perform it, though he anxiously anticipated it. Nor did he develop posttraumatic stress disorder. But if Darren didn't have PTSD, what had happened to him?

Darren was physically abused as a boy. This source of trauma—many studies have shown—increased the chances that he would be prey to health problems when he grew up. I mentioned this research in connection with Carol. The greater the number of unexplained symptoms, say researchers, the greater the likelihood that the person was abused early in life. Hypochondriasis and somatization are statistically associated with physical and sexual trauma in childhood. In addition, the military's own surveys show that its recruits may be abused at higher rates than civilian populations.

I didn't ask him directly. It came out in a conversation about Jackie, in which I remarked that she'd had a hard life, so I gathered.

"A hard life? My father beat the shit out of me with his fists for five years. 'Here, Darren, take that!' When I told Jackie, she asked me why I didn't tell my mom about it. Well, I didn't want to my *mom* to get beat."

He said that his older brother and sister left home early—"to get away"—leaving Darren and his younger sister. "After they left, *I* got to be the oldest," by which he meant the prime target.

I found it difficult to hear this, but Darren talked levelly, almost coolly, good cop that he was. "I was catching it all the time, the knuckles. You didn't try to beat the hell out of Dad, though I did take him on one time in later years." His brother and sister developed dangerously high blood pressure. "Mine's normal," said Darren, to show me that he was different from them, with his gulf war symptoms.

It was only after his father died that Darren made known the extent to which he'd been battered. "My brother and sister, they're still bitter," he said. "They see themselves as deprived children, beaten, by this hostile Jekyll and Hyde type. But I got past it. I chose a different path. I miss and love my dad. He was stern, yes, but he didn't know how to be loved. He *needed* the love, and they didn't show the interest in trying to give it."

Of late his siblings had asked Darren to take part in a family meeting about their father at which they would share their stories and feelings. So far he'd refused. "If they want to get together and get their anger out, that's fine for them. I'm not interested." Until I suggested it, Darren hadn't considered that the others might love their father also, just differently.

No one knows the biochemical basis by which abuse may set the stage for illness in adult life. Most theories center on the stress hormones that are released by the brain in response to traumatic events. A boy constantly on pins and needles because of an abusive parent would become hyper-aroused, hyperstressed—and then numb. Abnormally high levels of epi-nephrine and cortisol, the stress hormones, would sensitize the brain, and subsequent stressors would kick off the same process with much less provocation, leading to immune dysregulation and perhaps to the amplifi-cation of pain signals that Dan Clauw has proposed. The mechanism of cause and effect is speculative, given that in each individual there must be a myriad of variables. Yet the correlation between childhood abuse and adult symptoms is not speculative in the aggregate. It happens to too many people.

"They tell me a lot of my problems are because of my family's history," Darren said, unconvinced. He had taken a psychological survey, and on seeing the results, a VA psychiatrist had lit up. " 'Father cruelty,' she said. They isolated it down to one factor. There's other things I told her I wanted talk about. But she didn't ask me them. She zeroed in on the father cruelty."

The psychiatrist was offering Darren medication, not psychotherapy. But the VA would pay for sessions with a private psychologist close to his home, and therefore Darren went for counseling every couple of weeks. Another doctor-patient relationship had commenced, the first to explore areas beyond his physical symptoms. "He's been doing a lot of good," Dar-ren said of the psychologist. "We talk about my nightmares—my dreams, he insists I call them."

"What dreams?" I asked.

"Violent dreams, with science fiction monsters. I've been having dreams where I'm incapable of fighting off threats. Alien forms, monsters. Just a few weeks ago I dreamt about a family in a farmhouse. It was a two-story farmhouse. I didn't recognize it. We never had a two-story house. Anyway, the father in the house was shot. He was on fire. The mother was hurt, and the daughter had blood spurting out of her. All of it was happening in full color. . . ."

"You're in the dream too?"

"Yes, but I'm a standby observer. I can't do anything. I'm there, but I'm not touching or feeling anything."

Unable to stop people from getting hurt—not like the real Darren, as we both knew. From telling the dream he swung right into a true-life tale of blood, which had taken place within the past year, yet another time he'd come upon an accident and acted heroically. "I saved a little girl in a car wreck," he said. "I stopped her bleeding. They said she might have died without me. I felt really good. It put life back into mine. The girl's family still thanks me. They send me letters and pictures of her.

"That's why the nightmare about the farmhouse doesn't make sense to me. Why was I powerless? These are some of the things I've been trying to sort out with the doctor. He's identified some issues, like my not working and the pain that I have, physical and mental. But also there are some unresolved incidents from the war. . . ."

Hold on tight: It is February 1991, and Staff Sergeant Moreau is taking his customary evening run. A well-muscled man, who skirts the sandy airfield, picks up his pace, pushing himself. Hearing the noise of a helicopter, he turns. The craft, coming in, explodes in midair. The helicopter, coming apart before his eyes, tumbles to the ground.

He is the nearest person to the crash. Darren can hear the rolling and the thumping of the metal and the cries of the men inside. Awestruck, he lunges forward and then halts, because the helicopter is in flames. He's bare-legged, paralyzed, not knowing whether to run toward the fire or to run back to the post, raise the alarm, don his rescue gear, and hurry back.

Runway crews reach the scene. They've known the aircraft was in trouble. They are scrambling and equipped for the task, freeing Darren to move. He sprints for the post so fast he doesn't remember his feet touching the ground. Trained to prepare for the dead, he is responding as trained.

Only to be told, when he gets there, to let the British handle it because it's their zone. "That's final, Sergeant. That will be all, Sergeant."

"I couldn't get to the dead bodies. I was the standby. . . . Why didn't they set down earlier? Why did they try to come all the way in? Seeing the rotor blades going whoof-whoof! It seemed to drop to the ground in slow motion. Such a helpless feeling. I was powerless to be able to put flames out."

The incident was like a dry run for the war, he agreed. "My first death situation." In his mind, on the eve of the invasion, burned bodies many more than these were headed his way.

DARREN DIDN'T DIE, but he continued to suffer. His Social Security disability came through. "Being disabled has been the most difficult part of my life," he said. "It's not something you can quit or get fired from."

When the weather was good, he worked outside. "After the chores I can do maybe one to two hours on the cars. Then I get tired, come in and rest, and maybe go back out. . . . I'm down to forty-six."

"You're *down* to forty-six cars?"

"To restore the '57 is still the main goal," he said, a bit sheepishly. "That one's half done. The transmission and the exhaust are in.

"Restoring a car is like the birthing of a child," he went on. "It goes through a year's transition, learning to walk and such. All at once you turn the key, and it starts. You teach it to shine and glimmer and sparkle. It's a personal mark on yourself—it's a part of you. My taste and my style and my flair. It's my own kid. I'm substituting for not having any, sure.

"There's discipline too. A kid will be independent. And others'll look down on it maybe. A piece of shit, they'll say. But that's just one opinion."

"Why so many?" I asked him. "Why not just concentrate on fixing the '57?"

"I need to breathe life into as many as I can, so they won't go to the junkyard. It's worth putting off the '57 to save a bunch of cars."

Dear Darren [I wrote him],

On the subject of dreams, you probably have heard that dreams can involve puns. The names of people standing for something else, words that mean two things at once, that sort of thing.

For example, the bad dream you had about the "two-story" farmhouse that caught fire. We never lived in a two-story house, you said. But maybe you did, in the sense that two stories could be told about what was going on there. One story is the outside appearance, what looks like the happy life of a regular family. Inside, another story . . . Hence a two-story house.

For that I will only charge you $150.

Now, would you like my interpretation of the role of the '57 Chevy?

I inferred from his polite silence that he didn't want me for his psychoanalyst.

Dear Darren, what year were you born?

7

Tuite Agonistes

"I t's like being on rollerskates while holding on to the rear bumper of a car that's going a hundred miles per hour," Jim Tuite said. "Would *you* let go?"

He was describing how it felt—the rush, the danger—to be riding the fast-breaking political developments following Khamisiyah. We were having a drink in Cincinnati after attending a scientific meeting there. The time was the spring of 1997, the second of the two contentious periods during which Jim Tuite became prominent. The first was 1993–94, when his investigative reports on Capitol Hill fired the debate over the unknown illnesses. Although he had doubts about the epidemiologic value of Khamisiyah, since the blowup of the depot caused only local (and unnoticed) exposures to nerve gas, the belated news of the incident seemed to prove that the Pentagon concealed damaging evidence, as Tuite had charged all along.

"In '95 I had moved on," he recalled. "I'd moved on to the science, and I was not doing that much with the issue."

"What Khamisiyah did," I suggested, "was to vindicate you . . . lift you up. . . ."

"What Khamisiyah did was not a vindication of me, but a—

"Rehabilitation? It's some word with 're-,' anyway."

"Resurrection. Or maybe it was rehash."

Remarks like that made Tuite rewarding to reporters. He was, I repeat, the most important figure in the political history of the gulf war illnesses.

At the time I began to cover him, he was consulting with the producer and the screenwriter of a television movie. The movie, whose sarcastic title was *Thanks of a Grateful Nation*, was filmed in Toronto later that year, and I visited the set during the shooting. By then the fun was over between us.

The set on the day I came was an ornate judicial building, meant to represent a hallway off the U.S. Senate in 1994. In the scene the actor playing Tuite, Ted Danson, emerges from a crowd of dark-suited extras and confronts two other staffers. They get into a dispute over the amount of funding for research on the gulf war illnesses, and Tuite, who works for Senator Don Riegle, is stabbed in the back by the aides to Senator Jay Rockefeller. Not actually stabbed, although to murder the hero would not be unbelievable in a movie in which sick and dying veterans are so luridly betrayed.

The Senate scene was shot over and over, from different angles and with different intonations of dialogue, and at each take the dozens of extras, retreating to their marks, retraced their steps, nodded and smiled at one another, and pantomimed empty speeches. My thought as the cast circled was that when a public figure is brought to life on the screen, the deeds that have made the person important to history and attractive to Hollywood are finished. End of story: Roll camera. No third act for Jim. While veterans in the audience were still sick.

Two histories of the gulf war illnesses have been written, the one, ten years after the fact, that you're reading, and an earlier one, put together largely by Tuite in conjunction with the mass media. Both "authors" draw upon medicine, politics, and history; both mix facts and speculation. Both finally may be accused of scientism, not in the sense of having relied upon science exclusively but in the sense of dabbling in it, dressing up in it, in order to further their preconceptions. I do not normally depict my methods this way, but it's only fair if I'm going to analyze Tuite's.

The movie made him out to be a whistle-blower who brought dark documents to light, but that misses his importance. Jim's achievement lay in the tireless construction of information. I don't mean fabrication, but rather a conception of the gulf war illnesses that others could recognize and run with. Tuite's interpretation of the evidence from the battlefield was that pervasive, low-level exposures had occurred, especially to nerve gas, and that gas with other toxic substances was responsible for the illnesses. From his bases of support in Congress and the veterans' community—the latter instinctively believing, the former backing their constituents—Tuite extended the argument to journalists. As a source of information he posed an almost irresistible package: political consistency, technical detail, and, when needed, slashing quotations. In addition, he demonstrated the legwork of a reporter and deep commitment.

"What he did that hadn't been done," said David Brown, the medical writer for the *Washington Post*, "is to go and record the stories. Like a good investigator, he did the reporting. He gathered a couple dozen veterans and listened to what they had to say. He was the first person to interview them all. That report [the Senate Banking Committee report of May 1994], though it's a catalog of anecdotes, is primary source material and a very useful document."

"I think he *is* very important, a key figure," said Dr. Joyce Lashof, who chaired the Presidential Advisory Committee on Gulf War Veterans' Illnesses, "because of the Riegle connection and because he kept the whole question of chemicals as the cause alive."

Bernard Rostker, the top Pentagon official investigating the issue, conceded, "Tuite built a scenario, and the Defense Department wasn't prepared to question it." When the Pentagon and the CIA did challenge his analyses, Tuite only dug in harder. "Dogged" was the description I heard most often, from friend and foe alike. Indeed everyone seemed to admire him at one level or another.

"Jim discovered the issue," said a senior Democratic staffer, who wished to be unnamed. "Well, the reason I want to give him ninety percent of the credit is because of his due diligence."

Tuite and I didn't have an equal discourse, since my job as historian, starting later than he did, was to collect information, and his job was to distribute what he had already collected. He was helpful to me—voluminously. Bubbling over with self-assurance, he hectored me with his point of view. His lack of slyness was disarming. If I sent him an e-mail, he'd answer by e-mail, but I learned to stay by the telephone afterward, for he would follow up in a ninety-minute call, bursting with elaboration.

I once remarked to Jim that the veterans I was writing about were patients of his, after a fashion, because much of their medical understanding could be traced to his efforts. It was more than indirect. In his hospital room John Cabrillo kept a well-thumbed speech that Tuite had drafted for Riegle. Darren's Dr. Short referred to Jim's ideas and had Jim's fax number on a stack of papers about organophosphate chemicals.

Darren and Jackie had met Tuite when they testified before the Presidential Advisory Committee. They remembered him as friendly and concerned, although after they told Tuite they were of the Baumzweiger school of the illnesses, the conversation caught a chill. Having acquired his own medical theorist in Howard Urnovitz, an independent microbiologist, Tuite was critical of Baumzweiger and wrote off Darren and Jackie to boot, or so they felt.

He was a patriotic, high-minded person on a mission. The mission he chose was different from mine, obviously, and the best illustration of the difference I can offer is from the screenplay of *Thanks of a Grateful Nation*. Early in his struggle to understand the illnesses Tuite goes to the Vietnam Memorial in Washington. It is night. He is a Vietnam veteran himself. As he broods on the names of dead comrades, he is approached by a shadowy figure whom he never sees.

THE VOICE: Don't turn around.

TUITE: Are you kidding me?

THE VOICE: I know you were in the Secret Service and you could probably throttle me over your knee . . . but don't.

(and)

I'm doing this for me not you. If I'm found out, I'm gone. They're already suspicious. They know I'm trying to help—

TUITE: Who's they?

THE VOICE: I can't say any more.

TUITE: Oh bullshit.

THE VOICE: You think so?

TUITE: I don't know what I think about a lot of things, but I think this is bullshit.

THE VOICE: Forget the vets. Don't get caught up in the individual lives. I'll do that.

(and)

Track the alarms.

TUITE: I'm working on it.

THE VOICE: Track them.

(and now)

It gets worse.

TUITE: What do you mean?

THE VOICE: Follow the weapons.

TUITE: Which weapons?

THE VOICE: Did the Iraqis have chemical and biological capability?

TUITE: Of course.

THE VOICE: (softer) Where from?

Forget the vets. Don't get caught up in the individual lives. Tuite provided the line to the writer, I was told by the producer. The Deep Throat character didn't exist, but Tuite didn't mind the device, derivative though it was. He told me he saw it "as a metaphor for the several dozen individuals who provided me information, classified and unclassified, and for all of the work I did."

At any rate, from the Wall he goes off to uncover the embarrassing facts that might explain the illnesses, starting with the U.S. export of biological materials to Iraq before the war and thence to the possibility of theater-wide exposures from the bombing of chemical weapons factories. The movie follows him accurately. Tuite's interviews turned up numerous accounts of wartime incidents that were precursors, trial runs, as it were, for the Khamisiyah revelation. For chemical alarms had sounded, both on camp perimeters and during the march into Kuwait, and soldiers now sick claimed to have been tainted.

To secure the truth, a good investigator, like a good scientist, must avoid the snare of individual cases. He must stand back from the pain to observe the pattern, yes? But to me the individual life was the one place where the truth resided. If my rival's history is about a class of people, a group that he says was wronged by the government, mine is about scattered persons in pain. The challenge is to have compassion for people when they *don't* get screwed over.

AFTER RIEGLE RETIRED, at the end of 1994, Tuite left Capitol Hill and became an international security consultant. His résumé described his expertise as "relating to the proliferation of, and exposure to, chemical, biological, and radiological materials."

Educating himself in epidemiology and toxicology, Jim pondered the gulf war illnesses and the wartime exposures from a more academic perspective than he had done previously. He wrote an interesting essay in 1995 titled "When Science and Politics Collide." The setting was "a world in which the hazards of the political battlefield have become increasingly dependent upon our understanding of science."

The problem of the illnesses, Tuite decided, demanded the input of independent researchers. Why the need for outsiders? "The very same agencies and government who were responsible for providing protection against the hazardous exposures these individuals suffered during the Gulf War are now responsible for determining what is wrong with them. Here is where science and politics collide. We have asked the same government—whose actions may have resulted in the illnesses—to investigate itself."

His implication was that political requirements corrupted the scientific process. Of course the scientists for the government, not long launched on their research programs, would have disputed Tuite's charge. Whether salaried or contracted, they believed they had been given free rein to figure out the illnesses; they proceeded with professional (if sometimes maddening) caution. Interference from above wasn't the difficulty, as they saw it. It was the lack of data below.

The scientists, remember, were slogging on two tracks. There was health-based research, trying to fathom the sicknesses per se, including the psychological components, and exposure-based research, in which a smorgasbord of chemicals was compared with a battery of symptoms. But as I've said, the exposures were never measured, and the cases were never defined. It was as if a high-jump competition were being held in a swimming pool. What solid fact did you use to push off from?

When Khamisiyah put nerve gas back on the table, in the latter part of 1996, the federal research managers increased the assignments in the area of neurotoxicology. Robert Haley, for instance, got federal funding. At the same time all possible medical precedents had to be examined. Accordingly the Department of Veterans Affairs organized a conference in March 1997 on "Health Effects of Low-Level Chemical Warfare Nerve Agent Exposure." It was a brainstorming session about the organophosphate agents. Just starting my own work, I was eager to attend.

A biomedical meeting in Cincinnati, especially during a flood of the Ohio River, would not draw a lot of press, I knew, but given the consequence of the issue, I didn't expect to be the only observer. However, only 2 of the 150 attendees were not scientists, physicians, or government employees. The other one was Tuite. I realized then that he wasn't engaged in a Washington snow job.

Wearing his customary dark suit, he took a chair at the side of the conference room. James Joseph Tuite III is a burly, graying fellow, the son of a Pittsburgh construction worker. He was forty-seven years old. He has a serious presence, kind of standoffish, but an expressive, mobile face, which can grin broadly or frown deeply. Even before the session was under way, he looked coiled and ready to pounce. Tuite had retired from the Secret Service five years earlier, and alertness may have become habitual.

I made my way over. He gave me the latest on Khamisiyah. "We think that people in the Pentagon who said they had no documents were in fact holding them at the time," he said. I nodded, ignorant of the documents he meant. I didn't know who "we" was either, but Tuite was reputed to have a legion of sources.

A VA official named Frances Murphy walked by. A neurologist who used to treat gulf war veterans at the Washington (D.C.) VA Medical Center, Murphy currently directed the agency's Environmental Agents program. In essence she was the VA's top officer for the illnesses.

"You know what they call her?" he confided. "Satan in a skirt."

It was a slap that Tuite appeared to regret, for he added that he sympathized with Fran Murphy. But some things do tend to stick. The same line occurs in *Thanks of a Grateful Nation*, in reference to a cold and combative VA doctor who has a run-in with Tuite at the Washington hospital.

The conference began with rather gloomy remarks from John Feussner, the VA's chief of research. "If we're careful, it will be years before we have answers," he said. "All we need is ideas, energy and time. . . . All I'd say is, good luck to us and good luck to the vets who are ill."

In the preceding chapter I discussed the organophosphate insecticides. Chemical warfare agents belonging to the OP family, such as sarin and soman, are as lethal to humans as the pesticides are to bugs. Organophosphates knock out an enzyme called acetylcholinesterase, whose function is to control a neurotransmitter called acetylcholine. In OP poisoning, the acetylcholine molecules, uninhibited, "run amok and overstimulate the nervous system," as one speaker put it, until the nervous system collapses.

As I have noted, the conventional wisdom was that in the absence of sharp and timely symptoms there was no reason to worry about long-term health problems from exposure to an OP agent, be it a pesticide or a nerve gas. Conversely, argued the Pentagon, no symptoms in the field meant there had been no exposures in the field. Khamisiyah shot a big hole in this argument. The ensuing question was whether nerve gas in amounts too low to cause physical reactions might prompt a chronic illness months and years later, and if so, how.

The research literature on sarin and human beings, unlike that on insecticide exposure, was meager. Between 1955 and 1975 the U.S. Army ran a series of tests of various OP nerve agents on hundreds of volunteers. The doses were high enough for soldiers to have exhibited acute effects. Years later researchers surveyed the subjects, analyzed some of their hospital records, and didn't find any unusual health problems among them.

This study doesn't provide much to go on, observed Peter Spencer, a neurotoxicologist who gave the first presentation at the Cincinnati conference. Spencer had taken part in the follow-up work on the army test subjects. He said the study couldn't have educed the subtle health damage of nerve agents, if there were any; it could have found only conspicuous medical conditions. Changes in brain waves hadn't been assessed, for instance. There was a study in the medical literature showing that sarin altered brain waves a year after exposure.

Spencer's opinion was important. Because of his expertise, his laboratory at the Oregon Health Sciences University in Portland had received several grants from VA to study the gulf war illnesses.

"Spencer thinks it's chemicals," Tuite said to me at the break.

Oh? Thereafter I paid closer attention to Spencer. It was true that he pushed harder than his colleagues for exceptions to the rule about nerve agents. He didn't seem to accept that unless exposures were high enough to cause symptoms at once, long-term changes weren't expected. A typical comment: "Are we certain that the hen studies reassure us that sublethal exposures to sarin don't lead to peripheral neuropathy?"

He was being a "provocateur," Spencer told me later, in an effort to stimulate the discussion. But when I told him Tuite's comment, he demurred. He and Tuite had conferred several times, yes, "but I imagine he may have misunderstood my enthusiastic interest in what he had to say." Later in an e-mail: "I parted company with Jim on his belief that 'chemicals are the cause of veterans' symptoms,' not as a judgement on whether this association is correct or incorrect, but because scientists should make statements of cause and effect on the basis of carefully weighed data." All right, so maybe Jim got ahead of himself with Spencer.

The next speaker was a doctor and epidemiologist named Sanford Leffingwell. Ten years before Leffingwell had helped set the U.S. standard for public exposure to sarin, the level that is permitted in the air around a nerve gas plant, for example, or a storage facility. He was familiar with the full range of sarin's effects on both humans and lab animals.

Leffingwell attempted to shut the door that Peter Spencer had opened. He warned the assembly to keep the dosage of the chemicals in mind when reading about gulf war syndrome. He gave a figure, an air concentration for sarin, that he said was too low to produce effects even after a lifetime of exposure. He suggested that if sarin had been present in the air of the Gulf, its concentrations would have been still lower than that. Moreover, the faint vapor couldn't have lasted; it would quickly break down. "You cannot prove a negative," he said, but he believed that "no surprises lurk" and that "without symptomatic exposures, a connection would not be found to the gulf war illnesses."

Now it happened that Leffingwell was consulted by Tuite when Tuite was preparing his first Senate report, in August and early September 1993. Already suspecting nerve agents and not trusting the Pentagon's experts to advise him, he found Leffingwell, who worked then for the Centers for Disease Control in Atlanta. Tuite told Leffingwell about the sharp physical sensations that some veterans had experienced during the war, in what the veterans claimed were chemical incidents. Could they have been exposed to nerve gas?

Leffingwell didn't think so. He explained to Tuite what the acute signs entailed: narrowed pupils, vomiting, runny noses, etc. The veterans' reports didn't match. Maybe a biological toxin was involved, Leffingwell hazarded, but probably not a nerve agent.

According to notes that Leffingwell made of their phone conversation, Tuite also asked about delayed neuropathy, the nerve damage associated with organophosphate poisoning. Leffingwell said that progressive symptoms this long after an exposure were more consistent with a chronic infection, say, than with injuries from chemicals.

"I was simply speculating with him about cause of the illnesses," recalled Leffingwell. "At the conclusion of our talk I said something like 'I don't think it's going to turn out to be [nerve] agent.'"

Six days later Tuite completed and handed his report to Riegle, and Riegle with some fanfare put it before the Senate. The report came to no categorical conclusions, but it laid the groundwork for chemical warfare agents, especially nerve agents, to be the sources of the illnesses. Tuite was proud of his early analysis; subsequent findings bore it out, he told me. In the footnotes Sanford Leffingwell was cited seven times in support of his arguments.

"My read on Jim," Leffingwell said, "is that he's not an expert but that he's been working hard to come up to speed. Still, that leaves gaps, and I think he's wrong.

"In science the evidence in support of a hypothesis doesn't carry the idea. You have to look at the arguments against it. For example, I can give you lots of evidence that the earth is flat. I can take you all around the Midwest and everywhere you stand it will look flat. But if I take you to the moon, it doesn't look flat. With Jim's hypothesis you run into problems when you look at the other side."

LET ME NOT give the impression that everyone at the conference was opposed. Dr. Mohammed Abou-Donia, for one, seemed to be of like mind to Tuite. Abou-Donia was an Egyptian-born pharmacology researcher at Duke University Medical Center. While other speakers were happy to entertain ideas on how organophosphates *might* lead to gulf war–like symptoms, Abou-Donia flatly stated his opinion that it was so.

The subject of his presentation was his experiments on hens using a combination of chemical agents. His results demonstrated a neurotoxic synergy. Injections of the insecticides DEET and permethrin and the drug PB were more toxic to the animals when administered together than when given singly. The combination of the three caused neuropathy. Abou-Donia suggested that a toxic overload similar to this had sickened the veterans.

The rebuttals, however, were by far the most extensive of the meeting. Speakers lined up to challenge Abou-Donia, saying his doses were too high to be meaningful. The damage could have been from the overload pure and simple, not from the synergy. The Duke researcher acknowledged that the interactions needed to be demonstrated at lower doses. Significantly, Abou-Donia's study was funded by Ross Perot, the backer also of Robert Haley, who recently had published his work on the neurotoxic theme.

The matter of toxic interactions, the group agreed, ought to be pursued. In some people there may have been greater than additive effects from multiple exposures. The guiding precedents here came mainly from pharmacology, patients experiencing adverse reactions to a combination of prescription drugs that they tolerated separately. Toxic magnification can also occur if the person smokes. Cigarettes plus asbestos exposure, cigarettes plus radon exposure: They make the risk of lung disease exponentially higher than you'd expect from the two insults together. But at lower doses, the unknown doses that wafted in the Gulf, the chemical interactions were hypothetical. Also, how would you go about testing them? Someone made the calculation that if you took the dozen most suspect substances, they made 479 billion possible combinations.

Tuite always allowed for chemical interactions to have triggered the illnesses, but the specific agents within the mix—apart from nerve gas, his prime suspect, blown downwind from Iraq—didn't concern him much. "You can't test all the permutations," he said to me afterward. "There is a matrix of exposures and an inability to reconstruct them all. That's why we've gone to the molecular level."

At the conference Tuite showed he had picked up a good deal of molecular biology. Coolly he stood up during a dense lecture by an Israeli scientist and asked the man something about the "phosphorylation of acetylcholinesterase," a thing I couldn't even pronounce, let alone understand. "Could only *some* of the enzymes be aged?" Tuite asked.

More impressive was that the Israeli responded crisply, as if to a peer. When I had a chance, I asked Tuite what he'd been after. In some veterans, he explained, those who may be genetically vulnerable, the low-level exposures may have compromised enzymes and sparked immune reactions. He referred me to his partner, Howard Urnovitz, for details. Between sessions Tuite himself was on the phone to Urnovitz, relaying information and receiving feedback.

In the scientific world Urnovitz was a hard figure to place. He headed a small biomedical company in Berkeley, California. He had credentials, having invented an important test, a urine assay, to detect the HIV virus. He had written and lectured on virology and immunology. On the other hand, he had no university or institutional affiliations, and his scientific publications were slim. During a brief conversation with me he launched caustic words at the establishment—"the morons who are called scientists in Washington"—for preventing his ideas from being recognized. He also suggested that I was not qualified to write about him.

In other words, Urnovitz was a maverick in the mold of Tuite. When they met, a couple of years earlier, they found they had similar ideas about the long-term dangers of chemicals in the environment. "Most of the gulf war syndrome story has already been written," Urnovitz advised me. "It's called *Silent Spring*."

Like other reporters, I had been drawn to Tuite because he was a tough and articulate advocate for the veterans, but in Cincinnati I learned that the role he most desired was to represent *all* sick people who suffered from chemically instigated illnesses. To that end Urnovitz had set up a foundation, the Chronic Illness Research Foundation, which Tuite joined as "director of interdisciplinary sciences." Funds permitting, the foundation was to study the genetic and immunologic mechanisms of cancer, AIDS, gulf war syndrome, chronic fatigue syndrome, and the autoimmune diseases. All these were probably linked, according to Tuite and Urnovitz, with the individual's susceptibility the unifying factor. The people who got sick were those whose DNA was most sensitive to the toxic compounds that we had loosed upon our world.

'You've opened one can of worms," I remarked to him, "and then opened a second can before the first was resolved."

"The second can of worms is the only way that I'll get back to resolving the first," Tuite replied. He was looking ahead and thinking big, as usual. "Gene therapy is controversial, but it may be able to help two out of the five people in the world who have these twentieth-century chronic diseases. So if you don't test veterans for DNA damage, and you write them off as psychological stress cases, you're never going to find out."

THE WEEKEND BEFORE Memorial Day I went to see Jim in Washington. At this busy point in his career Tuite was splitting his hours between science and politics, sometimes working the one as if the other didn't matter, at other times mining the one in order to advance the other. The place where the two intersected was the Gulf War Research Foundation, which he had established after going out on his own. (It was separate from the Chronic Illness Research Foundation.) When quoted in the press, Tuite was identified as the foundation director, as a consultant to it, or, in the *New York Times*, as "founder of the Gulf War Research Foundation, a group that has accused the Pentagon of a cover-up."

The group's sole staffer was Tuite operating out of his Georgetown condominium. His office was a high-tech war room whence issued a stream of faxes, e-mails, and reports and where journalists came for briefings. At one end of the room sat a gleaming curvilinear desk and a massive computer for crunching satellite imagery. The wall opposite was hung with his plaques and framed degrees.

Formal even when off duty, Tuite met me in a pressed short-sleeved madras shirt and neat slacks. Making coffee, he said, "That's the trouble with being an ex-cop—you drink a lot of coffee." (A quiz to the reader: How many of the veterans in this book either served or wished to serve as policemen? Counting him, four.)

Jim settled in at the helm of his console. He had a lot to say to me. "Six hundred and ninety-seven thousand people were exposed to genotoxic poisons," he declared, "and ten percent are sick."

The pièce de résistance of the Tuite briefing was the satellite picture of the "thermal plume." He brought the gray-banded image to the screen. It showed the area around Muthanna, a bombed Iraqi chemical weapons plant, early on the morning of January 19, 1991. The data was obtained from the publicly available files of U.S. weather satellites, and it was rendered on his computer, Tuite said, by means of a ten-thousand-dollar software program and was then interpreted by an unnamed contractor.

"There's the plume coming off to the south," he said, pointing. "That's debris! Or heat! Directly off a targeted facility and going to the area [in Saudi Arabia] where the Czechs detected chemicals."

The picture had been taken at night in the infrared, or heat, spectrum, which the eye can't register. I put my face close to it. He wasn't very pleased when I observed that infrared patterns weren't the same as air movements and that the wind could have been blowing in the opposite direction.

"Yeah, well, the wind *was* blowing south that day," Tuite said. He added, "Image interpretation is an art, not a science." He conceded, "The CIA denies it has any significance."

The Central Intelligence Agency maintained that the winds—those at the altitude necessary to move a toxic vapor hundreds of miles—were actually blowing away from the troop locations. Tuite's plume was said to be a fog bank or low stratus clouds. I could give you details of the CIA refutation, but more interesting is that the details were laid on for me by three analysts, no less, over the course of several hours at Langley. The arms of the federal government took Tuite's charges extremely seriously. He wasn't any crank with a fax machine. His words delivered weight and power—because of their content and because of their having been amplified.

So much for his text but what of the subtext? Tuite and I, who were about the same age, had incorporated into opposing outlooks the same material from the history of environmental health. His reference to "fallout," for example, when describing the downwind exposures to the troops. If you clicked on that word in his statements, you would be (figuratively) taken to Web pages that were generated in the fifties and sixties. Thus Tuite testifying to the presidential panel: "[H]ow to target Iraqi chemical weapons facilities and deny Iraqi access to the weapons without causing hazardous fallout? That's a serious problem, because we all know that the nuclear blasts of the 1950s caused global radioactive fallout, and we all have concerns about the industrial pollution from the Midwest causing acid rain and things like that. So somehow, we had to figure out a way to target facilities housing toxins that were a thousand times more powerful than the most powerful production pesticides safely and effectively without killing massive amounts of Iraqis, without hurting our own soldiers and at the same time deny Iraq use of the weapons. . . ."

Tuite believed that the military hadn't succeeded and that fallout of sarin had reached the Americans, having got up and over the Iraqi population by an atmospheric process that the military disputed. Rather than make an argument that I was doomed to lose, the question that I tried to raise with Jim instead was why he and I had turned out to be different thinkers. From the cloud of uncertainty about chemical exposures and human health, he and I had fallen out to dueling positions. I gave him my brief speech about the paradigm of chemically caused illness created by Rachel Carson, the depth of her influence on public attitudes, etc.

He would not go along. "I'm not a follower of a paradigm," he said. "If anything I'm a victim of it." I wasn't sure what he meant by that since his health was fine.

Shifting to politics, Tuite showed me a copy of the speech he would give the next day at the Lincoln Memorial. A group of Persian Gulf and Vietnam veterans was holding a rally.

"This is a *political* speech," he said.

"Is there red meat in it?"

"Well, I can't very well put up laser images of DNA," he said, smiling. "Is there inflammatory rhetoric in here? You bet. But these agencies need a kick in the butt. . . . All we need to do is presume exposure and the war is over."

Tuite was lobbying behind the scenes in Congress for a bill that would officially make the presumption that all sick vets had encountered toxic substances. Like the Agent Orange legislation, it would provide compensation without further squabble. No more investigations, no more waiting for research to come in. "We've learned about as much as we can about *that* war," he said. If such a measure passed, he wouldn't have to go after the CIA and Pentagon any longer, he said, for he was concerned about the damage the controversy was doing to the national defense agencies.

Standing ramrod straight and gesturing toward the army commendations and medals framed on his wall, he stressed he was not antimilitary, just opposed to the military's mendacity in this situation. "You tell me what the Pentagon has done to help these soldiers except to react to public and congressional pressure."

When we were done, I asked if he'd like to go get something to eat, and he declined, laughing, "You're just trying to get inside my head." It was true I hankered for biographical details. Initially he wouldn't provide any because the rights to his story, he said, were owned by the producers of *Thanks of a Grateful Nation*.

LIKE ME, TUITE was the oldest of six children; like me, he had four brothers and a sister who was the youngest. He and I were given the names of our fathers and grandfathers, though I no longer used III after mine. "You know they say that the first-borns are the strivers of the family," I wrote to him. "My experience of being the oldest, and the one carrying the patronymic, was that I felt a greater responsibility than my siblings to do the right thing, at an age when the right thing wasn't immediately clear. Nevertheless I had guilt when I fell short, and a more sober childhood overall." He had no comment.

In phone conversation, if you let Jim go on for ten or fifteen minutes with his technical material, he would wind down, and pause, and then he'd entertain a few personal questions, though he was still very uncomfortable. "You have to understand I spent twenty-seven years avoiding the press," he said. "I consider even the friendliest journalist hostile."

Vietnam and Catholicism seem to have affected his stance on a range of issues. He was eighteen when he enlisted, a kid from Maryland with a parochial school background and a strong sense of right and wrong. "I went into the army in 1967," he said, "because I didn't believe people should be able to pick and choose when it comes to supporting their country."

I said something to the effect that ethics was a bandied term in Washington but that when he used the word, it didn't seem for show.

"Are you asking me, Did I receive a moral direction as a child? Yes. Is morality shaping my view of the science? No." And: "Ethics are the responsibilities of all individuals. Do I have a responsibility to act when I see government heading down the wrong road?"

His notion of public service, he allowed, was connected to his Catholic upbringing. "I haven't been out there in business," he said, making a faint aspersion to "business" that a freelance writer could appreciate.

Getting Tuite to elaborate on his Vietnam service was like pulling teeth. Since he thought he might become a doctor one day, he had signed up to be a medical corpsman. Before long he was bandaging the wounded in the unsteady bay of a Huey helicopter. Tuite earned the Distinguished Flying Cross for—he tersely described it—"pulling people out of a firefight under heavy enemy fire."

"One thing Vietnam taught me," he said another time, "is to see things in life-and-death terms. You could say I'm still going in to pull people out, only now the population pool is larger."

THE RAGTAG GROUP of veterans, which called itself the Last Patrol, assembled in Arlington National Cemetery across the Potomac. Some of them had walked from as far as Florida, holding rallies along the way, heading for the capital for Memorial Day.

They formed a circle, held hands, and said prayers. One of the leaders, a Vietnam vet, boomed, "We raised some hell, and we raised our estimation of ourselves. We dropped a few pounds, and we dropped some bitterness." At the end of the ceremony the flags of the Last Patrol were symbolically passed from the Vietnam vets to the Persian Gulf vets in the company.

The day was hot and the sward was green. Chanting, about one hundred people made the final march across the bridge, with the flag-bearing veterans in the lead and family members and supporters and one grateful conscientious objector, notebook tucked away, taking up the rear.

The little band was swallowed up in the panorama on the other side. Throngs of sightseers and veterans of all eras drifted between the Lincoln Memorial, the Reflecting Pool, and the Vietnam Memorial. A heavy sun beat upon the bleached marble of the stairways. After a few minutes the speeches began. Two or three protesting veterans were heard, the loudspeaker hardly denting the dreamy holiday ambiance, and then Tuite was introduced to the crowd. No fatigues or colors, no patches or earrings on Jim, but rather a blue blazer and tie. A straight arrow, who was warmly applauded for his work on behalf of the veterans.

His speaking style was not stirring. Tuite came obliquely to the point, yet it was a very harsh point. He called every member of Congress who had served in Vietnam—and he named them individually—a coward, for having failed to support the Persian Gulf vets.

The accusations flowed seamlessly: "We have absolute proof that the Pentagon lied to the gulf war veterans about their exposures; absolute proof that Pentagon officials lied to Congress about the exposures; absolute proof that both exposure and medical records are missing; absolute proof that the Department of Veterans Affairs has responded to the needs of soldiers with a known history of toxic exposure by providing only psychiatric care, or worse, no care at all; and now evidence that our veterans are exhibiting signs of DNA damage."

Afterward, wearing an apologetic grin, he told me he'd toned it down. "I don't have the visceral outrage that some of these folks have. Really, I'm not an activist."

We chatted, music floating in the background. Without knowing where I was going, I summed up for Jim my experiences during the Persian Gulf War: skidding the white rental car through black pools of oil, dodging the guardposts, hash with Ahmed, crazy stuff like that. The thing was, while others struggled and died, I had a good time in Arabia. Guiltily I said this and added, "But now look at me."

"Why? Are you sick?" he asked, his brow wrinkling in concern. He looked me full in the face.

Oh no, not like the others. It was just that I was unsettled by the day, the Wall—the lability of emotion that Vietnam causes me. The guy who didn't go was not as together as the guy who did, wasn't that rich?

IN 1970, WHILE I fought the draft, Tuite was back from the war and enrolled as a chemistry major at American University in Washington. After two years he couldn't afford to be a full-time student, so he took a day job as a D.C. policeman and began night courses in a new major, administration of justice. He got his degree in 1976. By then he had undertaken a career in the Secret Service. Assigned to the Protective Intelligence Division, he conducted advance work for President Reagan's trips and investigated threats against the president from individuals and terrorist organizations.

In the late eighties, now the divorced father of two children, Tuite went back to school, again on a part-time basis. He acquired his master's degree in national security studies at Georgetown University in 1990. At work he applied his eclectic intelligence in a new direction, switching to the Forensic Sciences Division of the Secret Service. The move was "partly because of my expertise in computers and technology. I worked on systems to identify bad guys, fingerprint ID technology, handwriting ID systems."

Another part of his assignment was to develop a chemical hygiene plan for the agency's forensic laboratory. "I had to do a lot of boning up in a hurry. I studied the RCRA [Resource Conservation and Recovery Act] regulations [on disposal of hazardous wastes]. I had to develop policies for handling chemicals, to see whether our people could be protected. What were the direct consequences of exposures to substances in our lab?"

In the early nineties Tuite remarried, retired with a pension from the Secret Service, and started to work full-time for his Ph.D. degree at Catholic University. World politics was his area of concentration. The title of his thesis was going to be "Cognitively Constrained Learning in the Development of U.S. Strategic Nuclear Policy: The Reliability of Nuclear Missiles."

According to Tuite's faculty adviser, Wallace Thies, the idea he and Tuite devised was to use the records of civilian rocket launches to gauge the success of a massive first-strike launch of nuclear missiles, whether by the United States or the Soviet Union. Aimed at the other side's launch sites, five hundred ICBMs have to go off within a minute, said Thies, or else the first-strike strategy fails because a dragged-out attack gives the foe time to respond.

Yet most civilian launches cannot get off on time, or within a minute of schedule, even after careful preparation. How could military planners expect to do better in a crisis? It followed that the strategy of the first strike was flawed. A massive attack was very unlikely to work. Why hadn't the Pentagon noticed this terrible problem before? Because planners were "cognitively constrained." The thesis was provocative, contrarian, and technically demanding, and Jim Tuite grabbed it.

"Jim made outstanding progress in the early stages," said Thies. "He went to the NASA archives and he got the air force's cooperation. I think he gathered data on seven hundred missile launches. These were for weather satellites, space shuttles and the like. It was a large amount of unclassified material, and he put it all into a database. I believe he even wrote his own computer program that allowed him to analyze each launch—why it didn't get off on time. He showed extraordinary ingenuity and energy. I felt the dissertation would be publishable as a major book. I still do."

But?

"But he didn't finish. I am concerned that he won't ever finish."

Another opportunity intervened. In 1993 Tuite took what he thought would be a temporary job in Senator Riegle's office through a fellowship program. As the low man on the totem pole he was handed the complaints of Michigan constituents sick from the Persian Gulf War. In short order Jim had adopted another thesis that was provocative, contrarian, and technically demanding. All the skills of his restless mind were brought to bear: environmental chemistry, intelligence gathering, weather analysis, military policy, medical treatment. He believed he saw a terrible flaw in the Pentagon's argument about the illnesses. The military was "cognitively constrained," he stated, from recognizing the hazards of low-level nerve gas exposures.

This thesis Tuite actually wrote up and presented and promoted many times, but he never had to defend it before a panel of experts. I suppose that this chapter is as close as he will come to a review. In the meantime he graduated to the grander thesis of the global toxic insult.

THROUGH THE SUMMER of 1997 I labored him for specifics on his gulf war charges. Tuite's examples of Pentagon "lies" referred almost exclusively to the stormy period of his Senate service, when documents were demanded and not turned over, and when the government categorically dismissed the possibility of chemical weapons exposure. He complained that Bernard Rostker, the official now running the investigation, had never even called him. When I suggested that hurt feelings impelled him, he reacted vigorously.

"Say that about me if you want," he said, "but when you have individuals violating the law, plus people's health and lives hanging in the balance . . . Keep in mind what my experiences have been. When soldiers were on the ground, I went in after them. I have had to protect individuals because of their office. I'm not in this for me, believe me. It's got nothing to do with my feelings being hurt. It's a matter of duty, not of choice."

He battled both at the moral heart of issues and at the technical margins: Whether sarin burned, for instance, and, if so, at what temperature; and did sarin mix with water, or was it degraded? the answers to which would affect the transport of sarin in the atmosphere, which of course depended also on the dynamics of the boundary layer and the quotidian heating. . . . Keep in mind that it was unknown whether the January bombing had released sarin at all. I asked for more details.

Jim protested that I was conducting my research like a "hockey game" because I took his statements point by point to scientists and government officials and brought him back their counterpoints to reply to. I could slap the puck back and forth indefinitely. This wasn't his experience of reporters, who, because of deadlines, let things drop after one exchange.

"At every step," he complained, "they [officials at the Pentagon] tell lie after lie, and the only thing that happens is that the hurdle gets raised for *me*." I agreed he was outmanned. But rather than managing a sporting contest, I was more like a dentist, I suggested. "No one likes to go to the dentist, but now and then, to keep yourself healthy, you have to be checked for cavities." How smug of me, but Jim didn't wilt.

"The Pentagon slices everything into the smallest possible fragments and then does what it can to refute the results," he insisted.

Good, he had touched the chief difference between his method and the other side's. The difference is worth burrowing into. The distinction is between the reductionist and probabilistic approach to a scientific problem, which was the conventional procedure, and the holistic, revolutionary approach that he believed was required.

He cast it simply: "You're trying, and science tries, to make linear what is a dynamic issue. Almost every breakthrough that occurs is from someone who is an outsider. It's not done by myopic specialists and 'vertical' thinking."

Tuite had digested Thomas Kuhn's seminal work *The Structure of Scientific Revolutions*. Embracing the concept of the paradigm shift, whereby an old scientific framework is overturned by a new one, he challenged the biomedical model established by Robert Koch.

Koch, a German microbiologist, articulated the germ theory of disease at the end of the nineteenth century. That bacteria were the source of human morbidity was a wide-open, exciting new idea. Koch laid down rules for how to prove that a particular pathogen caused a particular disease. You must extract the germ from the host, culture it, reinfect a second host from the bacterial culture, observe the same disease, and then isolate the same germ from the second host. A strict, "linear," and redundant procedure, which medicine still honors, but Tuite and his partner, Urnovitz, declared it inadequate for the types of diseases arising a century later.

"Those at the cutting edge," Tuite wrote me, "those who make the breakthroughs, those who challenge Koch, long since dead and unapplicable, however, are being branded by those clinging to the past as revolutionaries." The chronic illnesses of the twenty-first century, he maintained, would never be reduced to a single organism or agent. The human body was host to a hurly-burly of factors—genetic, environmental, immunological, neurological, for starters—too many for the old experimental methods to sort out. Hence a new paradigm was needed. Tuite and Urnovitz didn't have their replacement built yet, but they believed it would start at the level of DNA.

In one respect their theory, with its fixation on environmental toxics, was not so different from the paradigm of environmental disease that prevailed before Koch and reductionist practice came along. In premodern medicine, vapors and miasmas were the agents of epidemics. Under the sway of malign atmospheres, human illnesses metamorphosed from one type to another; they overlapped like today's functional somatic syndromes. Contagion and pestilence carried a distinctly chemical karma. The proof of biological infection did not take hold until Koch discovered the cholera vibrio under the microscope and John Snow, the first epidemiologist, traced the pathways of cholera through tainted water supplies in London. By the end of the nineteenth century the new paradigm had demonstrated its power, and out went the old beliefs. But the paradigm of microinfection has failed to tell us why John, Carol, Pete, and Darren were sick, Tuite might say.

Or he might say if he were caught up in individual lives. You know my bugaboo. Where was the patient in all this? Reductionist medicine may have overshadowed him in the twentieth century, but the patient was missing altogether from Tuite's paradigm-in-waiting, which leaped from the macrocosm of the chemical exposure to the microcosm of the susceptible gene. The best doctoring, I was convinced, not only started with the sufferer but went round no corner, made no shift in scale or resolution without keeping the whole person in sight. My holism versus his.

"HAVE YOU EVER been in psychotherapy?" My preamble was that everyone who reaches middle age may have been in need of it.

"No," Jim said. "I have never felt I wasn't in control of my own destiny." (A weary edge to his voice: Where was *this* headed?) "I don't have anything against it, but I've always felt capable of dealing with my own problems. I've been fairly hardened to events that induce people to get that kind of help."

On a later occasion Tuite said, "This belief that Vietnam vets carry baggage—well, I didn't carry baggage. For many, the conflict was coming back to the uncertainty, and some had a tremendous burden, but I came back with none of that. I've always had a full plate, I've always been working, and I haven't had time for. . . ."

"Reflection?"

"Reflection . . . But I tell you, I've got no baggage. I'm not one of those people who are concerned with what people think. What Jeff Wheelwright thinks of me is not the be-all and end-all."

OK, no phobias there, but I wondered why he seemed to be so hostile to psychological expositions of the illnesses. Tuite opposed them as fervidly as he championed the genotoxic theory. The following is pulled together from a stream of his messages and comments:

"You are supposed to rule out medical conditions before making a psychiatric diagnosis. VA and the Defense Department are treating the veterans with Zoloft and Prozac when we should be looking at their DNA damage.

"We have come up with terms like 'posttraumatic stress disorder' to treat the physicians' inadequacies—not the patients'. The symptoms of PTSD are a subset of organic brain syndrome. It is easier to give the former rather than the latter diagnosis because the one involves a simple questionnaire and the other takes tens of thousands of dollars in testing.

"Now imagine yourself in a situation where you are in true physical pain, suffering from cognitive impairment because of organic brain damage from toxic exposure, priding yourself as a soldier on your independence, soundness, and reputation, and being told you are mentally ill. It's hanging the failure to cope on people who were trained to cope. Would you be depressed? Would you accept being told you were imagining your illness?

"In Vietnam there was a real reason for that type of stress. It came from a year of walking around in fear of what's behind that bush, and then you make it home and people call you a babykiller. Now *that's* stress. But the Persian Gulf vets had a four-day war, and they came back as heroes.

"The whole issue of stress and war is a very questionable one in itself because many of the wars after which these stress phenomena were observed were wars in which there were serious toxic exposures.

"Anyway, where is the article that shows stress as the cause of physiological disease? I want you to show me."

Tuite made some good points, except for claiming that PTSD stems from a toxic injury to the brain, which is not close to being demonstrated, and for suggesting that PTSD was the only alternative for the vets' problems within the sphere of psychology. As for research "showing" that stress causes disease, he was right that it didn't exist, because the criteria for cause and effect were too stringent. You can make lab rats sick by stressing them. But what research institution would allow an experiment in which people were subjected to constant pain, mental or physical, so that their rates of illness might be recorded? Besides, the experiments, if successful, would still leave the physiology unclear.

The strength of the stress argument rests on worldwide medical literature from both the wartime and civilian experience, many pages linking emotional distress to physical symptoms like those reported by the Persian Gulf vets. The association is too strong to deny; it's as strong as the association between smoking and human lung cancer, which has never been "proved" in a laboratory setting either. When you have something that walks like a duck and talks like a duck, why wouldn't you act on the assumption that it's a duck rather than strive to devise a brand-new creature? That said, my own case stories tell of illnesses far more complex than "stress."

IN NOVEMBER 1996 the VA's undersecretary for health, Dr. Kenneth Kizer, wrote a letter to the *New York Times* in which he complained that the paper's coverage of the illnesses "creates the illusion of a scientific schism rather than reflecting growing consensus" and "seems to focus on exploiting nuances instead of contributing to understanding." Merits of the complaint aside, the problem is unavoidable because journalism and science construe the world differently. When a complexity arises, a matter full of unknowns, scientific opinion can be described as a bell curve, which is a massing of outlook in the middle ground, with outlying opinions on the two tails of the curve. The graph makes two points about science: The more conventional views differ not by much, and they greatly outnumber the radical views. By contrast the journalistic graph of the same complexity would be drawn as two equal spikes. That is how, on controversial issues, the press is inclined to depict scientific disagreement. Tuite of course sharpened one of the spikes.

Some pages ago I referred to the method of science as "reductionist and probabilistic." The use of probability goes hand in hand in with reductionism. A scientist breaks down a problem to its component questions and tries to answer each unknown. Often the answer can't be determined directly or unequivocally, and consequently the investigator turns to probabilistic calculation of the parts. What is the likelihood, considering the evidence, for phenomenon X to be true or for process Y to have happened? I won't give examples of the math, but ninety-five chances in one hundred is considered tantamount to truth, whereas one chance in one hundred, though a poor likelihood, can nevertheless contribute to the master calculation of overall probability.

The exercise works best when the subproblems are linear yet independent, like a row of dominoes that won't touch one another if they fall. Look at the likelihood, for instance, for the bombing of a sarin plant in Iraq to have made a portion of the American troops sick. I've sketched some of the variables, starting with whether gas was released, ranging through vapor chemistry and weather physics, and terminating in a speculative process of disease. Ignore each of the individual probabilities; they can be as high or low as you wish. The concept I wish to communicate is that the overall likelihood must go down each time a new uncertainty is fed into the equation.

Tuite's method, by contrast, piling clue upon clue, suspicion on suspicion, drew his followers to the opposite conclusion. Where there was so much smoke, there had to be fire. John Graham, of the Harvard Center for Risk Analysis, calls it "the fallacy of layering plausible assumptions."

Suppose, says Graham, that a serious harm will occur if ten plausible assumptions prove to be correct (e.g., whiffs of sarin cause delayed symptoms; the winds from Iraq were right; the detections of gas by Czech technicians represented the regional conditions for the troops; insecticides do interact with sarin adversely). Even if each assumption is 60 percent likely to be correct, a generous prediction, the probability that *all ten assumptions* are correct is only six chances in one thousand, which is less than 1 percent for the full scenario.

If you're with me, you have done more work than the typical readers or watchers of news were asked to do during the decade of the gulf war illnesses. Each time that an unverified charge was raised, sick veterans and their supporters might have been advised, but were not, that they had no more reason for alarm than yesterday. They might have been advised—instead of by the calculation above—that a simple explanation is usually superior to a complicated explanation. This rule is known as Occam's razor. But the press wants answers in black and white, not as risks and probabilities, and the math it prefers is a zero-sum game.

The polarization was sharpest over Khamisiyah, and by no coincidence Khamisiyah marked the period of Tuite's most concentrated run in the press. Between late August and early December 1996 he was quoted or mentioned in seven front-page stories of the *New York Times*, with broad spillover into other outlets. His issue was the Pentagon's knowledge of nerve gas exposures before, during, and after the war.

Tuite's information for the press was astutely divided between politics and science, the latter lending authority to the former. Few reporters had the time or training to delve into his technical offerings, but they admired one who had. Some swallowed his presentations whole, others took only pieces, but all were reassured by Tuite's motivation, which was to stick up for the little guy, the generic little guy, who was sick. Really, what was science, anyway, but another means of delivering the facts? Facts conveyed through the political process were more useful to reporters, being more immediately powerful, than facts obtained by science.

News organizations looked to Jim much less often as a critic of the VA than of the Pentagon, even though the VA was to me the more important agency because it oversaw the majority of the cases and the sickest veterans. Tuite worked upstream of the illnesses, as it were, at the time and place they may have been instigated, rather than tangle with the VA over epidemiology and treatment. Besides, no treatments existed for the chronic illness that Tuite believed the veterans had contracted. Gene repair was still far off. For those who'd failed the Darwinian test posed by the toxic environment, it was probably too late. Their symptoms were "intermediary," he feared; what they'd die of would be cancer.

In the usual model of scientific instruction, the student starts with the basic tenets and gradually specializes, until he or she arrives at the boundary of what is known. Tuite by contrast had started his course in genotoxic disease at the boundary and backfilled with information from textbooks and research journals.

Naturally he denied it. He granted that "the more commitment you have, the more you want to prove yourself right" but insisted, "You don't find facts to support conclusions. You *know* that chemicals cause this kind of damage. . . . Yes, I am going back to research the conventional wisdom, but I am not adapting science to fit my paradigm."

I asked for references. I asked for his top ten citations from the "mainstream scientific literature" (a frequent phrase of his) that "chemicals cause this kind of damage" among the veterans.

Though near the end of his patience, Jim tried hard to satisfy me. Typically he was unable to limit himself to ten citations or to one list, saying it was not that simple. The publications he cited were about laboratory experiments and clinical cases involving pesticides and chemical warfare agents. "None will prove the picture," Tuite admitted in a cover note. "It would be difficult to classify research among individuals for whom no acute phase was noted." That is, the subjects got sick—reacted to their exposures—at the time of exposure. The same old story. How to extrapolate from the farm and factory workers who were poisoned accidentally, and from animals injected with sarin, to the slippery cases of the gulf war vets? Linear thinking wouldn't get you there.

"You know, you're an anomaly," he remarked. "You're schizophrenic on this stuff."

"Meaning?"

"Meaning you don't know what you think"—about the cause of the illnesses.

I'd allowed Tuite to misread me. I knew what I thought. Instead of replying that he was all wrong and destructive besides, I said nothing.

At this time he was preparing rebuttals—he called them annotations—to a recent Defense Department report on the re-creation of the Khamisiyah detonation at a firing range in Utah. How was their modeling done? How had they accounted for the different materials? And so forth, Jim attacking on the margins of science.

After hearing him out, I said that science was a collective enterprise that was forging ahead. Science was like a hiker on a difficult course, I said, and it carried a backpack that contained a number of uncertainties. The weight of these uncertainties was not insignificant but it was allowable, tolerable, for the purposes of the hike. I said that Jim was the sort of critic who stops science on the trail, peers into the backpack, and cries, "Look at all that!" His objections couldn't stop scientific progress, however, unless they were amplified by politics and the media.

Tuite fielded the metaphor. "Do you know the game Harrier Haze? It's about trying to get to the goal by diverse paths."

Dander up, he once again accused me of holding him to standards not held to critics of the goverment. He compared himself unblinkingly with Linus Pauling, the establishment-tweaking biochemist and Nobelist. He maintained he was able to walk the fine line (I said he couldn't) between science and politics, between objectivity and advocacy. "When I'm in the science world," he said, "I play by science's rules. When I'm in the political world, I play by political rules. I have to come at the problem from all sides."

When he went back again to the Pentagon's Khamisiyah re-creation, how it misrepresented the altitude of the cloud from the explosion, I lost my temper. "What the fuck does it matter whether gas on a computer went thirty meters into the air or three hundred," I shouted. "What does it do for the sick veterans *now*?"

"Keep your emotions in check," Tuite warned me. "I can't get tied up trying to save these guys one at a time. What I'm doing matters for the environment, and your children, and for people in the larger sense."

HE AND HIS wife moved to the Virginia suburbs. She commuted to her important job as the chief of staff for a U.S. senator. He studied molecular biology and continued to lobby for the veterans, expressing little interest in making money. His position was, he didn't have the moral right to walk away from his responsibility.

He promoted *Thanks of a Grateful Nation* on a five-city tour before it aired on cable TV. I thought Jim would have no third act, but I was wrong. Before Congress adjourned in 1998, it provided for yet another scientific review of the hazardous exposures reported in the Gulf. According to the bill, the Institute of Medicine, after considering possible associations between possible exposures and veterans' symptoms, would make recommendations to the VA secretary, who could then pay disability compensation on a looser standard. The compensation provisions were pushed through by the senator for whom Tuite's wife worked. You couldn't help but admire him, and I don't mean the senator.

By then he had stopped speaking or corresponding with me. The freeze was broken only once, indirectly. A public TV producer whom I had advised approached Tuite for an interview.

"You're not working with Wheelwright, are you?" he asked the producer. "Good—he's gone off the deep end."

8

The Mind-Body Shop

Q. What's the difference between a gulf war veteran and a Scud missile?
A. The missile stops whining when it hits the beach.

Told by a sick veteran who was getting well

A book about sickness ought to have a section about wellness. The Persian Gulf War degraded the health of roughly one in seven participants. The other six veterans of the conflict came home well, or well enough. For purposes of discussion I include in this group the worried well, who signed up with the health registries for precautionary reasons, and those who recovered from their infections, wounds, and injuries, and I set aside the few fatalities.

Within the large majority of the well enough, then, were there not some whose health actually improved, mentally and physically? When you stop and think, one person in seven, the same number as were sick, is not too many to have profited from the life-searing experience. Several veterans I spoke to put themselves in this category, and they in turn assured me they knew others who felt better for their wartime service, but the evidence has to remain anecdotal. No studies were aimed at these people, for they were not the ones in need.

To "feel better," health-wise, is more subjective than feeling ill because illness usually can be allocated to body parts. In general the health professionals who study subjective sorts of wellness are psychologists. You hear them use terms like resilience, robustness and posttraumatic growth. Surveys of this phenomenon have taken stock of World War II, Korean War, and Vietnam veterans, men whose reactions to combat were decidedly mixed. The veterans told of damage to their physical and mental well-being, but also, and often the same men, of positive developments, such as an increased sense of mastery in their lives. For many the positives outweighed the negatives, and their feelings of self-worth grew as they got older.

After the Gulf conflict VA psychologists were on the lookout for posttraumatic stress disorders, as I have reported, to the exclusion of other changes. Occasionally they commented on the unmeasured benefits of the war. "An appreciable segment of the sample reported anticipating many positive effects of their wartime service," noted Robert Rosenheck, chairman of the VA Persian Gulf Returnees Working Group in 1991. Patricia Sutker of the New Orleans VAMC, who that year made the first record of the strange physical symptoms, wrote that the majority of the veterans she saw had quiet strengths, enabling them to ward off "negative psychological sequelae," including PTSD and "exaggerated somatic concerns." Family and social supports and certain personal characteristics were known to be protective of individuals, Sutker observed, calling for a wider investigation. But not until 1998 did the Pentagon commission a study of factors that might make troops resilient to postwar health problems. (This study also searched for health vulnerabilities.)

Richard Tedeschi, a psychologist at the University of North Carolina—Charlotte, coined the term posttraumatic growth in the mid-nineties. Obviously he was talking about a more active response than hardiness to trauma. Tedeschi's research hasn't dwelt solely on soldiers but rather on various groups, including crime victims and parents grieving the deaths of their children, who have been through a physical or emotional event "that shakes up your worldview," he explained. Without having worked with Persian Gulf vets, Tedeschi estimated that up to one-half would have benefited from their trials in the desert, the proof found in strengthened relationships, spiritual depth, appreciation of life, seizing of new opportunities, and the like.

One reason I favor this line of inquiry is that it challenges the toxic hypothesis of the illnesses. Whether or not an uptick in health can be measured scientifically, it surely happened to some people after the war. Concurrently other vets fell ill, and if environmental chemicals were responsible, chemicals the crucial modifiers of health, it's fair to conclude that the exposures had salubrious outcomes too, vets better off from the alien materials they breathed or ingested, which makes no biological sense.

More earnestly, I embrace the notion of the war as a catalyst. The war was equally a fork or fulcrum or transistor—a mechanical, up-down intersection of life, dispatching some people toward illness and disability and others toward enhanced vitality, while passing most men and women through much as they were. The process, if I'm right, was independent of the war. It suggests that some who went, John, Carol, Pete, and Darren, were predisposed to flounder upon their return.

This story, my final story, is of two men who came home fit and well. One remained well, if somewhat less fit, and the other, though very fit, strained his health and slipped, until he sought the care of the first man.

CAPTAIN CHARLES CLIFFORD (Chuck) Engel, Jr., a psychiatrist in the U.S. Army, turned thirty-two on the eve of Desert Storm. Married, he had no children. College studies, medical school and a four-year residency having eaten up his twenties, Engel's career as a military doctor was barely under way when he was called to war. "I never in my wildest dreams could have imagined it," he said, "even though technically I knew it could happen." Desert Storm did not change his life so much as jump-start it.

Engel served with the 1st Cavalry Division, based at Fort Hood, Texas. When the unit deployed to Saudi Arabia, his major tasks were to dampen the anxiety along the front lines and prepare for the emotional casualties of the invasion. The heart of combat psychiatry is the critical incident debriefing, in which emotions are aired following battle deaths and other traumatic events. Because the ground fighting was fortunately brief, Engel and his colleagues had no large emergencies to contend with. In a probe of enemy fortifications, a sergeant was killed, and there were debriefings of men who had witnessed it. The same was done in the wake of a fatal accident. The most ticklish situation took place on Christmas Eve. A group of soldiers feigned illness because they resented having to work on the holiday. Engel's mental health unit helped the protesters back down from their stance.

He stayed in the theater for two months after the war ended. Having constantly extended his antennae to distress signals from others, Engel tuned in for the time to his own feelings and discovered a jumble. He was elated at having survived—so elated he realized he must have been depressed beforehand, in anticipation of massive casualties. "I felt euphoric, a new lease on life, as if I had been forgiven," the doctor recalled. "I felt like a guy who'd recovered from a terminal illness."

At the same time he felt "stupid" for believing he'd been in peril. The riskiest thing to happen to him was after the cease-fire, when he drove through a battlefield that was pocked with unexploded ordnance. In that he was like me on the beach in Kuwait when the mine didn't go off at my foot. Hairs stood up on the back of your neck when you thought about it, but stupid was the overriding sensation.

Engel started lifting weights. This won't seem marvelous unless you know professorial Chuck and can picture him sweating in the Saudi sun, muscling up. Back home at Fort Hood he continued to work on his body, lifting four times a week and losing twenty-five pounds. His wife was impressed by his V-shaped torso, never evident in seven years of marriage.

Their relationship was "renewed," Engel said, in part because his wife had been "so supportive" of him during the war. He didn't say they decided to have children because of it, but two were born in short order.

He powered up academically as well. It was satisfying to look after gulf war veterans, both during the conflict and back at the base, but he wanted to do more. Engel returned to the University of Washington, adding a master's degree in epidemiology to his M.D. from that institution. He also took a research fellowship in psychiatry. His mentor was Wayne Katon, under whom he studied the overlapping patterns of depression, anxiety, and physical pain. The university runs a nationally known clinic that teaches patients to deal with chronic pain. All in all he had an excellent platform from which to observe the efflorescence of the gulf war illnesses.

Next came a two-year tour at an army base in Hawaii, where Engel worked as assistant chief of the Inpatient Psychiatry Service. The Pentagon made him an adviser to its CCEP, the medical evaluation program for Persian Gulf veterans who were still in the service. In 1996 he was asked to take over a new treatment clinic for active duty vets, the Gulf War Health Center, at Walter Reed Army Medical Center in Washington, D.C. He became a major player in the health mystery, recrudescent after Khamisiyah, and was promoted to lieutenant colonel. "Being a gulf war veteran is part of my identity," he said, "and it has also opened doors for me."

Engel had more and more to do. His clinic was expanded and renamed the Deployment Health Clinical Center. He taught at the military's medical school in Bethesda; he advised research panels and Congress. By the end of the decade the V shape was gone from his body; he had little chance to exercise, let alone lift weights. "As time has gone on, I am more like I was before," he said ruefully, "working too hard, taking people for granted." In "excellent" health following the war, he rated it now as "very good." He turned forty years old, accelerating.

FOR FIRSTHAND KNOWLEDGE of the war, solid science, and unflappable empathy, Chuck Engel covers all the bases and whatever good I have laid out in this book. If Daniel Clauw was the leading theoretician of the gulf war illnesses, Engel was the leading clinician. His philosophy was that the mind-body distinction was irrelevant to the needs of chronic patients.

"Medicine's limitations," he wrote to me, before I visited the clinic, "are based on a professionalization process that dichotomizes (psychological versus medical) what is a completely tandem process. No medical illness exists apart from emotional ramifications and no emotional illness exists apart from physical effects."

Of the veterans referred to his care program, half carried somatoform labels, along with other diagnoses for their physical complaints, and the rest would have been considered somatoform patients had they pressed as hard for answers. Engel never used that word with patients, however; in fact he banned it from the program. He wrote:

> Understand clearly that I believe that somatization occurs and that "stress" is an important cause of physical symptoms (maybe the most important cause). So where am I coming from when I minimize the importance of pressing that point with patients? We know that a certain percentage of patients under stress describe stress-related symptoms. What is harder to do (I would argue impossible to do) is to determine exactly who those patients are. The reason is that the largest proportion suffer from idiopathic symptoms or symptoms from other causes.
>
> So on what basis do you differentiate the one person with physical symptoms due to stress from the two who have symptoms due to something (or nothing) else? Because a patient "overreacts" or "misreacts" to a symptom does not mean that the symptom itself is a psychiatric one. This is my point about medical uncertainty. I believe that biology explains all symptoms (we

don't experience anything without some concomitant change in our biology to mediate it). However, the ability of our technology to assess the cause of those biological changes remains far less than precise, and I don't think we will live to see the day when we can make it for individual patients.

Such was his reasoning for withholding judgment on the cause or causes of the illnesses. With the most rancorous question off the table, Engel and his staff concentrated on illness behavior. The treatment, or Specialized Care Program, was offered to groups of no more than eight outpatients per three-week cycle. It was a holistic therapy—military holistic, not New Age. There were seminars, physical workouts, nutrition and relaxation instruction, occupational therapy, individual medical counseling: an intensive package. The goal was not to cure vets but to have each one adopt a symptom management plan in lieu of illness behavior. When the program succeeded, which wasn't always, it was because the patient's regard for scientific medicine had been upset, a paradox that Engel put to the group on the first morning.

Five veterans—called participants rather than patients—gathered at 0830 hours in a conference room on the sixth floor of the medical center. Glass on three sides permitted leafy views of the Walter Reed grounds and city beyond, and sunlight flooded the room. The participants were outnumbered by the program staff, who in introducing themselves outdid one another in solicitousness. No one was in uniform. First names were the rule.

When the Specialized Care Program was launched, by General Ronald Blanck in 1995, each day began at 0600 with a stiff round of PT (physical training). The first director, Engel's predecessor, made it plain that the symptoms were stress-connected and that soldiers could work their way through them. Patients and staff often "squared off," according to Engel, setting back progress, and the word went out that the Walter Reed course was a heavy-handed head trip. Engel installed a more lenient, but perhaps more evasive program, in which the participant, the customer, was always right. The reputation of the place improved. Even Jim Tuite didn't knock it, shrugging, when I asked his view: "Oh, you mean Camp Cope."

In their casual clothes the five participants, four men and a woman, looked like a focus group brought together to comment on a new medical product. That they didn't appear to be sick or in distress was no guide. Sim-

ply to come here proved they were needy and demanding medical consumers. Engel looked on those who enrolled in the program as the tip of the
iceberg, the most prominent of the mass of veterans harboring gulf war
symptoms. But compared to my subjects from the VA's referral program,
these five were better off and closer to average. Being on active duty or active
reserve status, they still held jobs. They weren't disabled or embittered. But
they were determined and, beneath that, defensive.

You can appreciate that Engel dared not talk down to this group. "What
is it like to go to the doctor?" he asked. "What does he do first?"

"They check you out," answered a husky marine. "They look in your
lungs, then look in a book, to try to get a panacea for you."

Engel moved the talk to diagnosis. "You've each had, on average, sixty
different diagnostic tests. There's no question that you're suffering, but the
medical system seems to have failed you. . . . Did you know that twenty-
five to thirty percent of people when they go to the doctor don't get *any*
diagnosis? On the one hand, there's what I call the find-it, fix-it mentality
of the doctor. On the other hand, in this program people come in with ten
different symptoms that have not been fixed."

He reminded me very much of Dr. Mark Green on *E.R.*, the same head
and glasses, a guileless mien but nobody's fool. A fault lay in the biomedical
inquiry, Engel intimated, a fault bigger than the doctor and the patient.
The inquiry itself was the fault.

"Millions are being spent on research, OK. But while we wait for what
might be the major answer, what can you do to manage your symptoms?
When folks come here, they are in a find-it-and-fix-it mode. We're looking
for a diagnosis of *impairment* if we're looking for any diagnosis at all.
Rather than try to treat causes which we don't know about, we want to treat
impairment. If we can't make it go away, still, we are trained, and you may
be surprised by what you learn here.

"And we are not going to be conducting a fact-finding mission about
your childhood, so that we can tell you that your illness is your fault. The
psychologists and the questions they will have for you are part of the symptom management plan."

Engel made sure the participants knew he was a gulf war vet, but not
that he was a psychiatrist. "If they think we are out to psychologize, we're
done before we start," he told me. "The packaging is not to slip them a
mickey—i.e., give them a psychological treatment without them know-

ing—so much as it is to find something that seems reasonably 'medical' and legitimate that won't feel quirky to the average soldier."

Each veteran gave a short account of his or her health and expectations of the program. Some themes were voiced in common: Participants worried more about their health in the future than at present; they felt increasing pressure to perform in a downsized military; they sought treatment when many of their peers, who also had symptoms, didn't dare. Individually, though, their cases were different. I am going to sketch four of the patients, condensing my reporting on each, so that I can get to the man who interested me most, the husky marine, who became the de facto leader of the group.

Two participants came from the military reserves. Charles, a postal worker in Queens, New York, was fifty-three, African-American, and a Vietnam vet. He was surprised and alarmed to have been called up by the army for the Persian Gulf War. His blood pressure shot up. "I was stressed out over there, working in the Transportation Division," Charles said. Heartburn, memory problems, pain in his shoulder and hypertension continued to concern him. "Yeah, I think it's getting worse," he said amiably. Sleepy-eyed, he didn't pay close attention to the instruction or talk much in the discussions. Did still waters run deep? With Charles I couldn't tell.

Mark, thirty-four, Asian-American, an air force reservist, also was from New York City, where he was employed by the Housing Authority. He was a plump, owlish, good-humored fellow. "I can hold a job," he said, "but I'm not functioning as well as I could." While at work he mostly looked forward to getting home and stretching out under the fan. A former medic, Mark was the most medically knowledgeable of the group, and in the seminars he piped up with jocular comments. His case file was loaded with diagnoses, among them diabetes, a liver condition, irritable bowel syndrome, and PTSD, for which he took a host of medications. Well aware that being overweight was a risk factor for disease, he had difficulty, as the course went along, committing to do anything about it. In an odd way he seemed comfortable with his illness. Toxic environmental exposures could have injured him, Mark told me, but he was not all that angry at the government.

There were two participants who were longtime army sergeants, both white. Larry, forty-seven, from a post in upstate New York, was an avid student of his symptoms. Perhaps because his job was in supply and logistics, Larry perceived his body like a Rube Goldberg machine, where a breakdown in one area had tripped a train of failures. The constriction in his breathing, as I understood it, was the master symptom, and the first to have been noticed, when "almost overnight" he found he couldn't run his daily eight or nine miles. His chest pains could easily be related to his constricted breathing, Larry thought, and the headaches were probably because his brain wasn't getting enough oxygen—his O^2 intake was measurably low, he claimed. His gastric reflux disorder would affect his breathing too if the acid from his stomach were inflaming his windpipe. The acid in turn might be due to his diarrhea medicine if the medicine, an antibiotic, had knocked the "virus" in his system down but not out. "Personally I think it's a chain reaction, a one, two, three kind of thing," Larry said, pleased by the sense of it.

Larry was scheduled for several advanced tests at the hospital outside the Specialized Care Program, and until he had the results, he wouldn't buy into Engel's argument that further testing for veterans at this stage was probably a wasted effort. The point in general might be sound, Larry admitted, but "I'm not ready to throw in the towel."

He was resisting a job reassignment on the base and unspoken pressure to retire. "No allowances are cut for the older guy," he said unhappily. "It's a way of saying we want new blood in here. But *I* ought to be the one to say when I retire." His two decisions were actually one, I proposed, and Larry agreed: To quit his medical pursuit would be to quit the army and change his life.

Joan, the sole woman, was a platoon sergeant. Less than five years before she could retire, she didn't want anything in her army record suggesting that she couldn't hack it. She was a high-strung person, crossing and uncrossing her legs during the first day's sessions, scratching discreetly at itches—she had sensitive skin, she informed me. During the war she'd worked in air traffic control, thriving on the busyness. Her bones ached on her return with the unit to North Carolina. Joan tried to tough her way through, ignoring the fatigue, "and eventually I'm a couch potato. I'm on the sofa, putting on pounds. I knew something was wrong."

Her attitude toward the program was the most enthusiastic of the group. "I want info or tools that will make the difference in my life," she declared. "Something to help me not become pathetic, that's what I hope to learn. I don't want to be fifty years old and in a wheelchair." The way she took to the lessons about relaxation and graduated exercise, it seemed she was a good bet to succeed, although she would have to overcome a couple of negative indicators. There was a whiplash injury in her past and a history of back pain. Also, her husband wasn't sympathetic. Joan did the housework in addition to her full-time job for the army. "When you're tired, you don't want to hear from him, 'Get up,'" she said.

The husky marine was Sergeant Paul Johnson, an African-American, twenty-nine years old. He was the most skittish at first about my presence, asking me, after I introduced myself to the group, "*Why* are you doing a book?"

Paul was a top-rated Marine Corps recruiter in the Northeast. Highly dedicated, he'd missed only one day of work because of sickness during the past six months. In speeches at urban high schools, he imparted the mythos of Semper Fi through periodic bouts of dizziness, forgetfulness, stomach cramps, and tingling in his arms. Every day and night Paul felt tired.

"It took me awhile to come in here," he said to the group. "I believed that exercise can cure everything. I don't want to be here today. But I have children, and I don't want to be a burden to them when they get older."

Remember Sir Thomas Lewis's remark that effort syndrome (irritable heart) existed "in the borderland between health and disease"? Sick soldiers in World War I responded to exercise with much the same symptoms as healthy ones, the difference being that the sick felt something terribly wrong in their racing hearts and burning muscles and so shrank from all strain, while healthy soldiers considered these reactions normal, transient, not to be feared. In the modern analogs to effort syndrome—i.e., fibromyalgia, chronic fatigue syndrome—and gulf war syndrome, clinicians have found the same resistance to exercise because patients complain it makes the pain and fatigue worse.

Paul, however, had turned the borderland between health and disease upside down. He almost could be counted among the worried well of the veterans, because his diagnostic tests were negative and his symptoms never slowed him down. In physical function and fitness he was far ahead of most healthy people. He felt sick only when he *wasn't* being strenuous.

THE RAH-RAH AND regimentation that had soured Pete Timmons on life in the Marine Corps was tonic to Paul Johnson. A high school football star, he enlisted in 1986, and to him the challenge of military service included physical improvement. About the only time he eased off on his body was during the war, not because he had no opportunity to work out but because the oil smoke and whatever else was in the air had deterred him. "You'd blow your nose and black stuff'd come out," he said. "We tried not to PT too much, because we'd be pulling that stuff into our lungs."

Paul's unit supported the combat engineers, "the ground pounders," he called them, near the front in Kuwait. He took no direct fire himself, but since the enemy sprayed missiles about, the troops were jittery and on several occasions were ordered to put on their MOPP suits. After the invasion Paul handled prisoners and casualties; he traveled the so-called Highway of Death, north of Kuwait City, where the Iraqi tanks and corpses lay.

"How did you perform?" I asked Paul.

"I was commended. Most definitely I did my job well. I had outstanding fitness and combat reports."

He came back physically well and mentally charged, "having been through the shit," and it took awhile for his accomplishment to sink in. He remembers the awed reactions of kids he was trying to recruit: "'Wow, you were in the war? Like on TV?'"

In 1994, three years later, Paul started feeling "run down" and "out of it." He had some dizziness and stomach flu and an episode of blood in his urine whose source was never identified.

"I heard about this gulf war crap, but I never met anyone with it. Then, right after New Year's in '96, I had bad flu symptoms. I rested for a week and a half. Then, in February, the dizziness came, with the same flulike symptoms. It was obvious that something was wrong. I couldn't even *fake* being well, which is what I usually do. That's how sick I was."

Out of work for weeks, his blood pressure "going through the roof," Paul lost thirty pounds and most of his hard-won muscle. At one point he stopped eating so as not to vomit. But he didn't connect the illness to the war until the doctors became "spellbound" by it, he said. "When they couldn't find the cause, then I got concerned." Though the acute phase had passed, Paul for more than a year had engaged in a hunt to explain his lingering symptoms, undergoing tests of ever-greater complexity, while he recaptured his physical tone and bore down on the job.

Now he was at Walter Reed and confused. The academic lectures and wellness discussions were not what he'd had in mind. He stared down at his brawny hands; sometimes he got up and paced in the back of the room. The relaxation tapes, however, wafting soft music over the vets as they reclined with their eyes closed, made for a new and pleasing daily "activity." He liked the gym time best, naturally, and permitted the exercise therapist to fine-tune his workout.

On the one hand, Paul Johnson was an ideal candidate for the program's message because he was already skeptical of medical testing. "OK, to vent some more," he said during a group venting session, "Phase One and Two [the Pentagon's gulf war exams] are a joke because they can't find out what's wrong. It's a big loop that's going nowhere." About being sent from specialist to specialist, he said, "You need someone following these patterns from beginning to end!"

On the other hand, he resolutely denied there could be any psychological aspects to his health problem. When rating himself on the intake questionnaire, he stated he was not depressed, anxious, angry, or isolated; had never seen a psychologist or psychiatrist; was in almost total control of his symptoms. Yet he felt "calm and peaceful" only rarely. (Perhaps this was why the relaxation sessions were a treat.)

"My symptoms—I'm controlling it now," he told the group. "But if your body starts to deteriorate, it's gotta be something in your body. Your mind couldn't do this." On the contrary, he said. "The power of the mind is what is keeping me *on top* of this. Whenever I get a bout, I got to keep busy—do something else and don't think about the pain. Like we're taught in survival training, you block it out. Put the pain to the side and keep going."

Paul's image of his illness was not merely organic; it was a parasitic thing living within him. To beat it demanded all his force. "Everything's a battle," he said. "To slack off and diminish your activities, that's the worst thing to do. What's inside could take root and grow if you did that."

Since his many doctors had failed to eradicate it, Paul had devised his own treatments, led by exercise, "to heat the blood, get it flowing, get it mixed"; water by the quart, which helped alleviate dizziness and stomach cramps; a low-fat diet and vitamins. "I figure things out, though I'm not a scientist. If it works, I keep on doing it."

His regular workout consisted of three sets of pull-ups, eight to ten reps each, sets of push-ups until 150, scores of sit-ups, and running four miles.

Weighing 195 pounds, 10 pounds heavier than before he got sick, he claimed that he needed the extra bulk to pass the Marine Corps physical standards, but really it was ammunition for his interior war. "If something hits me, I counter it. Like when I had pain in my legs, I did squats with weights and I countered it. If I have pain in my shoulders, I change my workout to emphasize my shoulders. I exercise, I feel better. I don't want to take medication for it."

It's said that boot camp tries to break down recruits by shearing the outsides of their heads of hair and the insides of woolly ideas, in necessary preparation for the planting of military values. Similarly, Chuck Engel had to disabuse participants of what he called the biomedical model before they would be receptive to his new approach to their symptoms. The biomedical model was created and driven by reductionist scientific procedure. Engel was in league with Tuite and other critics of the government in questioning it, but the alternative that Engel put forward was a far cry from theirs.

For the first week of the Specialized Care Program the teardown was in progress. Engel's colleague, a psychologist named Roy Clymer, took the academic route in a presentation to the group. The germ theory of disease, Clymer explained, was at the foundation of the mainstream model. Despite its successes—namely, the control of infectious disease, "the cardinal achievement of mankind,"—biomedicine was incomplete. For instance, it couldn't tell you why acupuncture worked. It had no solid answers for the major killers in America today, heart disease and cancer, whose causes were much more complicated than infections. As for bacteria, people were subject to bacteria all the time, and only a few of them were made sick. Why? There was much about the body that biomedicine didn't know.

Although he encouraged questions and feedback, Clymer's talk may have been aimed a bit too high, I thought. Paul, in a green and gold Marine Corps T-shirt, looked somber. Several vets were taking notes, but he did not. He rolled his head to loosen his neck muscles.

"It's not that the old model is wrong, it's just that it needs improving," continued the doctor. "Since we want to have something new, let's call it the biopsychosocial model, or the mind-body model, or the holistic model." Clymer broached "stress" for the first time since the program began and quickly added: "I don't believe that stress causes gulf war illness. But next time I want to talk to you generally about how stress operates in the body. For example, immune suppression. We have strong indications that a body under stress not only takes longer to recover from an illness but also is more susceptible to it."

In the afternoon Engel took a turn. His approach to the veterans was by case study and close example. Going to the whiteboard with a purple pen, he drew five boxes across the top, which he labeled "History," "Exam," "Tests," "Diagnosis," and "Treatment."

"The goal is for you to become critical learners about Persian Gulf issues," he said, "and also to become better medical consumers. . . . All right, what happens when you meet with the doctor?"

As he spoke, Engel drew arrows connecting the boxes. "First the doctor takes a history—your story. Then the exam—that's *his* story." He moved to the Tests stage, made a large important arrow to Diagnosis, and lastly came to Treatment, under which he drew a smiley face. "You walk away feeling better, right?"

He faced the class. "Where does this break down? It's not just at the testing and treatment phases. The wrong diagnosis leads to the wrong treatment. Chronically ill people go to the doctor more. Sometimes that can be to your detriment. More medical care is not necessarily better medical care."

"You're saying that can hurt us," Larry said.

Paul put in, "I don't take any medications because it causes other problems."

"All tests are wrong some of the time," Engel said. "When they're wrong, either they're a false positive or a false negative." He explained the difference. A false negative test was the more familiar. It fails to catch an actual condition, an error of omission. A false positive, an error of commission, provides signs of a condition that doesn't exist, which might even be worse for a patient yearning for discrete answers and treatment.

"When you work up the patient over and over, and you finally get a positive, more than likely it's a false positive," he explained. "And tests are not free, whether to society or to the patient who suffers because the procedures are invasive." He gave an example of a doctor who acts on hunches about a diagnosis. "He 'shotguns' tests, even if the exam or history doesn't support the risk factor quotient. Let's say the test is positive—but a false positive, and they decide to operate."

The group had been following him more or less, but "operate" made everyone perk up.

"Now you have to undergo anesthesia, and your chances of dying under anesthesia are one in a thousand. Those are the statistics. So you see, having more medical care can be harmful."

Engel brought up another point: "Why do doctors order so many tests? One reason is, under fee-for-service medicine they are reimbursed for it. Under managed care the physician has less interest in testing. The military system is more like managed care as far as the doctors are concerned [because earnings were fixed], but for the patients, it's 'leave no stone unturned.' That's why the average SCP participant has had sixty tests.

"Doctors tend to order tests at the end of the exam, which doesn't leave you much time for discussion. But take time to ask the following questions: One, is it necessary? Two, what are we looking for? What are the chances that I have it? Three, how will the results change what we do for me? If the doctor says to you, 'We want to do this test in order to rule out something,' it's a red flag. The doctor is saying he thinks it's unlikely you have this condition, but let's do the test anyway. And four, what are the alternatives?"

I have left out most of the interchange with the veterans. A few times Larry objected, denying he'd had too many tests and vouching for their results. Mark made extraneous observations. Joan was intently listening, Charles less so. I thought about the biomedical cornucopia that had spilled over on John, Carol, Pete, and Darren.

Paul Johnson was the most discerning. He told how one of his doctors had missed a high white blood cell count. In other words, he wanted Engel to pay more attention to the risk of the false negative.

"Probably it meant nothing," said Engel. "But you have to repeat the test."

He went to the whiteboard for a set piece he titled "The four R's." "At the breakdown point of diagnosis, what happens if there are no answers from the primary care doctor? Well, the doctor can *refer* you to someone else or he can *reject* you—'It's stress, go elsewhere.' He can *retest* you. You know what that's about. And he can—putting *Rx* on the board—"prescribe pills, which is to say, treat you anyway." Engel then told them about the overprescription of antibiotics: Patients with cold and flu viruses were often given pills just because they demanded pills. The medicine not only was ineffective but also aggravated the long-term danger of antibiotic resistance.

"What are other examples of 'rejection'?"

"'It's old age,'"said Larry.

"'It's probably not serious,'" said Paul.

"That response is not so bad," commented Engel.

The doctor turned to the story of the Helicobacter pylori bacterium. This was a good story to tell because it undermined physicians' omniscience as well as hit a shibboleth about psychological stress. H. pylori is the germ responsible for most peptic ulcers. Prior to its discovery, in the early 1980s, doctors thought that ulcers were caused by spicy foods or by an anxious personality. "To give someone an ulcer" stems from that belief. Now people with ulcers are treated with antibiotic drugs as well as with acid-suppressing medication, a combination that can cure.

"Medicine thinks it has all the answers, but in that case it's not just 'stress' or 'psychosomatic,' " Engel concluded, putting quote marks around the distasteful words with upraised fingers. Left unsaid was that H. pylori infects many more people than have ulcers. Something else happens in company with the germ that Clymer, his colleague, might call biopsychosocial. Anxiety is still a risk factor for the stomach condition.

Then Engel put two more boxes on the board, headed "Illness" and "Impairment." "OK, if that's the model for ninety-five percent of America, what do we do here that's different? The traditional model treats illness." He made an arrow from one box to the other. "But what factors resulting from illness lead to impairment?" With the group's help, he wrote down "inactivity," "worry," "other medical problems. . . ."

"Given the absence of consensus about the illness, we are going to work with you on managing impairment. The answer is no longer in a test or a silver-bullet treatment but in looking within and forward to beat whatever it is bothering your body."

In a sense that's what Paul had been doing.

"A million push-ups can't help your memory," the marine fretted. After fatigue, forgetfulness was the symptom troubling Paul the most. This morning he was headed to the hospital's Occupational Therapy clinic to practice his concentration and memory skills.

It was not hard duty to play games for an hour with two smiling young women. The two occupational technicians showed him a game they called Rapid Recall, in which you bet chips on whether you could remember a fact given to you earlier. Or when cards were spread facedown, you picked up one and tried to find or remember another card with the same number. Paul—a man with a large round head, big eyes, big teeth—bent studiously over the card table, playing against one of the techs. He knew to start at the corners of the game because cards at those locations were easier to remember. He picked up more matches than she, and seemed pleased. She was laughing lightly, happy to lose because one of the goals was to boost the veteran's confidence.

When working at the recruiting station, Paul said, he used yellow stickies for marking papers, the better to remember them. The therapists suggested other compensatory tricks: making daily lists; putting the car keys in the same place every day when you came into the house; visualizing the route you were going to drive before you set out and why you were going. "Yeah," said Paul excitedly. "One time I was supposed to pick up a sergeant major at the airport, and I forgot and went to a high school instead. I mean, that's ridiculous. I was on my way there!"

MARK AND PAUL were in the gym together. Paul in his sweat suit, pounding on the treadmill, criticized Mark, who was pedaling the exercise bike at the lowest setting. "The discipline level's just not there," he said. Paul made certain he could match the physical fitness of anyone he recruited, even though the kids he worked out with were ten years younger. "It's hard to keep this up," he admitted, aware that his body was aging. "Your scores will go down if you don't work harder."

Others might cut themselves some slack, he conceded, and still meet the minimum PT standards. Not Paul. His illness, though it was known to his commanders, would not block his career as long as he could help it. "I'm not wimping out. I'm keeping up with my production of recruits. I give 'em what they want. I've always exceeded what's been expected of me."

1400 HOURS. Skill-building class. Today's topic: "Identifying Triggers." The instructor, Suzanne Des Marais, started by asking each of the five, "What do you ruminate about? Where does your mind go?"

Charles said: "My job."

Mark: "Going home to rest. Wanting to relax."

Larry: "Job hassles."

Joan: "The job. Generally I don't have control, and they still expect me to perform. Doing more with less."

But Paul's first thoughts were of his health: "How long is this going to last? Recovery time takes longer and longer. My chest hurts. . . ."

Recovery from working out, he meant. Muscles fibrillating, Paul walked back and forth in the corner of the conference room.

Next Des Marais had them write for three minutes. They could vent, or ruminate, or put down anything they chose. "Our thoughts have some kind of emotional charge, whether positive, negative, or neutral," the instructor said. "Some things may raise your blood pressure. Some may give you a good feeling."

When they were finished, she asked the vets to rate their thoughts in terms of the effects on them. Charles produced a list of household chores, but he claimed it was a positive list because chores were items he could control.

"My wife is a list person like Charles," said Paul.

Joan had understood the drill completely. Her composition was about hawks soaring and the wind in the trees and leaves changing and how "I can't change my health and can't change the army, so I don't want to hold on to that stuff."

Des Marais beamed. "In cognitive-behavioral therapy this is what we call reframing your thoughts. Now, what 'feeling' words come to mind about what Joan read?"

They answered, "Relaxation . . . peaceful . . . pleasure." Even Paul got into it and said to Joan, "When you said the leaves are changing, I'm feeling what you're saying. You're accepting that change is constant."

The instructor asked them write down the things in their lives they were grateful for.

"I'm not feeling too grateful right now," cracked Mark, but he got busy nonetheless.

Paul offered to read his list first: "My family, being able to get up in the morning, sanity, strength . . . career . . . patience . . . being loved and needed . . . clothes, and food." He confessed he wasn't as "poetic" as Joan. Surprisingly he pulled out a book of love notes for his wife, which he'd been writing since his stay at the clinic.

Paul had a growing family. Though he was stationed in the Northeast, his wife and children lived in the D.C. area. Not until his recruiting stint was up would he be able to join them full-time.

Looking to his future after the Marines, he seemed to be in a hurry—"I want my bachelor's degree, and I don't have that much time"—even though his retirement was nine years off. With his job, extended family, and symptoms to manage, Paul Johnson's days were full of knots, yet from his intake questionnaire I gathered he did not confide in anyone, not even his wife. Later, when I pointed out the lack of personal support, he said, "I don't want to be a burden on anyone. I don't want a shoulder to cry on when I'm not crying on my own shoulder. Do you know what I mean?"

TWO GRADUATES OF the Specialized Care Program came to talk to the group. The man and the woman had nothing but praise for the program. Frank, formerly an extreme fitness buff and weight lifter, said he had learned to engage in gentler exercise. Bicycling, for instance, instead of roadwork, and on a recumbent bike, which was easier on his neck.

"I don't beat my limbs up trying to run anymore," Frank said. "And now I make time for myself to relax." He spoke rapidly and gestured with his tattooed, muscular forearms. "I don't believe stress caused it [his illness], but also I know that stress doesn't help me none."

Paul's only question for Frank was about medications. Had he cut back on those? Frank said yes, he had scaled back, except for Tagamet for his stomach—"Otherwise it'd be on fire"—and steroids that were injected into his sore hip. This was Frank *after* the program, a veteran still wired, and riding his special bike for seventeen miles at a clip.

FINISHED WITH THE biomedical model, Roy Clymer spoke to the group today on the new-fashioned specialty of psychoneuroimmunology. "It is the physiological basis of the biopsychosocial model," he announced. The keys for the new lock. Where the psyche interacted with the nervous and immune systems, opening direct communication between mind and body.

If there were some people who had gained from the pressure of war, the one in seven veterans I proposed, their psychoneuroimmune systems may have acted to *reduce* their risk of illness. However, the focus of the field and of Clymer's lecture was the unhealthy consequences of stress, starting with the overloading of the fight-or-flight response.

The fight-or-flight response is an evolutionary adaptation that was useful to the caveman, who was surrounded by natural enemies, but in today's world it is commonly expressed as road rage. The response is powered by the hormones epinephrine (adrenaline) and cortisol. A perceived threat leads to a state of arousal and vigilance, an aggressive eyeballing of the situation, and as the individual chooses whether to fight or flee, his heart rate increases, his blood vessels contract, and his sensitivity to pain lessens. Subsequently, his immune system is throttled back, perhaps because the body is borrowing energy, as Clymer put it, from an energy-hungry function that is not needed during stressful episodes.

Human beings pay a price if the stress response is turned on and off too often. The internal seesaw, as glands work to restore equilibrium, is called allostasis. A timely article on the subject in *Chemical and Engineering News* states:

> In humans, high allostatic loads can suppress the immune system, decrease bone mineral density, weaken muscles, promote atherosclerosis (leading to heart disease), hike insulin resistance (leading to diabetes), and accelerate memory loss. Some Gulf War veterans suffer symptoms that are known to result from too much stress hormone. On the flip side, low allostatic loads—the failure to produce enough stress hormone—can result in elevated autoimmune and inflammatory responses, some of which also are being found in some Gulf War veterans.

Moreover, according to Dan Clauw, an underperforming stress response is associated with fibromyalgia, chronic fatigue syndrome and allied conditions. Here the person's sensitivity to pain is not blunted but heightened.

Before Clymer resumes, I shall offer the final iteration of what I think of the gulf war illnesses. Was it chemicals or was it all in their heads? It was chemicals in their heads, of course. "Brain chemicals" set them up for idiopathic physical reactions to X (any of numerous triggers), and then other chemicals magnified the symptoms and promoted illness behavior. There was even a place, to give a nod to Tuite, for genetics, if vets were born to a biochemical overload. It was all chemicals in the end, and you needn't look outside the body to find them.

Clymer proposed to the class not that psychological stress caused their illnesses—"I wouldn't argue that"—but that "stress will aggravate whatever you have." His examples were about laboratory animals and electric shocks.

"A monkey is subjected to a shock, it hurts, the monkey screams. Its heart rate goes up, with adrenal secretions. The classic fight-or-flight response. . . . After a few weeks of shock, though, the monkey is lethargic. It won't eat or sleep. And it won't jump when it's shocked anymore. What would you call a *person* who acted like that?"

Paul said, "Lazy."

"That's depression," said Joan.

Clymer nodded at her. "If I do this long enough, I can kill this monkey, though the precise cause of death will vary." With fewer white blood cells on patrol in the immune system, the animal was more vulnerable to infections. The circulating hormones themselves were noxious. "Cortisol, a natural steroid, is there to help you cope with stressful situations, but long-term use of a steroid will mess you up."

Paul got up, walked to the back, then returned to his seat. Impatience? Or stomach cramps, which a few days ago in occupational therapy had caused him to bolt from the room?

"Depression is an adaptive response to perceived helplessness. Is the monkey wrong, or lazy, or immoral, for getting depressed? No. Depression turns down the amps, making the monkey nonreactive. It turns off sensors. He'll survive better than if he's highly charged all the time. But he will still be depressed even if you move him to a box where he can control the shock with the lever. It's too late, he won't try. He's already learned it's no use."

"So what's the relation?" Paul interjected. "What's the parallel?"

"I hope you're noticing some," said Clymer. "This lying-there is called avoidance response. We learn ways of coping by avoiding, and then we don't notice when the world has changed."

The psychologist recounted another behavioral experiment, this one involving a dog in a box. The animal learns to expect a shock when a light comes on, and avoids it by jumping over a barrier. The dog will jump over the barrier whenever the light cues him, even if no shock is delivered.

"The adaptive behavior of depression," Clymer repeated, "is such that we don't notice when conditions have changed. If the dog keeps jumping at the light, with no memory of the shock, and he can't feel the shock, what would you say about him?"

Paul: "He's crazy!"

Clymer paused. "Right . . . In therapy this dog will be anxious if he sees a light and *doesn't* jump. The first time he is faced with a change, he will be anxious. . . . Our minds are far more complicated than dogs'. We construct reality. We have *perceptions* ruling our stress response, symbolic representations that we make."

Next he described the placebo effect, sick people who felt better on dummy pills, and its converse, an experiment in which new cancer patients were given a dummy chemotherapy. A third of them lost their hair. Clymer's examples went back and forth among the animals. Caged rabbits live longer if their owners cuddle and stroke them. Married men live longer than bachelors. Zebras, which do not feel road rage, recover from stress so quickly that they can graze right beside the lions that were chasing them a minute earlier. "Again, this illness is not all in your mind, but please appreciate how the power of your minds can help you."

Wearing a blue warmup outfit with red and white stripes, Paul scowled and paced in the corner like a caged lion.

Clymer came to the nub: "Enough about stress in the abstract. Our stance is that you have a chronic illness—no, symptoms—and that the biomedical model has failed you. This chronic illness can be exacerbated by stress. Psychotherapy's role is to change those perceptions that lead to stress, or to calm the response, and that's also where medication and distractive techniques and exercise are valuable."

The psychologist stopped talking at the end of the hour and exited the room, a few snickers trailing him, not for what he'd said but because he always came and went on the dot.

"I could see right through it," said Paul. "He's trying to say it's all in your head."

"Well, instead of the dog in the box," I suggested, "it's you doing PT and working long hours."

"Yeah, he was trying to say that if I didn't do that, I'd feel better. But stress is making it worse? Then why am I still tired now? I've been here two weeks and getting a lot of rest. I'm not working a long day now."

0800. DR. ENGEL wrote five headings on the whiteboard: "Symptoms" . . . "Evaluation". . . "Diagnoses" . . . "Treatment" . . . "Impairments." He turned to Paul.

The session was called Medical Systems Review Group. For an hour the staff and the other participants would deal with one veteran's case. It was similar to the reviews that I had conducted with Carol and Darren and their doctors, but Engel's was structured and skillful. No one went away mad.

As Engel questioned Paul, the columns under "Symptoms" and "Evaluation" filled up with the history I gave you earlier—Paul's "run-down" period in 1994, the acute dizziness and stomach problems of '96, which mystified the doctors and launched a procession of scans and tests—but as before his "Diagnoses" column received few entries.

"The best thing they could come up with was that I had an inner ear syndrome," Paul said. "That's a swelling that causes your equilibrium to go out of whack." Drugs were prescribed for his vertigo and high blood pressure, "but that just about exploded my heart, so I stopped."

He took things into his own hands, changing his diet, dosing himself with water, herbal energy supplements, and vitamins instead of the prescribed medications. Engel noted these under "Treatment."

"And when my blood pressure got back down, they said, 'Oh, it [the medication] must be working.' " Paul rolled his eyes. "Am I hooked on the vitamins now? I don't know."

Engel asked about the 1996 attack. "What made you think it was a stomach virus?"

"That's what they said—'It's just a virus. You got kids? Oh, well, they bring it home.' . . . I had no clue what was going on with the testing. It was repetitious. But I thought it was something they were missing. I didn't know about this Persian Gulf syndrome."

"How much weight lifting and calisthenics do you do?"

"An hour to an hour and a half a day," Paul replied. "I exercise six days a week, but with alternating days for weights and aerobics."

"Does anything other than exercise help your symptoms?"

"No. That's why I'm here."

Moving to the right side of the whiteboard, Engel asked Paul to list his impairments. Paul had to think a moment about this.

"My wife thought I was being lazy for not helping with the housework. I was on the couch or in the bed." Second, he didn't want to go out anywhere. Third, he couldn't get organized to pay the bills, so his wife had to do it. Fourth, he couldn't do any cooking and forgot tasks around the house.

Having recorded these impairments, Engel said, "How do you reconcile that you exercise an hour and a half a day and yet you can't do household chores?"

"The exercise *has* to be done. To keep up with U.S. Marine Corps standards. I don't want to be kicked out if I can't meet the standards."

For once I gladly sat back and kept quiet.

"Any more impairments you can think of?" Engel asked.

"I didn't mention the memory loss. I'll be giving a speech in a [high school] auditorium, and it'll be hard to remember what I'm going to say. I don't want go, 'Uh, uh.' So I pause. . . . I forget to mail a letter for my wife, and we get in an argument. . . . Driving on the road, you forget where you're going." Paul told the story of driving to the high school instead of the airport to pick up a superior.

"So there's a sense on your part that your work is impaired?"

"Yeah, at work they will joke about it. They say, 'Oh, you got the Saudi syndrome.' But thank God, I still get the numbers [recruits]. So my evaluations aren't affected. In fact they're still excellent."

Engel wrote "work impair" on the board with a plus-minus sign in front of it, indicating yet another equivocal finding of the gulf war illnesses, because the veteran believed he was impaired but the official data didn't show it.

"Any other concerns?"

"Yes, I'm worried about my wife and kids," said Paul. "All the problems she's been having, chronic pains in the shoulder and upper back. She's had an MRI and steroid shots at one point. Headaches and fatigue. I've got her going to the gym. . . . Looking back, when she said, 'I think you gave me that Saudi syndrome,' and I said, 'Yeah, right.' But now I don't know. She's weaker than I. Maybe I've been able to ignore the same thing—you know, ward it off."

"These sorts of symptoms are common," said Engel, "and people can have them at the same time, even in the same family." I was thinking of Darren communicating mind-body symptoms to Jackie. But as it turned out, Paul's wife had sickle-cell anemia, or at least she got back a positive test result in that area, as Paul told me later, so you never know.

He was unloading everything. "Oh—every time I get behind the wheel, I nod off. My eyes probably shut. That went on for about three or four years. I did have an accident in '94, but I don't think it will happen again." For unknown reasons gulf war vets have been found to have more auto accidents than other soldiers. Paul went on to have two more mishaps on the road, one requiring neck surgery. The more serious was not his fault, but it occurred late at night while he was coming home from a second job.

After Engel had finished taking the information, he threw open a discussion of the case. In the cross talk Mark said something about Paul being a "workaholic."

Engel, innocently: "What about this workaholic notion? Is that relevant?"

Reluctantly, Paul allowed that he worked from 7:00 a.m. until 9:30 p.m. "Yeah, about a 14-hour day, even on Saturday. But in an earlier job, when I was managing the PX, I worked hard but I still could do my duties at home."

"Paul," a staff internist put in, "compare the stress of recruiting to the stress of the earlier job."

"Stress on your body? What do you mean?"

It was explained—he already knew—that stress acts upon the whole person.

"Oh, yeah, recruiting takes more out of me. There is some stress in getting the numbers. But a fourteen-hour day, that's a normal day."

Charles shook his head. "That's a lot of hours!"

Larry said, "Yeah, but that's right across the military. Twelve-hour days. The mission hasn't gone away, but there's less personnel to do it with."

Clymer: "If these guys were machines, wouldn't they break down?"

Paul: "Well, for six months in '96, I had an easier tour, from eight-thirty to five, and I *still* felt the symptoms."

Engel: "You're giving most of your energy to work, but your impairments are mostly at home."

Paul resisted. "Two Saturdays a month I take off, and I try to go home early. I guess since I already made my quota for the year, I could do nothing. But I'm supposed to help others get their numbers—the station's quota."

The review session ended. At the elevator Paul said forcefully, "It's ridiculous that this thing could be the stress of work. I know my own body and what it's capable of. They're leading up to saying it has nothing to do with the Gulf.

"What if they told you to cut back your hours by one-third?" I asked.

"No way," he said grimly.

FOR ITS COSTLY and well-founded efforts, the Walter Reed Specialized Care Program has reached, as of this writing, just three hundred veterans and effected in them only modest improvements.

Analyzing a batch of three-month follow-up surveys, Engel declared the results "underwhelming." He added, "We tell them right up front that they are not likely to experience dramatic effects on their physical symptoms, and they don't. They report going from ten bothersome symptoms to nine."

On more abstract measures, such as levels of emotional distress and fears about physical function, the SCP participants did show gains from the program. They became, on average, less worried about succumbing to a serious, undiagnosed ailment. The women reported greater benefits than the men. Of the group I observed, Joan seemed to gain the most.

"This kind of patient," Engel said, "doesn't give you a great big hug and thank you for what you've done. If you say to yourself, If this guy doesn't get better, I'm going to be grumpy, well, you'll be grumpy."

I said I was disappointed that the lessons of the program didn't appear to have altered Paul Johnson. Principally he had learned to take regular naps and time-outs. Paul had arrived with a symptom management plan already, a hand-hewn and strictly physical plan, which he had softened with a few breathers. That was hardly a breakthrough.

"It's like a light flickering on and off," Engel said. "That's the best you can hope for. Our main message to him was: You only have so much energy to give. Pace yourself. You can afford to give less to recruiting and more to your family. It seemed to resonate with him at the end. . . . Be content with small gains."

Paul shook my hand good-bye and took the elevator down. I deliberated for a minute, then followed him.

He was walking across the Walter Reed compound with Charles. I kept forty yards behind, waiting for Charles to peel off. Although in one sense I was coming after him with all the pages of this book, what I intended to give, when I caught him, was the helpful example of my depression.

About twelve years ago, upon concluding an intense period of work, I drifted into a clinical depression. Drift, because it took all spring and summer to attain the bottom. As my spirits sank and my sleepless nights lengthened, my mind started to fog. I couldn't remember, and I couldn't make decisions effectively. I didn't want pills. Only aerobic exercise seemed to pick me up. So I hit upon the strategy of putting off all choices and actions until the afternoon, and in the middle of the day I would go to the gym. With a brief spike of brain chemicals and a surge in my heart from the workout, I was able to return to the office and cope. For several months this slender symptom management plan carried me along, until I fell hard through the floor.

Charles turned to the right, and Paul turned left around a corner. Out of view I scooted ahead and closed the gulf between us. But when I rounded the corner, Paul was not there. He was far ahead of me down the straight blacktop path. He was *sprinting*! Small in the distance, he couldn't have known I was tracking him, could he? Godspeed, Paul.

Acknowledgments

This book would not have been possible without a grant from the Alfred P. Sloan Foundation, which takes an interest in scientific controversies of national importance. I thank Doron Weber at the foundation for launching me. He believed that I could do justice to the stormy topic of the gulf war illnesses. Esther Newberg, my literary agent, and Starling Lawrence, my editor, signed on and proved stalwart and wise during the voyage.

To the subjects of my chapters, all veterans, I thank you for the offer of yourselves. I bow before your bravery—in sickness and in health.

I can't acknowledge all the physicians and medical researchers who talked to me and provided me with reprints of their work. But five with a deep sense of the illnesses extended themselves to my project. Profound thanks to Charles Engel of the Deployment Health Clinical Center, Walter Reed Army Medical Center; Timothy Gerrity of the Office of Research and Development, Department of Veterans Affairs (since moved to Georgetown Medical Center); Ronald Hamm of the West Los Angeles VA Medical Center; K. Craig Hyams of the Naval Medical Research Center; and Terry Jemison of the VA Office of Public Affairs.

The following men and women, of various affiliations, helped me at critical junctures. My gratitude to Ross Anthony, Harry Becnel, Jim Benson, Ronald Blanck, Daniel Clauw, Bob Currieo, Albert Donnay, Dan Fahey, Jennifer Freedman, Tom Gilroy, Gregory Gray, Jack Heller, Craig Hicks,

Chris Kornkven, Kurt Kroenke, Joyce Lashof, Dian Lawhon, Les Line, Dean Lundholm, Erika Lundholm, Mac Macfie, Frances Murphy, Bob Newman, Jackie Olsen, Jon Palfreman, Matt Puglisi, Dan Quinn, Gary Roselle, Joe Rosenbloom, Bernard Rostker, Fred Sidell, Peter Spencer, Mike Sullivan, Ahmed Turkestani, Jim Turner, Molly Wheelwright (for artful medical advice), Peter Wheelwright (for pointing me to the philosophers).

I celebrate my loving wife, Mia. She sustains me through each day, work or play, fog or shine, and she knows the right word for what I want to say.

I close this book as it began, with a note about my father, Henry Jefferds Wheelwright, who died in 1999. He was a doctor, a wonderful doctor. He always stood up for the right thing while being kind to every person, a balance of high qualities that I shall never master.

Notes and Sources

Chapter One

Page 18 Further discussion of irritable heart can be found in chapter 6. See p. 280 and also pp. 405–406.

Pages 18–19 Details of the postwar relationship between the Atomic Energy Commission, UCLA Medical School, and the Veterans Administration can be found in the administrative files of Dr. Stafford Warren, University Archives, University of California at Los Angeles. Warren, the first dean of the medical school, served as the chief medical officer of the Manhattan Project, the agency that built the atom bomb during World War II.

For analysis of the VA radioisotope program, see "Advisory Committee on Human Radiation Experiments: Final Report," U.S. Government Printing Office, Washington, D.C., October 1995, pp. 29–32, 283–319. For background on the atomic veterans and VA concerns about disability claims, see "Advisory Committee on Human Radiation Experiments: Final Report," op. cit., pp. 454–505.

Recently the Institute of Medicine, an arm of the National Academy of Sciences, confirmed the slight increase in leukemia deaths among Nevada Test Site atomic veterans, compared to military personnel who were not exposed. But the overall rates of mortality in the two groups was no different. Source: *The Five Series Study: Mortality of Military Participants in U.S. Nuclear Weapons Tests*, Institute of Medicine, National Academy Press, Washington, D.C., November 1999.

Page 19 I discuss Agent Orange in more detail in the following chapter. See pp. 69–71 and also pp. 365–366.

Page 20 For the criticisms of the VA Referral Program, see: "Final Report—An Oversight Evaluation of the Department of Veterans Affairs' Response to Health Care Issues Relating to Military Service in the Persian Gulf War," Report Number 5HI-A28-011, assistant inspector general for healthcare inspections, DVA, December 29, 1994; "Presidential Advisory Committee on Gulf War Veterans' Illnesses: Final Report," U.S. Government Printing Office, Washington, D.C., December 1996, p. 22 (the PAC report is also available at www.gwvi.ncr.gov); "Observations on Medical Care Provided to Persian Gulf Veterans," Statement of Stephen P. Backhus, director, Veterans' Affairs and Military Health Care Issues, U.S. General Accounting Office, Testimony before the Subcommittee on Health, Committee on Veterans' Affairs, U.S. House of Representatives, Washington, D.C., June 19, 1997; Statement by Matthew L. Puglisi, assistant director for gulf war veterans, the American Legion, before the Subcommittee on Health, Committee on Veterans' Affairs, House of Representatives, June 19, 1997.

According to the VA, by the end of 1997, 471 veterans had been evaluated at the referral centers; by the end of 1999 the number was 630. The program slowed because local VA facilities began to offer their own in-depth evaluations.

Page 21 The multiple investigations of chemical exposures are summarized in "Gulf War Illness: Public and Private Efforts Relating to Exposures of U.S. Personnel to Chemical Agents," U.S. General Accounting Office, Report to the Ranking Minority Member, Committee on Veterans' Affairs, U.S. House of Representatives, Washington, D.C., October 1997.

Page 28 Compensation for undiagnosed illness was part of the Persian Gulf War Veterans' Benefits Act of 1994 (P.L. 103-446), signed on November 2, 1994. The final rule on compensation payments was published in the *Federal Register* on February 3, 1995. In March 1997 the VA extended the presumptive period, the time in which a veteran's undiagnosed condition would be presumed to be service-connected, from two years to ten. In practical terms this meant that veterans could come forward with disabling but undiagnosed symptoms until the year 2001 and still be entitled to compensation. As of 2000, about three thousand veterans were granted compensation on the basis of an undiagnosed illness, but many more claims in that category were turned down.

Page 29 Regarding his Social Security payments, there is a difference between the SSD program under which John was paid and the SSI program. According to an information booklet published by the Social Security Administration (SSI, Publication No. 05-11000): "We pay disability benefits under two programs: the Social Security disability insurance program and the Supplemental Security Income (SSI) program. The medical requirements for disability payments are the same under both programs and a person's disability is determined by the same process. While eligibility for Social Security disability is based on prior work under Social Security, SSI disability payments are made on the basis of financial need."

Page 31 The Riegle speech that John had is from the *Congressional Record*, vol. 140, no. 12 (February 9, 1994), pp. S1196–S1201. References to Tuite's Senate reports may be found in the notes to chapters 3 and 7.

All official reports since have disallowed the possibility that biological weapons were used during the war. See, for instance, K. C. Hyams et al., "The Navy Forward Laboratory during Operations Desert Shield/Desert Storm," *Military Medicine*, vol. 158, November 1993, pp. 729–732; "Report of the Defense Science Board Task Force on Persian Gulf War Health Effects," Office of the Under Secretary of Defense for Acquisition and Technology, U.S. Department of Defense, Washington, D.C., June 1994, pp. 28–29; "Presidential Advisory Committee on Gulf War Veterans' Illnesses: Final Report," loc. cit., p. 38; "Gulf War Illnesses: Improved Monitoring of Clinical Progress and Reexamination of Research Emphasis Are Needed," U.S. General Accounting Office, GAO/NSIAD-97-163, Washington, D.C., June 1997, pp. 62–63. The GAO report, the least categorical on the question, notes that there could have been asymptomatic exposures to biological weapons. Low concentrations of agents would not have registered on the detection equipment.

Pages 33–34 Haldol is a brand name. John's information sheet on the drug was by McNeil Pharmaceutical, Spring House, Pa., dated March 31, 1992.

Page 36 Although the Defense Department blood ban for gulf war vets was withdrawn in December, 1992, potential donors continued to be warned about leishmaniasis. The official guideline deferred donors who reported "diarrhea, significant fatigue that impairs work, night sweats, fever greater than 101F, or sore or aching joints." Except for the elevated temperature, such symptoms might apply to the emerging phenomenon of gulf war syndrome. In 1993, however, since the cases of leishmaniasis identified were so few, the reference to its symptoms was dropped from the blood donor form. Yet the two issues became confused in the minds of many veterans, such as John, who were developing puzzling symptoms. "DoD Blood Donor Leishmaniasis Sequence," an unpublished Pentagon account of these events written in 1994, was provided to me by Captain Bruce Rutherford, Office of the U.S. Army Surgeon General.

Pages 42–43 As for unusual neurological conditions that have been called "neurotoxic," see the passages in chapters 3 and 6 on the work of Dr. Robert Haley, an independent investigator who did the most credible research in this area.

In 1999 Haley testified to the Special Oversight Board for Department of Defense Investigations of Gulf War Chemical and Biological Incidents that "we have some veterans—in our sample of 26 cases, we have three that have developed Parkinsonian-like tremors, a couple that are fast, fine tremors, unilateral, and one that is a unilateral gross tremor. And these are in fellows pretty young to have Parkinson's. As well, we have one other veteran in our VA sample that is among our small group of cases of controls, who has what appears to be a chorea-form thing with ticks, uncontrollable jerks, and so forth. And what is more important, the absence of any neurological localizing signs and the absence of MRI abnormalities." The transcript of the board hearing that was devoted to Haley's research is available at www.oversight.ncr.gov/hal.htm.

Chapter Two

Page 58 Here are examples of the dueling paradigms of the wartime conditions:

The government report best embodying what I call the toxic hypothesis is "Gulf War Illnesses: Improved Monitoring of Clinical Progress and Reexamination of Research Emphasis Are Needed," U.S. General Accounting Office, GAO/NSIAD-97-163, Washington, D.C., June, 1997. The first page of the report states: "U.S. troops might have been exposed to a variety of potentially hazardous substances. These substances include compounds used to decontaminate equipment and protect it against chemical agents, fuel used as a sand suppressant in and around encampments, fuel oil used to burn human waste, fuel in shower water, leaded vehicle exhaust used to dry sleeping bags, depleted uranium, parasites, pesticides, drugs to protect against chemical warfare agents (such as pyridostigmine bromide), and smoke from oil well fires. DoD acknowledged in June 1996 that some veterans may have been exposed to the nerve agent sarin following the postwar demolition of Iraqi ammunition facilities."

See also, in the same vein, "Gulf War Veterans Illnesses: VA, DoD Continue to Resist Strong Evidence Linking Toxic Causes to Chronic Health Effects," Report 105-388, Committee on Government Reform and Oversight, U.S. House of Representatives, Washington, D.C., November 1997.

As for the opposing point of view, two reports appearing in 1994 underlined the role of psychological stress. The first was a summary of a workshop held under the auspices of the National Institutes of Health, "The Persian Gulf Experience and Health," NIH Technology Assessment Workshop Statement, April 27–29, 1994. (The summary was published in the *Journal of the American Medical Association*, vol. 272, no. 5, 1994.) The report's section on "plausible etiologies and biological explanations" began: "The Persian Gulf War was an experience of unprecedented stress for our military and their families. Reserve and National Guard units were rapidly mobilized to join 500,000 active-duty troops in southwest Asia. The military command anticipated that chemical and/or biological weapons would be used. Detectors signaled the presence of chemical weapons on several occasions that caused increased anxiety. As many as 50,000 casualties were expected in a full-scale 15-day war with Iraq. Tactical strategy demanded secrecy. Troops could not be informed about the timing and objectives of their actual assignments. Public knowledge that Iraq had stockpiles and capabilities of delivering chemical and biological weapons contributed to mass anxiety."

The other report favoring this point of view was "Defense Science Board Task Force on Persian Gulf War Health Effects," Office of the Under Secretary of Defense for Acquisition and Technology, Department of Defense, June 1994. Under the heading "Stressors of Deployment" the report listed desert snakes, scorpions, heat injury, nighttime cold, fine penetrating sand, soot and oil residue from oil fires, high winds that could turn tent pegs into "missiles," social isolation, lack of privacy, long hours, prohibition of alcohol. The combat stressors listed were friendly fire incidents, anxiety about chemical and biological weapons, fear of capture and death, sight of dead bodies. Personal stressors included separation from family and friends, shock at being called up, postwar financial problems, shifting of domestic roles.

Finally, for the most nuanced and balanced descriptions of the wartime conditions, see *Health Consequences of Service during the Persian Gulf War: Recommendations for Research and Information Systems*, National Academy of Sciences, Institute of Medicine, National Academy Press, Washington, D.C., 1996; "Presidential Advisory Committee on Gulf War Veterans' Illnesses: Final Report," U.S. Government Printing Office, Washington, D.C., December 1996; and "Report of the Special Investigation Unit on Gulf War Illnesses," Report 105-39, Committee on Veterans' Affairs, U.S. Senate, Washington, D.C., September 1998.

Page 59 I found a reference to "Agent Oil" on p. 3 of the Defense Department report "Illness and Injury among US Marines during Operation Desert Storm," 5 U.S.C. 552 (b)(6), dated January 18, 1993 and authored by the Naval Aerospace Medical Institute with help from other agencies. The report was available at: www.gulflink.osd.mil/declassimages/bumed/961230/123096_sep96_decls1_0001.html. See also the March 15–17, 1991 (weekend), edition of *USA Today* for a story headlined "Kuwait Blazes Compared to Agent Orange."

Page 59 King Hussein's quote about the likely effects of the oil fires is taken from United Press International, "King Hussein Cites Possible Enormous Gulf Environment Damage," November 6, 1990. Carl Sagan's prediction was made on the ABC News program *Nightline* on January 22, 1991. See *Nightline* Transcript #2522, p. 13. The Friends of the Earth statement is from a press release, "Environmental Consequences of a War with Iraq," F.O.E., Washington, D.C., December 22, 1990.

Pages 60–62 My account of the oil spill and fires in the Persian Gulf is based on my own reporting for *Audubon* magazine and on several other sources. Of the latter, the most valuable is a special issue of *Marine Pollution Bulletin*, "The 1991 Gulf War: Coastal and Marine Environmental Consequences," ed. A. R. G. Price and J. H. Robinson, vol. 27, Pergamon Press, Tarrytown, N.Y., 1993. My information on the wind direction and the deposition of oil droplets is taken from pp. 334–335, and on the terrestrial impacts of the war from pp. 312–313.

Conflicting contemporary accounts of the environmental damage of the spill are: "Dead Sea in the Making: A Fragile Ecosystem Brimming with Life Is Headed for Destruction," Michael D. Lemonick, *Time*, February 11, 1991, pp. 40–41; "The Gulf Isn't Dead," Donald R. Leal, Op-Ed page, *New York Times*, February 9, 1991; "Wartime Oil Spill Not as Big or Bad as Feared: Toll for Wildlife Heaviest," Rae Tyson, *USA Today*, April 9, 1991; "Aramco Ecologist Fears Oil Slick Will Produce a 'Dead Gulf,' " Philip Shenon, *New York Times*, February 9, 1991.

My evaluation of the shrimp fishery is taken from "The Post-Gulf-War Shrimp Fishery Management in the Territorial Waters of Kuwait," M. S. Siddiqui and K. A. Al-Mubaraq, *Environment International*, vol. 24, no.1/2, 1998, pp. 105–108. The current state of the beached oil is from Jacqueline Michel, Research Planning, Inc., personal communication, July 1998.

Page 66 The March 2, 1991, *Washington Post* story was "Gulf War Leaves Environment Severely Wounded," by Thomas W. Lippman. On the job of extinguishing the fires, see "Amid Ceremony and Ingenuity, Kuwait's Oil-Well Fires Are Declared Out," Matthew L. Wald, *New York Times*, November 7, 1991, p. A3.

Regarding the Pentagon's approach to the health threat of the smoke, see "Kuwaiti Oil Fires—Chronic Health Risks Unknown but Assessments Are Under Way," U.S. General Accounting Office, GAO/RCED-92-80BR, Washington, D.C., January 1992.

Pages 66–68 The two reports I cite on the behavior of the oil smoke in the atmosphere are: "Kuwait Oil Fires: Interagency Interim Report," U.S. Environmental Protection Agency, Washington, D.C., April 3, 1991, and "Report of the Second WMO Meeting of Experts to Assess the Response to and Atmospheric Effects of the Kuwait Oil Fires," World Meteorological Organization, Geneva, Switzerland, May 25–29, 1992.

A sense of the perceived threat of the smoke is contained in a report by the federal Interagency Health Group, which met at the EPA's Emergency Operations Center in Washington on April 5, 1991. The purpose of the meeting was to "develop health effect assessments of populations affected by the Kuwait oil well fires situation." A packet of information, including the memo by Thomas Baca, deputy assistant secretary of defense (environment), was put together on April 18. For more on the DoD's concerns about liability, see "Efforts to Address Health Effects of the Kuwait Oil Well Fires," U.S. General Accounting Office, GAO/HRD-92-50, Washington, D.C., January 1992, p. 8.

Page 68 The Holsinger statement is from "Readjustment Problems of Persian Gulf War Veterans and Their Families," Hearings before the Committee on Veterans' Affairs, U.S. Senate, July 16 and 25, 1991, U.S. Government Printing Office, Washington, D.C., p. 69.

Pages 69–71 The health questions posed by Agent Orange have been exhaustively analyzed by the Institute of Medicine, a unit of the National Academy of Sciences. See: *Veterans and Agent Orange: Health Effects of Herbicides Use in Vietnam*, National Academy Press, Washington, D.C., 1994; *Veterans and Agent Orange: Update 1996*, National Academy Press, Washington, D.C., 1996; and *Veterans and Agent Orange: Update 1998*, National Academy Press, Washington, D.C., 1999.

For easier reading I recommend three less technical accounts, which I list according to their points of view. Arguing strongly for the chronic health hazards: "Report to the Secretary of the Department of Veterans Affairs on the Association between Adverse Health Effects and Exposure to Agent Orange," Admiral Elmo R. Zumwalt, Jr., Department of Veterans Affairs, Washington, D.C., May 5, 1990. Taking more or less the middle ground: "Agent Orange Briefs," Environmental Agents Service, Department of Veterans Affairs, Washington, D.C., January 1997. Arguing strongly against the health threat: *Science Under Siege*, Michael Fumento, William Morrow, New York, 1993, pp. 144–181.

The Alsea study: "Report of Assessment of a Field Investigation of Six-Year Spontaneous Abortion Rates in Three Oregon Areas in Relation to Forest 2,4,5-T Spray Practices," U.S. Environmental Protection Agency, Epidemiologic Studies Program, Human Effects Monitoring Branch, February 1979.

The Institute of Medicine's findings of statistical associations (epidemiologic links) have guided the VA compensation criteria. Thus, according to the IOM, there is "sufficient evidence" of an association between Agent Orange and soft-tissue sarcoma, non-Hodgkin's lymphoma, Hodgkin's disease and chloracne. There is "limited suggested evidence"—a weaker link—to five other conditions contracted by Vietnam veterans: respiratory cancers, prostate cancer, multiple myeloma, porphyria cutanea tarda, peripheral neuropathy. There is also "limited suggested evidence" of a link to spina bifida, a birth defect, which affected some of the children of veterans.

Recently a link has been established between Agent Orange and diabetes. According to one study, "Serum Dioxin and Diabetes Mellitus in Veterans of Operation Ranch Hand," G. L. Henriksen et al., *Epidemiology*, May 1997, pp. 252–258, there has been a statistically significant increase in the risk of diabetes among the veterans with highest dioxin levels. In March 2000, an update by the air force on the Ranch Hand group declared the evidence for a diabetes connection to be "particularly strong," although obesity, which can cause diabetes, was a complicating factor. The IOM has since taken up the first question, and eventually the VA may add diabetes to the list of compensable conditions. See: "Air Force Report Links Agent Orange to Diabetes," Philip Shenon, *New York Times*, March 29, 2000, p. A23. The air force review is posted at www.brooks.af.mil/AFRL/HED/hedb/afhs/97report.shtml.

Pages 72–73 The work conducted by Jack Heller's team is summarized in "Final Report: Kuwait Oil Fire Health Risk Assessment, Report No. 39-26-L192-91, 5 May–3 December, 1991," U.S. Army, Environmental Hygiene Agency, February 1994. An interim report was released in June 1992. Heller's 1996 testimony to the Presidential Advisory Committee on Gulf War Veterans' Illnesses is available at www.gwvi.gov/0806gulf.html.

Page 74 The DoD health registry was called for in PL 102-90, the National Defense Authorization Act for Fiscal Years 1992 and 1993, which became law in December 1991. Its Section 734 dealt with the "Registry of Members of the Armed Forces Exposed to Fumes of Burning Oil in Connection with Operation Desert Storm."

Page 75 The absence of health effects in firefighters was reported by G. K. Friedman, of the Texas Lung Institute, Houston, Texas, at the National Institutes of Health Technology Assessment Workshop on the Persian Gulf Experience and Health, April 1994. Separately it was demonstrated that firefighters absorbed volatile hydrocarbons in greater amounts than did the troops. See: "Volatile Organic Compounds in the Blood of Persons in Kuwait During the Oil Fires," R. A. Etzel and D. L. Ashley, *International Archives of Occupational and Environmental Health*," vol. 66, 1994, pp. 125–129. The two findings indicate the typical gap between measures of toxic exposure and records of illness.

For an academic overview of the health risks of the smoke, see "Oil Well Fires, A Review of the Scientific Literature as It Pertains to Gulf War Illnesses, vol. 6," Dalia M. Spektor, prepared for the Office of the Secretary of Defense by RAND's National Defense Research Institute, Washington, D.C., 1998, and "Environmental Exposure Report: Particulate Matter," Office of the Special Assistant for Gulf War Illnesses, Department of Defense, Washington, D.C., July 2000.

Page 76 The VA medical report on the aftermath of the Scud attack is "Unit-Based Intervention for Gulf War Soldiers Surviving a SCUD Missile Attack: Program Description and Preliminary Findings," Stephen Perconte et al., *Journal of Traumatic Stress*, vol. 6, no. 2, 1993, pp. 225–238.

Pages 77–78 The statistical distinction between PTSD and the poorly defined somatic symptoms of the Persian Gulf War is made clear in a 1997 analysis by the Pentagon. See: "A Comprehensive Clinical Evaluation of 20,000 Persian Gulf War Veterans," Stephen C. Joseph, *Military Medicine*, vol. 162, no. 3, March 1997, pp. 149–155. The analogous analysis by the VA is

"52,835 Veterans on the Original Department of Veterans Affairs Persian Gulf Registry," Han K. Kang et al., Environmental Epidemiology Service, Department of Veterans Affairs, Washington, D.C., February 1997.

The best overall reference on PTSD and Vietnam vets is *Trauma and the Vietnam War Generation: Report of Findings from the National Vietnam Veterans Readjustment Study*, R. A. Kulka, W. E. Schlenger, J. A. Fairhank, R. L. Hough, B. K. Jordan, C. R. Marmar, D. S. Weiss, Brunner/Mazel, New York 1990.

The specific criteria for PTSD are listed in *DSM-IV: Diagnostic and Statistical Manual of Mental Disorders*, 4th edition, American Psychiatric Association, Washington, D.C., 1994. For a review of the widespread application of PTSD diagnoses after the disorder's 1980 codification, see "Psychosocial Research in Traumatic Stress: An Update," Bonnie L. Green, *Journal of Traumatic Stress*, vol. 7, No. 3, 1994, pp. 341–362.

Pages 78–79 My account of the agencies' prewar mental health planning is taken from "Preparation for Psychiatric Casualties in the Department of Veterans Affairs Medical System," Arthur S. Blank, Jr., M.D., and Laurent Lehmann, M.D., in *Emotional Aftermath of the Persian Gulf War*, ed. Robert J. Ursano and Ann E. Norwood, American Psychiatric Press, Inc., Washington, D.C., 1996, pp. 251–281. In addition, I interviewed Dr. Lehman, who was associate chief consultant to VA for mental health and PTSD; Dr. Matthew Friedman, director of the VA's National Center for Post-Traumatic Stress Disorder; and Joe Gelsomino, Ph.D., southeast regional manager, Readjustment Counseling Service, Department. of Veterans Affairs, Bay Pines, Fla.

On the management of psychiatric risk during Operation Desert Shield, see: "Combat Psychiatry the 'First Team' Way: First Cavalry Division Mental Health in Operation Desert Storm," Spencer J. Campbell and Charles C. Engel, Jr., in *The Gulf War and Mental Health: A Comprehensive Guide*, ed. J. A. Martin, L. R. Sparacino, G. Belenky, Praeger Publishers, Westport, Connecticut, 1996; and "Mental Health Professionals Find Fewer Problems Than Expected in Desert Storm," Phil Gunby, *Journal of the American Medical Association*, February 6, 1991, pp. 559–560.

On the number of casualties feared: "Report of the Special Investigation Unit on Gulf War Illnesses," Report 105-39, Committee on Veterans' Affairs, U.S. Senate, Washington, D.C., 1998, p. 107. The overall number of dead and wounded was projected to be as high as fifty thousand, according to "The Persian Gulf Experience and Health," NIH Technology Assessment Workshop Statement, April 27–29, 1994," loc. cit.

The quotation about the preinvasion anxiety is taken from "Operation Desert Shield/Desert Storm: A Summary Report," Kathleen Wright, David Marlowe, et al., Walter Reed Army Institute of Research, WRAIR/TR-95-0019, Washington, D.C., 1995, p. 46.

Colonel Joe G. Fagan, a U.S. Army psychiatrist who coordinated mental services in the theater of operations during the Persian Gulf War, told Congress: "[D]uring this conflict, we probably had more soldiers, sailors, and airmen voluntarily seeking mental health services than in previous wars. Within the Army, well over 1 per cent of the force was seen by a mental health professional during the course of Desert Shield and Desert Storm.

"Despite that, the people who required psychiatric evacuation out of the theater were only about 3 per 1,000 per year, which is almost the residual rate for psychoses and actually was lower than the rate for similar populations back in CONUS [the United States]. From: "Readjustment Problems of Persian Gulf War Veterans and Their Families," Hearings before the Committee on Veterans' Affairs, U.S. Senate, July 16 and 25, 1991, U.S. Government Printing Office, Washington, D.C., p. 82.

Page 81 Regarding the "excellent" medical support during the war, see: "The Impact of Infectious Diseases on the Health of U.S. Troops Deployed to the Persian Gulf during Operations Desert Shield/Desert Storm," K. C. Hyams et al., *Clinical Infectious Disease*, vol. 20, 1995, pp. 1497–1504. Also, by the same lead author, "The Navy Forward Laboratory during Operations Desert Shield/Desert Storm," *Military Medicine*, vol. 158, 1993, pp. 729–732. The latter report is posted on GulfLINK, the Pentagon Website: www.gulflink.osd.mil/medical/med_lab.htm.

As for the uneven Pentagon response to mental health needs after the fighting, see: "The Psychological and Psychosocial Consequences of Combat and Deployment with Special Emphasis on the Gulf War," David H. Marlowe, prepared for the Office of the Secretary of Defense by RAND's National Defense Research Institute, Washington, D.C., 2000.

Another good picture of vets' postwar stress is contained in "Readjustment Problems of Persian Gulf War Veterans and Their Families," Hearings before the Committee on Veterans' Affairs, U.S. Senate, July 16 and 25, 1991, U.S. Government Printing Office, Washington, D.C.

The stipulation by Congress that PTSD should be assessed was included in PL 102-25, a.k.a "Persian Gulf Conflict Supplemental Authorization and Personnel Benefits Act of 1991," which was enacted on April 6. Instead of producing a comprehensive report on PTSD, the Defense Department belatedly surveyed a sample of veterans in Hawaii and Pennsylvania: "The General Well-Being of Gulf War Era Service Personnel from the States of Pennsylvania and Hawaii: A Survey," U.S. Army Medical Research and Materiel Command, Walter Reed Army Institute of Research, Washington, D.C., 1994. This work was later published as "Physical Health Symptomatology of Gulf War–Era Service Personnel from the States of Pennsylvania and Hawaii," Robert H. Stretch et al., *Military Medicine*, vol. 160, March 1995, pp. 131–136. Note the shift in emphasis to physical symptoms, which had been included in the original survey and had in retrospect become more significant than PTSD.

Page 82 Harry Becnel's unpublished report on his counseling for the army was "Readjustment of the Ex-Combat Soldier: A Proposed Model Program to Prevent Combat Stress Disorder," H. Becnel, Department of the Army, Fort Benning, Ga., May 1991.

The extensive VA mental health program is described in "Returning Persian Gulf Troops: First Year Findings," Robert Rosenheck, M.D., et al., VA Northeast Program Evaluation Center, National Center for PTSD, Department of Veterans Affairs, West Haven, Conn., March 31, 1992. The report consists of contributions from a number of PTSD teams. A common theme of investigators is the vets' reluctance to seek mental health care. For example, the Little Rock VAMC group (Daniel Rodell et al., p. 87), which found that up to 10 percent of reservists had symptoms of PTSD (a typical finding), discussed why the veterans might be "wary of admitting psychological distress." Among the suggested reasons were the fear of being discharged from the reserve unit and the belief that "heroes don't have problems," especially since this wasn't a "real war" like Vietnam and since "real men" didn't have such problems anyway.

Page 83 Dr. Robert Haley, an independent investigator, challenged the PTSD findings that were reported by Pentagon and VA researchers in 1992–1994. Haley argued that the surveys measuring PTSD symptoms had been incorrectly analyzed. See: "Is Gulf War Syndrome Due to Stress? The Evidence Reexamined," R. Haley, *American Journal of Epidemiology*, vol. 146, no. 9, 1997, pp. 695–703. The Haley paper has a bibliography of the VA and DoD publications.

Page 83 A good overview on the connection between PTSD and physical health complaints is "The Relationship between Trauma, Post-Traumatic Stress Disorder, and Physical Health," Matthew J. Friedman and Paula P. Schnurr, in *Neurobiological and Clinical Consequences of Stress:*

From Normal Adaptation to PTSD, ed., M. J. Friedman et al., Lippincott-Raven Publishers, Philadelphia, 1995. Most of the affected populations that I cite are taken from this chapter. See also: "Health Status of Vietnam Veterans," Centers for Disease Control Vietnam Experience Study, *Journal of the American Medical Association*, vol. 259, no. 18, May 13, 1988, pp. 2701–2719.

As for the relationship between PTSD and bodily symptoms among gulf war vets, see: "Relationship between Posttraumatic Stress Disorder and Self-Reported Physical Symptoms in Persian Gulf Veterans," Dewleen G. Baker, M.D., et al., *Archives of Internal Medicine*, vol. 157, 1997, pp. 2076–2078, and "Psychiatric Syndromes among Persian Gulf War Veterans: Association of Handling Dead Bodies with Somatoform Disorders," Lawrence Labbate et al., *Psychotherapy and Psychosomatics*, vol. 67, no. 4, 1998; pp. 275–279.

The prescient Hobfoll paper is "War-Related Stress: Addressing the Stress of War and Other Traumatic Events," Stevan E. Hobfoll et al., *American Psychologist*, vol. 46, no. 8, August 1991, pp. 848–855.

Pages 84–86 For Patricia Sutker's work with older veterans, see: "Cognitive Deficits and Psychopathology among Former Prisoners of War and Combat Veterans of the Korean Conflict," Patricia B. Sutker et al., *American Journal of Psychiatry*, vol. 148, no. 1, January 1991, pp. 67–72. Her "review paper" that I quote is "Clinical and Research Assessment of Posttraumatic Stress Disorder: A Conceptual Overview," Patricia B. Sutker et al., *Psychological Assessment*, vol. 3., no. 4, 1991, pp. 520–530.

Sutker's early snapshot of gulf war syndrome, though not identified by her as such, can be found in "War-Zone Trauma and Stress-Related Symptoms in Operation Desert Shield/Storm (ODS) Returnees," Patricia B. Sutker et al., *Journal of Social Issues*, vol. 49, no. 4, 1993, pp. 33–49.

Pages 86–87 My selections from the Senate testimony are taken from "Readjustment Problems of Persian Gulf War Veterans and Their Families," Hearings before the Committee on Veterans' Affairs, U.S. Senate, July 16 and 25, 1991, U.S. Government Printing Office, Washington, D.C. The Robertson quote appears on p. 5, Anderson on p. 19, Embry on p. 34.

Page 87 There is more discussion of leishmaniasis on p. 36 and pp. 362–363.

Page 88 The newsletter cited is *Newswire*, Military Families Support Network, vol. 2, no. 1, February 1992, Milwaukee, p. 1.

Chapter Three

Page 89 Epigraph: "The Journalist and the Murderer" by Janet Malcolm was first published in *The New Yorker* on March 13, 1989.

Page 99 The EPICON report: "Investigation of a Suspected Outbreak of an Unknown Disease among Veterans of Operation Desert Shield/Storm, 123d Army Reserve Command, Fort Benjamin Harrison, Indiana, April, 1992," Major Robert F. DeFraites, Major E. Robert Wanat II, Major Ann E. Norwood, Major Stephen Williams, Major David Cowan, Specialist Timothy Callahan, Epidemiology Consultant Service (EPICON), Division of Preventive Medicine, Walter Reed Army Institute of Research, Washington, D.C., June 15, 1992.

Pages 100–102 My references for the Legionnaires' disease investigation were "Legionnaires' Disease: Description of an Epidemic of Pneumonia," D. W. Fraser et al., *New England Journal of Medicine*, vol. 297, no. 22, December 1, 1977, pp. 1189–1196; "Legionnaires' Disease: Isolation of a Bacterium and Demonstration of Its Role in Other Respiratory Diseases," J. E. McDade et al., *New England Journal of Medicine*, vol. 297, no. 22, December 1, 1977, pp. 1197–1203.

For HIV/AIDS epidemiology: "Classification and Staging of HIV Disease," Dennis H. Osmond, in *The AIDS Knowledge Base*, 2d edition, ed. P. T. Cohen, M. A. Sande and P. A. Volberding,: Little, Brown, New York, 1994; "1993 Revised Classification System for HIV Infection and Expanded Surveillance Definition for AIDS among Adolescents and Report 41," Centers for Disease Control and Prevention, December 18, 1992, pp. 1–19.

My discussion of the problem of defining the gulf war illnesses drew upon three excellent commentaries: "Developing Case Definitions for Symptom-Based Conditions: The Problem of Specificity," Kenneth C. Hyams, *Epidemiologic Reviews*, vol. 20, November. 2, 1998, pp. 148–156; "Resolving the Gulf War Syndrome Question," Kenneth C. Hyams and Robert H. Roswell, *American Journal of Epidemiology*, vol. 148, no. 4, 1998, pp. 339–342; and "Invited Commentary: How Would We Know a Gulf War Syndrome If We Saw One?," David H. Wegman, Nancy F. Woods and John C. Bailar, *American Journal of Epidemiology*, vol. 146, no. 9, 1997, pp. 704–712.

Pages 106–107 Norwood raised the possibility of psychological contagion among the Indiana reservists. Because in later years sick gulf war vets were unfairly accused of succumbing to "mass hysteria," a short essay on this phenomenon is in order.

The formal name for the condition is mass psychogenic illness, MPI. A good text on the subject is *Mass Psychogenic Illness: A Social Psychological Analysis*, ed. M. J. Colligan, J. W. Pennebaker and L. R. Murphy, Lawrence Erlbaum Associates, Hillsdale, N.J., 1982. The authors give a history of MPI, starting with the frenzied movements of St. Vitus' dancers in fifteenth- and sixteenth-century Europe. Such episodes were tied up with beliefs about demonic possession. The victims of the "witchcraft" in colonial Salem, who felt their bodies under attack, were probably suffering from MPI. In twentieth-century episodes, the demons said to cause MPI attacks are food poisons and industrial chemicals, which are experienced by people working or living in close quarters.

Mass psychogenic illness is diagnosed only after environmental explanations for the characteristic fainting, nerves, and dizziness have been investigated and ruled out. The MPI trigger need not be imaginary—in most cases it's probably real. A minor exposure to chemical odors may escalate into MPI contagion. But all tests for various toxins come back negative. After being informed that there is no medical danger, the affected workers or children usually are able to return to the factory or school without further complications. Therapists suggest separating the victims, if possible, because symptomatic people collectively reinforce the belief in the toxic threat. Stress in the workplace has been found to increase the risk of MPI, with females more vulnerable than males.

One night in September 1988, at a navy base in San Diego, a psychologic epidemic broke out among young male recruits. The weather had been hot, and the air smoky from wildfires in the area. After supper a group of recruits began to cough and complain of pain in their lungs. As superiors investigated, men in other units began to cough, and soon an evacuations of the barracks was ordered. Word spread about some sort of gas or airborne toxin.

Before the night was over, eighteen hundred men had been rousted, with one thousand reporting symptoms of sore throat, nausea, dizziness and coughing. To protect themselves, individuals sat outside with their heads under blankets; some recruits, having hyperventilated and fainted, lay sprawled on the ground, increasing the sense of emergency. Almost four hundred men were taken from the base in ambulances, and dozens hospitalized. But no gas or infectious agent was ever uncovered, and all the victims felt better by morning. Source: "An Epidemic of Respiratory Complaints Exacerbated by Mass Psychogenic Illness in a Military Recruit Population," Jeffrey P. Struewing and Gregory C. Gray, *American Journal of Epidemiology*, vol. 32, no. 6, 1990, pp. 1120–1129.

Page 111 Norman Teer's statement about Type A individuals is from "Diagnosis Unknown: Gulf War Syndrome," David Brown, *Washington Post*, July 24, 1994, p. A1. Jim Simpson's statement was obtained by PBS's *Frontline* in an interview with the Indiana veteran on October 5, 1997. A transcript is posted at the Website: www.pbs.org/wgbh/pages/frontline/shows/syndrome/. The *Frontline* program, "Last Battle of the Gulf War," was produced by Jon Palfreman and broadcast on January 20, 1998.

Type A traits may be characteristic of chronic fatigue syndrome as well. See, for instance: "An Anthropological Approach to Understanding Chronic Fatigue Syndrome," Norma C. Ware, in *Chronic Fatigue Syndrome*, ed. Stephen E. Straus, Marcel Dekker, Inc., New York, 1994, pp. 85–95. Ware writes: "Interviewees' descriptions of the months and years before their illness began suggest that they saw themselves as extremely busy people. Their accounts overflow with references to how intensely involved they were in the wide range of activities that defined the scope of their lives. . . . Not content to focus on just one or two responsibilities, respondents reported being involved in 'a million things at once.' "

Page 114 The ABC program was "What Happened over There?," *20/20*, ABC News, August 14, 1992. The wartime experiences and health problems of the 24th Navy Seabee reservists were covered in a series of articles in the *Birmingham* (Ala.) *News* beginning in October 1992. The reporters were Dave Parks and Michael Brumas.

As for the National Guard unit in New Jersey whose members believed they were dangerously exposed to depleted uranium, see: "Operation Desert Storm: Army Not Adequately Prepared to Deal with Depleted Uranium Contamination," U.S. General Accounting Office, GAO/NSIAD-93-90, Washington, D.C., January 1993, p. 23.

Page 115 The VA established a fourth referral center, at the Birmingham, Ala., VAMC, in June 1995.

Pages 116–117 Before testifying to Congress, General Blanck reported on the cases of the gulf war illnesses in a statement. See: "The Possible Adverse Health Effects of Service in the Persian Gulf; and H.R. 5864, To Establish a Persian Gulf War Veterans Registry," Hearing before the Subcommittee on Hospitals and Health Care of the Committee on Veterans' Affairs, U.S. House of Representatives, September 16, 1992, Serial No. 102-49, U.S. Government Printing Office, Washington, D.C., 1992, p. 87. At the same hearing Blanck submitted a report on the effects of the oil fires, "Consensus Statement, Expert Panel on Petroleum Toxicity." See: ibid., Attachment 6, p. 198.

The exchanges between Blanck and Representative Joe Kennedy, who has since retired, and between the epidemiologist Lewis Kuller and Kennedy, are taken from the hearing transcript, loc. cit., pp. 1–74. Blanck's endorsement of Claudia Miller is on p. 43.

Blanck's earlier comments dismissing the Agent Orange precedent are from "Veterans Groups Call for Study of Possible Desert Storm Illnesses," Sandra Evans, *Washington Post*, April 29, 1992, p. A11.

Pages 117–121 There is no end of information in the public realm on the condition called multiple chemical sensitivity. See, especially: *Chemical Exposures: Low Levels and High Stakes*, Nicholas Ashford and Claudia Miller, 2nd edition, Van Nostrand Reinhold, New York, 1998. In addition to published work by Miller, I recommend the research of Iris R. Bell, M.D., which has appeared in mainstream professional journals as well as in the more passionate literature of MCS advocates.

Among the most informed and trenchant of the MCS advocates are Dr. Grace Ziem and Albert Donnay of MCS Referral and Resources, Inc. (www.mcsrr.org). The definition of MCS that Donnay and advocates espouse can be found at www.heldref.org/html/Consensus.html.

A medically conservative overview of MCS is "Experimental Approaches to Chemical Sensitivity," *Environmental Health Perspectives*, vol. 105, Supplement 2, National Institute of Environmental Health Sciences, U.S. Dept. of Health and Human Services, Washington, D.C., March 1997. The profile of the "typical MCS patient" comes from the paper by Nancy Fiedler and Howard Kipen on p. 410 of this volume. See also their earlier paper, "Neuropsychology and psychology of MCS," N. Fiedler, H. Kipen, J. DeLuca, K. Kelly-McNeil, B. Natelson, *Toxicology and Industrial Health*, vol. 10, 1994, pp. 545–554.

For an account of the governmental response to MCS, see: "A Report on Multiple Chemical Sensitivities (MCS), Predecisional Draft," produced by the Interagency Workgroup on Multiple Chemical Sensitivity, August 24, 1998. The lead agency of the group was the U.S. Dept. of Health and Human Services, and requests for this report should start there.

The term "MCS" and the initial criteria for the condition were proposed in "The Worker with Chemical Sensitivity: An Overview," M. R. Cullen, in *Occupational Medicine: State of the Art Reviews*, vol. 2, ed. M. R. Cullen, Hanley and Belfus, Philadelphia, 1987, pp. 655–662.

The 1991 skeptical statement of the American College of Occupational Medicine is taken from "Multiple Chemical Sensitivity—What is It?," Roy L DeHart, in *Multiple Chemical Sensitivities: A Workshop*, National Research Council, National Academy Press, Washington, D.C., 1992. The college changed its name in the early nineties to American College of Occupational and Environmental Medicine. For more information: www.acoem.org.

A good magazine article on the subject of MCS is "Breather Beware?," Sophie L. Wilkinson, *Chemical & Engineering News*, September 21, 1998. A good book is *Allergic to the Twentieth Century: The Explosion in Environmental Allergies—From Sick Buildings to Multiple Chemical Sensitivity*, Peter Radetsky, Little, Brown and Co., Boston, 1997.

Page 123 The legislation establishing a VA health registry and an expanded Pentagon health registry for the Persian Gulf vets was part of the Omnibus Veterans' Health-Care Improvements Act of 1992, PL-102-585, signed on November 4, 1992.

Pages 124–125 For a statistical breakdown of the VA's diagnoses in the PGHR, see "The Health Status of Gulf War Veterans: Lessons Learned from the Department of Veterans Affairs Health Registry," Frances M. Murphy et al., *Military Medicine*, vol. 164, May 1999, pp. 327–331, and also *Adequacy of the VA Persian Gulf Registry and Uniform Case Assessment Protocol*, Institute of Medicine, National Academy Press, Washington, D.C., 1998, pp. 23–26.

For an analysis of the diagnoses in the Defense Department registry, particularly the diagnoses in the SSID category, see "Signs, Symptoms, and Ill-Defined Conditions in Persian Gulf War Veterans: Findings from the Comprehensive Clinical Evaluation Program," Michael J. Roy et al., *Psychosomatic Medicine*, vol. 60, 1998, pp. 663–668. A more general treatment of the CCEP diagnoses is contained in *Adequacy of the Comprehensive Clinical Evaluation Program: A Focused Assessment*, Institute of Medicine, National Academy Press, Washington, D.C., 1997.

Page 125 Representative Kennedy's "guinea pig" charge at the June 1993 hearing raised questions about the vaccinations and drugs administered to the troops during the war. Most of the vaccines and drugs that were used by the military were standard, but some were not. As the health controversy mounted, three agents came under suspicion.

According to the Final Report by the Presidential Advisory Committee on Gulf War Veterans' Illnesses, 150,000 of the troops received anthrax vaccinations during the war, and 8,000 troops got botulinum-toxoid (BT) vaccinations. The two shots were meant to defend against Iraqi biological weapons. In addition, approximately 250,000 of the troops took pyridostigmine bromide (PB) pills as a protection against nerve gas, more about which on p. 149 and pp. 384–386. Because record keeping was poor, the exact number and amount of the doses of the three medicines are unknown.

At the time of the conflict the anthrax shots had full approval from the Food and Drug Administration. However, PB and BT were classed as "investigational new drugs." Obtaining a waiver of procedure from FDA, the Pentagon was able to order its soldiers to take the latter two medicines without their informed consent—hence "guinea pig." The Pentagon was supposed to follow up with the FDA about the effects of medicines, but did not.

Although the presidential panel and other scientific reviewers concluded that the injections and the pills were unlikely to be factors in the veterans' illnesses, doubts have persisted among the veterans and their supporters. One result was that throughout the 1990s numerous incidents of active duty personnel refusing to submit to anthrax vaccinations.

Basic resources on this question: For the Kennedy hearing: "Persian Gulf War Veterans and Related Issues," Hearing before the Subcommittee on Oversight and Investigations of the Committee on Veterans' Affairs, U.S. House of Representatives, First Session, June 9, 1993, Serial No. 103-17, U.S. Government Printing Office, Washington, D.C., 1994. On the administration of shots and pills: Presidential Advisory Committee on Gulf War Veterans' Illnesses: Final Report, U.S. Government Printing Office, Washington, D.C., December, 1996, pp. 18, 98, 112–117. On the FDA-Pentagon arrangement: "Changing the Consent Rules for Desert Storm," G. J. Annas, *New England Journal of Medicine*, vol. 326, 1992, pp. 770–773 and "Military Use of Drugs Not Yet Approved by the FDA for CW/BW Defense: Lessons from the Gulf War," Richard A. Rettig, prepared for the Office of the Secretary of Defense by RAND's National Defense Research Institute, Washington, D.C., 1999.

As for toxic interactions, the idea that the medicines in combination with environmental chemicals may have caused harm, a scientific review, *Interactions of Drugs, Biologics, and Chemicals in U.S. Military Forces*, the Institute of Medicine, National Academy Press, Washington, D.C., 1996, stated that little was known about the interactions between the prophylactic drugs and other Persian Gulf exposures, but that there was no basis for "extraordinary concern." A much tougher assessment is contained in "Gulf War Veterans' Illnesses: VA, DOD Continue to Resist Strong Evidence Linking Toxic Causes to Chronic Health Effects," Second Report by the Committee on Government Reform and Oversight, U.S. House of Representatives, Report 105-388, Washington, D.C., November 1997.

Finally, a persistent allegation about the vaccination program is that an adjuvant called squalene was in the vaccines and caused auto-immune reactions. The Pentagon has long denied that squalene, a natural substance, was used as a vaccine adjuvant, or booster, before the Persian Gulf War deployment. But in 2000, after a Tulane University researcher claimed to have found antibodies to squalene in veterans' blood, the Pentagon promised to review the issue. See the 1996 official report on squalene at www.gulflink.osd.mil/finalrpt.html, and the subsequent review proposal, "Development and Validation of an Assay to Test for the Presence of Squalene Antibodies,"

Department of Defense, Washington, D.C., January 1, 2000. For darkly suspicious reporing on the squalene affair, see: "The Pentagon's Toxic Secret," Gary Matsumoto, *Vanity Fair*, May 1999, and numerous articles by Paul M. Rodriguez of *Insight Magazine* (www.insightmag.com).

Page 126 Blanck's statement about CFS is from the June 1993 House Veterans' Affairs subcommittee hearing, op. cit., p. 119.

Pages 127–129 My treatment of chronic fatigue syndrome is based upon three texts: *Fighting and Facing Fatigue: A Practical Approach*, Benjamin H. Natelson, Yale University Press, New Haven, 1998; *Osler's Web: Inside the Labyrinth of the Chronic Fatigue Syndrome Epidemic*, Hillary Johnson, Crown Publishers, Inc., New York, 1996; and *Chronic Fatigue Syndrome*, ed. Stephen E. Straus, Marcel Dekker, Inc., New York, 1994. If Straus and Johnson represent two ends of the spectrum of opinion on the nature and causation of CFS, Natelson is at the center.

Also, I recommend any publications on this subject by William Reeves, M.D., of the U.S. Centers for Disease Control; Dedra Buchwald, M.D., of the University of Washington; and the British psychiatrist Simon Wessely. These three not only are recognized for their expertise on CFS but also have explored the connection between CFS and the gulf war illnesses (as has Natelson).

For CFS prevalence in America see the estimates posted on the CDC Website (www.cdc.gov/ncidod/diseases/cfs/cfshome.html) and the research paper "A Community-Based Study of Chronic Fatigue Syndrome," L. A. Jason, J. A. Richman, A. W. Rademacher, et al., *Archives of Internal Medicine*, vol. 159, 1999, pp. 2129–2137.

Here are the 1988 (a) and 1994 (b) case definitions of CFS as promulgated in the medical literature, summarized by Natelson, op. cit., and edited by me for clarity.

(a) "Chronic Fatigue Syndrome: A Working Case Definition," G. P. Holmes et al., *Annals of Internal Medicine*, vol. 108, 1988, pp. 387–389.
• Major criteria for diagnosis:
1. Persisting or relapsing fatigue or easy fatigability that does not involve bed rest and is severe enough to reduce daily activity by at least 50 percent.
2. Other chronic clinical conditions have been excluded, including preexisting psychiatric diseases.
• Minor criteria:
Report of at least eight of the following symptoms, which must persist or recur for at least six months:
1. Mild fever (99.5 degrees to 101.5 degrees oral) or chills
2. Sore throat
3. Painful lymph nodes in front or back of the neck or under the arms
4. Unexplained, generalized muscle weakness
5. Muscle discomfort or myalgia
6. Prolonged (more than twenty-four hours) generalized fatigue following previously tolerable levels of exercise
7. New, generalized headaches
8. Pain in more than one joint without redness or swelling
9. Neuropsychological symptoms (one or more of the following)
   a. Photophobia [a painful sensitivity to strong light]
   b. Brief periods of blind spots in vision
   c. Forgetfulness

d. Excessive irritability

e. Confusion

f. Difficulty in thinking

g. Inability to concentrate

h. Depression (following illness onset)

10. Sleep disturbance (hypersomnia or insomnia)

11. Illness onset occurring over hours to a few days (sudden onset)

(b) "The Chronic Fatigue Syndrome: A Comprehensive Approach to Its Definition and Study," K. Fukuda et al., *Annals of Internal Medicine*, vol. 121, 1994, pp. 953–959.

• Diagnostic criteria:

Medically unexplained, persistent or relapsing chronic fatigue that is of new or definite onset; that is not due to exertion and is not relieved by rest; and that results in substantial reduction in previous levels of occupational, educational, social, or personal activities.

• Reported along with four or more of the following symptoms, which must have persisted or recurred for at least six months and not have predated the fatigue:

1. Severe impairment in short-term memory or concentration

2. Painful lymph nodes in front or back of the neck or under the arms

3. Sore throat

4. Muscle pain

5. Pain in more than one joint without redness or swelling

6. Headaches of a new type

7. Unrefreshing sleep

8. Postexertional malaise lasting more than twenty-four hours

As in the 1988 definition, other chronic physiological and psychological conditions must have been ruled out, including major depression (past or present) and substance abuse. Note that in the 1994 definition five of the eight minor criteria refer to pain in some way, reinforcing the connection to the pain-based syndrome called fibromyalgia.

Page 130 The information paper by Blanck and his staff on the Czech detections of nerve gas was entered into the record of a Senate hearing chaired by Alabama's Shelby on June 30, 1993. See: "Department of Defense Authorization for Appropriations for Fiscal Year 1994 and the Future Years Defense Program: Force Requirements and Personnel, May–June 1993," Hearings before the Committee on Armed Services, U.S. Senate, No. 103-3-3, Part 6, May–June 1993, U.S. Government Printing Office, Washington, D.C., 1994, p. 549. A month later came the newspaper revelation: "Czech Claim of Gulf Gas Confirmed," Dave Parks, *Birmingham News*, July 29, 1993. According to Parks (personal communication), the very first mention of the Czech detections was in January 1991, in a column by Arnaud de Borchgrave in the *Washington* (D.C.) *Times*. Given the other news from the ongoing war, the significance of the detections was missed.

James Tuite's report was "Gulf War Syndrome: The Case for Multiple Origin Mixed Chemical/Biotoxin Warfare Related Disorders," staff report to U.S. Senator Donald W. Riegle Jr., U.S. Senate, Washington, D.C., September 9, 1993.

Page 132 About the critics of the Persian Gulf Health Registry: Pentagon adviser Dr. Lewis Kuller was chair of the Department of Epidemiology, School of Public Health, at the University of Pittsburgh. His statements can be found in "The Possible Adverse Health Effects of Service in the Persian Gulf; and H.R. 5864, To Establish a Persian Gulf War Veterans Registry," Hearing before the Subcommittee on Hospitals and Health Care of the Committee on Veterans' Affairs, U.S. House of Representatives, September 16, 1992, Serial No. 102-49, U.S. Government Printing Office, Washington, D.C., 1992, pp. 15, 25. The IOM comments on the registry are from *Health Consequences of Service During the Persian Gulf War: Initial Findings and Recommendations for Immediate Action*, Institute of Medicine, Committee to Review the Health Consequences of Service during the Persian Gulf War, National Academy Press, January 1995, p. 8. See also pp. 22–23. The criticism by Dr. Robert Haley is from a prepared statement that he submitted to the Subcommittee on Human Resources of the Committee on Government Reform and Oversight (since changed to the Subcommittee on National Security, Veterans' Affairs and International Relations), U.S. House of Representatives, prior to his appearance before the subcommittee on Feb. 24, 1998.

Pages 133-134 Regarding the number of malignant lymphomas in the PGHR, the VA public affairs office told me that the agency has three diagnostic categories covering this condition: "lymphoma and reticulosarcoma," "Hodgkin's disease," and "other lymphomas." Through June 1998 the registry recorded a total of 57 cases among 68,726 participants. Hence 0.08 percent. My source for the national incidence of lymphoma is the Leukemia Society of America, Washington, D.C. Informed that the number of cases in the United States was 450,000, I figured them as a percentage of the U.S. population of 270 million. Hence a figure of less than 0.2 percent.

As for the overall cancer incidence in gulf war vets, the General Accounting Office, the investigative arm of Congress, issued a report in March 1998. The GAO noted: "The number of registry veterans with a primary diagnosis of a malignant or benign tumor is very small, less than 1 percent." However, in keeping with the GAO's persistent skepticism of VA and DoD findings, the report's authors added: "The suitability of the registries for assessing cancer incidence is extremely limited. As designed, the registries are not intended to be used to determine the frequency and causes of illnesses among the general Gulf War veteran population." Source: "Gulf War Veterans: Incidence of Tumors Cannot Be Reliably Determined From Available Data," U.S. General Accounting Office, GAO/NSIAD-98-89, Washington, D.C., March 1998.

Nick Roberts's account of his cancer is taken mainly from his prepared statement to the Subcommittee on Human Resources and Intergovernment Relations of the Committee on Government Reform and Oversight, U.S. House of Representatives, at a hearing in Washington, D.C., on September 19, 1996. That his disease was missed by the VA was confirmed in a personal communication by a VA doctor who wished to be unnamed.

Two examples of the media attention to the Roberts case: The veteran was featured in the *Hartford Courant* on October 6, 1993. The story, by Thomas D. Williams, was titled "Gas Mask Effectiveness Questioned." He was also the main character in a *GQ* magazine article, "Dying for Their Country," Mary A. Fischer, May 1994.

Pages 134–135 The IOM committee's final report was *Health Consequences of Service during the Persian Gulf War: Recommendations for Research and Information Systems*, Institute of Medicine, National Academy Press, Washington, D.C., October 1996. The quotation that contrasts individual stories with epidemiologic analysis appears on p. 5.

Not just journalists favored the individuals' stories. Congress, and particularly the House committee headed by Connecticut Representative Christopher Shays, championed the veterans' explanations of their illnesses over the scientific accounts. According to a report by the Shays committee: "Absent precise exposure data which can never be recaptured, the best evidence linking toxic exposures to chronic effects lies within the bodies and minds of Gulf War veterans. That evidence has been too long ignored." Source: "VA, DOD Continue to Resist Strong Evidence Linking Toxic Causes to Chronic Health Effects," Second Report by the Committee on Government Reform and Oversight, U.S. House of Representatives, Report 105-388, November 1997, p. 3.

Pages 136–138 Three reports inform my analysis of the demographics of gulf war veterans: "Unexplained Illnesses among Desert Storm Veterans: A Search for Causes, Treatment, and Cooperation," Persian Gulf Veterans Coordinating Board, *Archives of Internal Medicine*, vol. 155, February 13, 1995; pp. 262–268; "Consolidation and Combined Analysis of the Databases of the Department of Veterans Affairs Persian Gulf Health Registry and the Department of Defense Comprehensive Clinical Evaluation Program," Environmental Epidemiology Service, Department of Veterans Affairs, March 1998; and "Gulf War Veterans' Health Registries: Who Is Most Likely to Seek Evaluation?," Gregory C. Gray et al., *American Journal of Epidemiology*, vol. 48, no. 4, 1998, pp. 343–349. Where the statistics in these reports differ, I have used those provided by Gray et al.

In addition to Gray, Richard Miller of the Medical Follow-up Agency, Institute of Medicine, National Academy of Sciences, collected data on "Illness and Health Care Seeking in Persian Gulf War Veterans Prior to Deployment." At an Institute of Medicine workshop in July 1998, Miller reported his preliminary findings: "Persian Gulf War veterans who sought health care . . . in the 12 months prior had a higher risk of being on the Persian Gulf health registry with unexplained illnesses."

Gray found the risk of illness (as measured by health registry participation) to be greatest for those who served during combat, but a smaller study by VA-funded researchers of veterans in the Pacific Northwest found no differences in gulf war symptoms according to the time of deployment. Those who were posted pre- and postcombat had as many unexplained illnesses as combat-phase soldiers. The authors noted that this finding weakened the argument that chemical exposures made veterans sick because, since most such exposures occurred during the combat period, one would expect that troops posted during that period would be sicker. Instead, those who served afterward, like Carol, tended to be more symptomatic. See: "U.S. Gulf War Veterans: Service Periods in Theater, Differential Exposures, and Persistent Unexplained Illness," Peter S. Spencer et al., *Toxicology Letters*, vols. 102–103, 1998, pp. 515–521. A similar finding—that time of deployment made no difference to the risk of symptoms—was derived by Centers for Disease Control researchers. Their paper: "Deployment Stressors and a Chronic Multisymptom Condition among Gulf War Veterans," R. Nisenbaum et al., *Journal of Nervous & Mental Disorders* (in press).

Pages 139–142 Much of my treatment of fibromyalgia (FM) is based upon the transcript of a 1997 meeting of an Institute of Medicine committee advising the Pentagon on the gulf war illnesses. The committee heard presentations from experts on chronic fatigue syndrome and multiple chemical sensitivity as well as on fibromyalgia. The speakers on FM specifically were Frederick Wolfe, M.D., of the University of Kansas; Robert Simms, M.D., of Boston University School of Medicine; and Daniel Clauw, M.D., of Georgetown University in Washington, D.C. The unpublished transcript: *Committee Meeting on Difficult to Diagnose and Ill-Defined Conditions*, Committee on the Evaluation of the DoD Comprehensive Clinical Evaluation Program, Institute of Medicine, National Academy of Sciences, Washington, D.C., March 3, 1997.

The case definition for FM can be found in "The American College of Rheumatology 1990 Criteria for the Classification of Fibromyalgia: Report of the Multicenter Criteria Committee," F. Wolfe et al., *Arthritis and Rheumatism*, vol. 33, 1990, pp. 160–172.

Other instructive medical articles, some by FM skeptics: "Fibromyalgia Syndrome: New Research on an Old Malady," M. B. Yunus, *British Medical Journal*, vol. 298, 1989, pp. 474–475; "Comorbidity of Fibromyalgia with Medical and Psychiatric Disorders," J. Hudson et al., *American Journal of Medicine*, vol. 92, 1992, pp. 363–367; "Fibromyalgia Syndrome, a Problem of Tautology," Milton L. Cohen and John L. Quintner, *Lancet*, vol. 342, October 9, 1993, pp. 906–909; *Evaluation and Treatment of Myopathies*, Robert C. Griggs, Jerry R. Mandell and Robert G. Miller, F.A. Davis, Philadelphia, 1995, pp. 395–398; "Fibromyalgia: More Than Just a Musculoskeletal Disease," D. J. Clauw, *American Family Physician*, vol. 52, 1995, pp. 843–851; "The Prevalence and Characteristics of Fibromyalgia in the General Population," F. Wolfe et al., *Arthritis and Rheumatism*, vol. 38, 1995, pp. 19–28; "Problems with Myofascial Pain Syndrome and Fibromyalgia Syndrome," editorial, Thomas Bohr, M.D., *Neurology*, vol. 46, March 1996, pp. 593–597.

Page 142 Here is a sampling of the research on the overlap of the FM, CFS, and MCS conditions: "The Chronic Fatigue Syndrome: Definition, Current Studies and Lessons for Fibromyalgia Research," Anthony L. Komaroff and Don Goldenberg, *Journal of Rheumatology*, Supplement 19, vol. 16, 1989, pp. 23–27; "High Frequency of Fibromyalgia in Patients with Chronic Fatigue Seen in a Primary Care Practice," D. L. Goldenberg et al., *Arthritis and Rheumatism*, vol. 33, 1990, pp. 381–387; "Fibromyalgia, Chronic Fatigue Syndrome, and Myofascial Pain Syndrome," Don L. Goldenberg, *Current Opinion in Rheumatology*, vol. 5, 1993, pp. 199–208; "Comparison of Patients with Chronic Fatigue Syndrome, Fibromyalgia, and Multiple Chemical Sensitivities," Dedra Buchwald and Deborah Garrity, *Archives of Internal Medicine*, vol. 154, Sept. 26, 1994, pp. 2049–2053; "Chronic Fatigue, Fibromyalgia, and Chemical Sensitivity: Overlapping Disorders," letter, Grace Ziem and Albert Donnay, *Archives of Internal Medicine*, vol. 155, 1995, p. 1913; "A Controlled Comparison of Multiple Chemical Sensitivities and Chronic Fatigue Syndrome," Nancy Fiedler, Howard Kipen et al., in *Psychosomatic Medicine*, vol. 58, 1996, pp. 38–49; "Chronic Pain and Fatigue Syndromes: Overlapping Clinical and Neuroendocrine Features and Potential Pathogenic Mechanisms," Daniel J. Clauw and George P. Chrousos, *Neuroimmunomodulation*, vol. 4, 1997, pp. 134–153.

The increasing recognition of the overlap has boosted the stature of MCS in medical circles. In April 1999 the American College of Occupational and Environmental Medicine, which took a hard line against MCS in 1991, modified its stance as follows: "Research has noted overlap between MCS, chronic fatigue syndrome, fibromyalgia and other historic non-specific conditions. Survey data suggest that odor related symptoms are common in the general population. Less clear from these studies, however, is the extent and prevalence of disability associated with these symptoms. The prevalence of pre-existing and concurrent psychiatric disease remains highly controversial. Research suggests an excess of symptoms of psychological distress consistent with anxiety and depression in many, but not all MCS patients. One of the best-designed studies points to an excess of premorbid somatic complaints in some MCS patients. Evidence also supports an etiologic role for conditioned response. MCS research, however, will not finally dissect psychologic and physiologic effects. Indeed, modern medicine no longer supports a mind-body dichotomy." See the full ACOEM position statement at: www.acoem.org/paprguid/papers/mcs.htm

Page 143 Of the "odd or rare" conditions associated with gulf war syndrome, the oddest, if not the rarest, was burning semen. Couples reported that the male veteran's semen burned the woman's skin or greatly irritated her vagina, and sometimes the man felt it too, so that intercourse became difficult or impossible. It was feared that the semen had been made toxic. Eventually the Defense Department funded a University of Cincinnati immunologist, Jonathan Bernstein, to look into the problem. Couples were solicited for a study of "burning semen syndrome" through the Internet and other means.

Bernstein suspected that burning semen syndrome was a variant of seminal plasma hypersensitivity—an allergic reaction to proteins in the seminal fluid. It occurs in the civilian populace and affects both men and women. The physician enlisted a dozen civilian couples reporting hypersensitivity symptoms and compared them to ten gulf war couples, testing the skin for sensitivity and the blood for antibodies to the proteins and performing other examinations. The results from the two groups were not identical but were close enough for him to conclude that symptoms of the gulf war pairs were not unique. Vaginal infections and vulvar pain, in addition to the hypersensitivity problem, occurred in both groups. See: "Localized Human Seminal Plasma Hypersensitivity: A Potential Model for Gulf War 'Burning Semen Syndrome,' " J. A. Bernstein et al., *Fundamental and Applied Toxicology*, vol. 36, 1997, p. 201, and "Specific Antibody Responses in Civilian Couples with Seminal Plasma Protein Hypersensitivity and Gulf War Couples with Burning Semen Syndrome," J. A. Bernstein et al., Program and Abstract Book, Conference on Federally Sponsored Gulf War Veterans' Illnesses Research, Research Working Group, Persian Gulf Veterans Coordinating Board, Washington, D.C., June 23–25, 1999.

If burning semen represented a direct transmission from the sick person to his spouse, other symptoms were said to be conveyed also—such as fatigue and pain and confusion—but no one could tell how. The government said there was no evidence for the infectiousness of gulf war illness, but the matter was never studied directly, probably because the government had a hard enough time identifying the condition in the vets themselves. Outside investigators, led by Garth Nicolson (see pp. 387–388), proposed infectious agents, but at this writing none have been confirmed.

At the behest of Congress, the VA and Defense Department invited the spouses and children of sick veterans to come in for health exams, and over the years about two thousand have done so. Analysis of the pattern of their symptoms is still pending. As part of its much-delayed National Health Survey, the VA investigated whether gulf war veterans' families had more sickness than the families of other military personnel. Analysis of the data is still out. Meanwhile, the concern over contagiousness within families has faded.

The question of birth defects in the newborns of veterans was a more straightforward issue, it seemed, since birth defects could be counted, categorized, and compared to occurrences in other groups, both military and civilian. However, the incidence of birth defects "normally" was between 3 and 6 percent, depending on the kinds of malformations that were included, and what prompted them was unclear. To tie a birth defect to an environmental exposure in the Gulf was a tall order. Proven teratogens (agents known to cause malformations in humans, such as thalidomide and ionizing radiation) were few, and the exposure, whatever it might be, had to be high.

When the reproductive health issue first arose, in 1993, the Pentagon looked at the outcomes of pregnancies at several military hospitals and found no differences in miscarriages and birth abnormalities between the deployed and nondeployed veterans. In 1994 the Mississippi Department of Health, working with the federal Centers for Disease Control, found "no evidence of increase in birth defects and health problems among children born to Persian Gulf War veterans in Mississippi." A scientific paper with that title appeared later in a medical journal. (Op. cit., Alan Penman and Russell Tarver, *Military Medicine*, vol. 161, January 1996, pp. 1–6.)

Journalists published their own investigations. For example, in November 1995 *Life* magazine ran a sensational article, "The Tiny Victims of Desert Storm," depicting several families torn by the births of damaged children. The Mississippi study, which was the only epidemiology that was then available, was not mentioned in the article.

Also in 1995, several large reproductive surveys were commenced under the direction of Navy epidemiologist Gregory Gray at the Naval Health Research Center in San Diego. The results were slow in coming but consistent. The first study to appear, "A Records-Based Evaluation of the Risk of Birth Defects among Children of Gulf War Veterans" (D. N. Cowan et al., *New England Journal of Medicine*, vol. 336, 1997, pp. 1650–1656), examined records of sixty thousand births in military hospitals through the fall of '93, and found no increase in the risk of defects in the gulf war group.

In the *Life* article and elsewhere, cases of Goldenhar syndrome, a particularly unfortunate disfigurement, were reported to be excessive. The claim about Goldenhar prompted an inquiry by the navy researchers, and the results were equivocal. Among seventy-five thousand births sampled, there were five cases of Goldenhar syndrome reported in offspring of the war-deployed group and two cases in the nondeployed group, which, for a Persian Gulf parent, amounted to a threefold higher risk of producing a child with this deformity. Yet because the cases overall were so few, the results of the study were not "statistically significant," and the risk could have been due to chance. See "Goldenhar Syndrome among Infants Born in Military Hospitals to Gulf War Veterans," Maria Rosario G. Araneta et al., *Teratology*, vol. 56, 1997, pp. 244–251. Recently the same team published "Birth Defects Prevalence among Infants of Persian Gulf War Veterans Born in Hawaii, 1989–1993," Maria Rosario G. Araneta et al., *Teratology*, vol. 62, 2000, pp. 195–204. Higher rates of birth defects were not found.

The cases of amyotrophic lateral sclerosis (Lou Gehrig's disease), a ravaging and fatal neurological condition, were not epidemic but appeared to make a cluster in the wake of the war. Families of the sick pressed forward with their stories, and more than one veteran with ALS was brought to Capitol Hill to testify. By 1999, the Pentagon and VA had ascertained that at least twenty-eight veterans had contracted ALS. Twenty-eight cases in seven hundred thousand people was at the upper threshold of the background rate of ALS, and the veterans contracted the condition at a younger age than others. Was it because of toxic exposures?

The VA and Pentagon eventually assigned the problem to an epidemiologist at the Durham (N.C.) VA Medical Center, Dr. Ron Horner, who sought to determine whether the rate of ALS in veterans was truly unusual. Not being able to track down and quiz everyone who had gone to the war, Horner had to rely on reports of ALS that were relayed to him. Announcements of the study were disseminated, and cases additional to the twenty-eight, if any were out there, were solicited. The plan was to compare all the verified cases to those of ALS in a comparable military population. Horner hoped to have results sometime in 2001. A preliminary review of the records of active duty military members found that the rate of ALS in the component that served in the Gulf was not elevated. For accounts of the ALS controversy, see: "Lou Gehrig's Disease Claims Gulf Veterans," David Brown, *Washington Post*, August 3, 1999, p. A3; "Veterans Link Lou Gehrig's Disease to the Gulf War," John Hanchette and Norm Brewer, Gannett News Service (*USA Today*), December 11, 1998; "Persian Gulf Veterans with ALS: Report of a Review Panel," Department of Veterans Affairs, Washington, D.C., January 18–19, 1999.

Death was the bottom line of the gulf war health issue, if not publicly discussed. Because many veterans thought their health was only getting worse, they looked down the road fearfully. Statistically it was found that the veterans were not dying at higher rates than normal. In fact, gulf war vets were proving to be hardier than most Americans. Some epidemiologists disputed the comparison, saying that military personnel were inherently healthier than average Americans because the standards for enlistment and service were stricter than in other walks of life. A better comparison was to other groups of military personnel. Given that restriction, those who *hadn't* served in the Gulf showed a lower likelihood of death in the postwar years than the deployed group did.

The reason that gulf war vets died unusually was that they had more fatal auto accidents than their peers, not because of any wasting disease or mysterious syndrome. Moreover, the female veterans had a higher risk of suicide than their military counterparts. A number of researchers noted that in prior wars, particularly the Vietnam War, there was a significant increase in the rates of fatal auto accidents and suicides. Homicides were also more frequent among female vets than among males. Still, I must emphasize that death was a rare development because the cohort on the whole was young.

See on this question: "Mortality among U.S. Veterans of the Persian Gulf War," Han K. Kang and Tim A. Bullman, *New England Journal of Medicine*, vol. 335, no. 20, November 14, 1996, pp. 1498–1504; "Mortality among U.S. Veterans of the Persian Gulf War: First Update through December, 1995," Kang and Bullman, Environmental Epidemiology Service, Department of Veterans Affairs, Washington, D.C., February 1998; "Mortality Among U.S. Veterans of the Persian Gulf War: Update Through December, 1997," Kang and Bullman, Environmental Epidemiology Service, Department of Veterans Affairs, Washington, D.C., June 1999; "Gulf War Illnesses: Causation and Treatment," Michael J. Hodgson and Howard M. Kipen, *Journal of Occupational and Environmental Medicine*, vol. 41, no. 6, 1999, pp. 443–452.

Page 144 General Blanck did not find comparable illnesses when he went abroad in late 1993 and early 1994, but illnesses were starting among troops belonging to the allied coalition. The phenomenon was spotty. The British, Canadians, Danes, Czechs, and Slovaks eventually reported gulf war symptoms, while the French and the Arabs did not.

Czechoslovakia, which had sent military technicians to Saudi Arabia, split into two countries following the war. The Czechs and Slovaks became concerned about illness because their personnel had made detections of chemical warfare agents. Several hundred men were rumored to be sick. Bernard Rostker, special assistant to the deputy secretary of defense for gulf war illnesses, visited the Czech Republic in 1997. Subsequently he told reporters that 150 men from the detection units had been examined, and "about six" had unexplained illnesses—about the same proportion as in the much larger U.S. force. See: "Coalition Chemical Detections and Health of Coalition Troops in Detection Area," Department of Defense, August 5, 1996, www.gulflink.osd.mil/coalitn.html; "Slovakia Joins in Screening of Its Gulf War Veterans," *New York Times*, November 30, 1996, p. 7; DoD News Briefing (Rostker statement), January 8, 1998, www.defenselink.mil/news/Jan1998/t01121998_t0108gwi.html.

In Britain the Ministry of Defence started a medical assessment program for its fifty-three thousand veterans at the end of 1993. British troops reported the most illnesses after the Americans, but the government denied the need for epidemiologic studies until late 1996. Then, with funding from the U.S. Defense Department, a research team took a measure of the problem.

In a random survey, about three thousand British veterans were compared to two other military groups of similar size: personnel who were not deployed to the Gulf and peacekeepers sent to Bosnia between 1992 and 1997. As in the U.S., the gulf war vets reported symptoms and disorders more frequently than their peers. They had more headache, chest pain, fatigue, anger, depression, sleeplessness, etc., among the symptoms, as well as more arthritis, back problems, migraines and ear infections. Gulf vets in the U.K.were three times more likely than those who were not deployed to fulfill criteria for CFS, PTSD and the multisystem illness proposed by the U.S. Centers for Disease Control (see p. 187). They were twice as likely meet those criteria as the Bosnia servicemen were. Men who were sick remembered being exposed to oil smoke; they recalled side effects of multiple vaccinations; they said they had been in chemical warfare incidents. In short, the British experience remarkably paralleled the U.S. experience. Sources: "Health of UK Servicemen Who Served in Persian Gulf War," Catherine Unwin et al., *Lancet*, vol. 353, January 16, 1999, pp. 169–178; "Is There a Gulf War Syndrome?," Khalida Ismail et al., *Lancet*, vol. 353, January 16, 1999, pp. 179–182; "Britain to Check Veterans for Gulf War Problems," Warren Hoge, *New York Times*, December 11, 1996; "A Review of Gulf War Illness," W. J. Coker, *Journal of the Royal Navy Medical Service*, vol. 82, 1996, pp. 141–146.

In 1997 Canadian epidemiologists surveyed nine thousand veterans, attempting to contact all who had served during the war for Canada. Deployed troops had about twice as many symptoms as nondeployed troops. There were significantly higher rates of fibromyalgia symptoms, chronic fatigue, depression, PTSD, MCS, asthma, cognitive dysfunction and respiratory conditions—again, all by self-report.

The Canadian researchers concluded that psychological stress was a more important factor than any toxic exposures in the theater. Their study had included a de facto test of the possible effects of the special pills, shots, oil smoke, etc. Two navy crews addressed by the survey had served on the same warship during the conflict. The first crew returned home before Christmas 1990, during the buildup phase of the war, and the second crew, replacing the first, served during the period of combat. Only the second group of men received special shots and pills; only they were exposed to oil smoke and whatever else was in the air, possibly even traces of nerve gas. Yet there was no difference between the two groups in their increased prevalence of symptoms. Their health reports looked alike. The one exposure that the two groups had in common was psychological stress. See: *Health Study of Canadian Forces Personnel Involved in the 1991 Conflict in the Persian Gulf*, vol. 1, Goss Gilroy Inc., Ottawa, Ontario, April 1998. The naval task force analysis is summarized on pp. 58–59.

Danish researchers, in a series of papers on the health experience of their troops, determined that deployed veterans were more symptomatic than nondeployed. Danish vets had the same fatigue, pain, diarrhea, etc. as the Americans, British, and Canadians. But most Danish troops were posted after the war as peacekeepers, when the environmental hazards were much reduced. To the study authors this suggested "risk factors independent of war action." See: "The Danish Gulf War Study," T. Ishoy, P. Suadicani et al., *Danish Medical Bulletin*, vol. 46, no. 5, November 1999, pp. 416–427 (three papers).

On the world stage the French often act contrariwise to the Americans and British. So too with the gulf war illnesses. For years the French Ministry of Defense insisted that none of its Persian Gulf veterans had symptoms that might be connected to chemical exposures during the war, nor did their troops report any unusual illnesses. Critics in the United States argued that this was because French soldiers did not take pyridostigmine bromide pills, the nerve gas prophylactic. But two U.S. officials, Rostker and Rear Admiral (Retired) Alan Steinman, said they were told by

French military authorities that some of their personnel did in fact use the PB pills. See: "Coalition Chemical Detections and Health of Coalition Troops in Detection Area," Department of Defense, August 5, 1996, www.gulflink.osd.mil/coalitn.html; DoD News Briefing (Rostker statement), January 8, 1998, www.defenselink.mil/news/Jan1998/t01121998_t0108gwi.html; Hearing of the Special Oversight Board for Department of Defense Investigations of Gulf War Chemical and Biological Incidents (Steinman statement), Arlington, Va., June 22, 1999, www.oversight.ncr.gov/hal.htm.

As for the Arab nations allied with the U.S., medical officials in Kuwait told Rostker in late 1997 that there were no unusual conditions being reported by their population. But there was said to be a rise in asthma and other respiratory conditions, presumably as a consequence of the oil smoke. Egypt reported no health problems among its troops, although all since had left the military. Source: "Middle East Trip Provides Useful Information Exchange," Department of Defense news release, Washington, D.C., January 27, 1988, available at www.gulflink.osd.mil.

Nor did the Saudi Arabian forces attest to any health problems. In 1998 the Saudis permitted U.S. epidemiologists to review hospitalization records of the Saudi National Guardsmen who were on duty during the gulf war. Since these records antedated the war, the object was to see whether changes had occurred following the conflict in hospital admissions or diagnoses. Results of the study are pending.

From Iraq came numerous anecdotal reports that people were suffering more diseases and birth defects because of toxic substances loosed by the war. None of these reports could be confirmed.

In early 2000 Australia announced that it was commencing a health study of its eighteen hundred veterans of the gulf war. The study was prompted by veterans' concerns.

Finally the French succumbed. In September 2000, according to a news report by Reuters, the French defense minister announced the creation of a panel to study the health of its gulf war soldiers. About eighty veterans had come forward and were said to be suffering from "mysterious illnesses ranging from flu to chronic fatigue and asthma."

Page 144 The first veterans acquiring the CFS, FM, and MCS labels were from the VA's referral center population. Fewer than one hundred vets had gone through the special program as of early 1994, but diagnoses of CFS, FM, and MCS had been made in almost half the cases. The MCS quotient stemmed from Claudia Miller's affiliation with the Houston VAMC referral center. See: "Veterans Seeking Answers to Syndrome Suspect They Were Goats in Gulf War," Paul Cotton, *Journal of the American Medical Association*, May 25, 1994, and the minutes of the February 22–23, 1994, meeting of the Persian Gulf Expert Scientific Committee, Department of Veterans Affairs, Washington, D.C.

The VA had the dual task of defining CFS and FM for its practitioners and formulating regulations to govern compensation claims for the conditions. In November 1993 VA Secretary Jesse Brown said that CFS would be compensable if it was found to be connected to gulf war service. The department published a diagnostic code for CFS in the fall of 1994, and for FM a little later, but the regulations on service-connected compensation did not appear until 1996. The Defense Department passed along definitions for CFS and FM to its clinicians in March 1995.

Pages 144–145 For the official report of the NIH conference, see "The Persian Gulf Experience and Health," NIH Technology Assessment Workshop Panel, *Journal of the American Medical Association*, August 3, 1994, pp. 391–396. The anticipatory story in the press was " 'Agent Orange All Over Again,' Veterans Charge," John Ritter, *USA Today*, April 27, 1994.

Dr. Grace Ziem, who treated MCS patients and had added gulf war vets to her practice, contacted General Blanck and Jay Sanford on the eve of the NIH conference. "Of greatest concern to me," Ziem wrote, "is that a new syndrome—Gulf War Syndrome, in this case—not be defined unless no other existing diagnosis can account for the symptoms. . . ." To Ziem the existing diagnosis that was available was MCS, and she recommended changes in the Sanford definition to make it conform with her construction of the condition. Her letter, available from MCS Referral and Resources (www.mcsrr.org), listed the many agencies of government that had recognized MCS, even if U.S. medical associations did not.

At the workshop itself Myra Shayevitz, an M.D. at the Northampton (Mass.) VAMC, reported some success in treating gulf war vets with methods similar to Ziem's. Also making strong presentations on behalf of MCS were Dr. Claudia Miller and the head of the Desert Storm Veterans Association, Betty Zuspann.

Pages 145–146 The Senate Banking Committee report was "U.S. Chemical and Biological Warfare-Related Dual Use Exports to Iraq and Their Possible Impact on the Health Consequences of the Persian Gulf War," a report of Chairman Donald W. Riegle, Jr., and Ranking Member Alfonse M. D'Amato of the Committee on Banking, Housing and Urban Affairs with respect to Export Administration, U.S. Senate, May 25, 1994. The comment about exposures that were not specific to the war is on p. 151. My transcript of the committee hearing was obtained from a Web page, the Tuite Reports, carrying postings by and about Jim Tuite: www.chronicillnet.org/PGWS/tuite/hearings.html.

Pages 146–147 The official name of the Lederberg report is "Report of the Defense Science Board Task Force on Persian Gulf War Health Effects," Office of the Under Secretary of Defense for Acquisition and Technology, Washington, D.C., June 1994.

Page 147 Tuite's third report for Riegle was "U.S. Chemical and Biological Exports to Iraq and Their Possible Impact on the Health Consequences of the Persian Gulf War, Committee Staff Report No. 3: Chemical Warfare Agent Identification, Chemical Injuries, and Other Findings," James J. Tuite, III, principal investigator, Committee on Banking, Housing, and Urban Affairs, U.S. Senate, October, 1994. My copy was taken from www.chronicillnet.org/PGWS/tuite/chembio. For news coverage of Tuite's survey of the transmission of symptoms, see, for example: "Gulf War Syndrome Appears Contagious, Survey Shows," Carol Viszant, Reuters, October 21, 1994.

Page 148 Regarding the gulf war studies: Starting in 1995, yearly summaries of the federal research program were produced in reports titled "Annual Report to Congress, Federally Sponsored Research on Gulf War Veterans' Illnesses for [year]" Persian Gulf Veterans Coordinating Board, Research Working Group, Washington, D.C. The Department of Veterans Affairs was the lead agency on the coordinating board.

Pages 148-149 More about pyridostigmine bromide: The quote about the acute effects of PB is taken from "Veterans Seeking Answers to Syndrome Suspect They Were Goats in Gulf War," Paul Cotton, *Journal of the American Medical Association*, 1994, loc. cit. The Pentagon expert cited was Dr. Fred Sidell of the U.S. Army Medical Research Institute of Chemical Defense. For a more typical example of the early news coverage of PB, see: "U.S. Gave Its Own Troops a Toxic Brew," Peggy R. Townsend, *Santa Cruz County* (Calif.) *Sentinel*, June 12, 1994, p. A1.

The Rockefeller report featuring PB was "Is Military Research Hazardous to Veterans' Health? Lessons Spanning Half a Century," Staff Report 103–97, prepared for the Committee on Veterans' Affairs, U.S. Senate, Washington, D.C., December 8, 1994. For an advocate's account of the PB controversy: "Credibility Gulf: The Military's Battle over Whether to Protect Its Image or Its Troops," Amy Waldman, *Washington Monthly*, December, 1996, pp. 28–35. But doubts about PB were expressed by the Presidential Advisory Committee (PAC): "Given the extensive cumulative experience with the use of PB in patients with myasthenia gravis and data collected by military personnel, the Committee concludes it is unlikely that health effects reported today by Gulf War veterans are the result of exposure simply to PB." Op. cit., 1996, p. 117.

Some background biochemistry: The pyridostigmine bromide pills were meant to protect the nervous systems of soldiers against the nerve gas soman, one of the Iraqi threats. PB does not help against sarin and VX, related nerve agents. The drug works by a somewhat similar mechanism as the chemical warfare agents themselves. Both substances bind to a vital enzyme called acetyl-cholinesterase: the pyridostigmine temporarily and the nerve gas irreversibly. If taken first, the PB shields the enzyme from the much more dangerous attack of the nerve agent and then "lets go" of the enzyme when the threat is over. But if something were to go amiss with the interaction—because of the presence, say, of other chemicals, overloading the system—unforeseen neurological changes might result. Such was the thinking, at any rate, of scientists who focused on PB.

If a nerve agent exposure doesn't kill the person, it can injure him and at the same time cause psychological and behavioral alterations—mood swings, fatigue, irritability, forgetfulness and more, indicating that the compound has penetrated the central nervous system. Such effects have been known to last weeks or months. Could PB, especially if in combination with other chemicals, have done something similar to the troops, over a longer period? If so, the psychological aspects of the gulf war ills might have a neurotoxic explanation. The arguments were waged using laboratory animals.

Experimental evidence for a toxic synergy in chickens had been announced by Duke University researchers in 1995 and published in the spring of 1996. Their paper was: "Neurotoxicity Resulting from Coexposure to Pyridostigmine Bromide, DEET, and Permethrin: Implications of Gulf War Chemical Exposures," M. B. Abou-Donia, K. Wilmarth et al., *Journal of Toxicology and Environmental Health*, vol. 48, 1996, pp. 35–56. The Abou-Donia work drew wide notice at the initial announcement, as in "Pills May Be Culprits in Gulf War Sickness," Associated Press, *Washington Times*, April 10, 1995, and again upon formal publication, as in "Chemical Mix May Be Cause of Illnesses," Philip J. Hilts, *New York Times*, April 17, 1996, p. A6. Also garnering attention was the work of James Moss, a scientist at the U.S. Department of Agriculture. In his research on cockroaches Moss found that when pyridostigmine was used in combination with a common insect repellent called DEET (diethyl-m-toluamide), the DEET became almost seven times as toxic as when used alone. See: "Synergism of Toxicity of N,N-Diethyl-m-toluamide to German Cockroaches (Othoptera: Blattellidae) by Hydrolytic Enzyme Inhibitors," J. I. Moss, *Journal of Economic Entomology*, vol. 89, no. 5, 1996, pp.1151–1155. When Jim Moss lost his job with the USDA, his cause was championed by Senator Rockefeller.

For PB to have caused injuries to vets' memories and concentration, the pyridostigmine must have passed from the bloodstreams of the subjects into their brains. The scientific understanding was that this drug normally could not cross the blood-brain barrier. But at the end of 1996 an Israeli team, funded in part by the U.S. Army, published an important paper, "Pyridostigmine Brain Penetration under Stress Enhances Neuronal Excitability and Induces Early Immediate Transcriptional Response," Alon Friedman et al., *Nature Medicine*, vol. 2. no. 12, December 1996, pp. 1382–1385. The paper described an experiment on mice that had been put under conditions of stress. When PB was injected, the drug affected their brains. The researchers also had survey information from Israeli troops who'd taken PB during the gulf war, clearly a stressful situation. Some of troops' immediate symptoms seemed to stem from their central nervous systems. The case against PB appeared stronger.

In October 1999 a Defense Department consultant made news with the publication of a lengthy scientific review of PB. Her conclusion was that the use of the drug by 250,000 soldiers "cannot be ruled out" as a source of the nagging illnesses. "Stressful or other special conditions may allow PB to breach the blood-brain barrier and penetrate the brain, producing effects that would not 'normally' occur." Since the previous reviews released through the Pentagon's Office of the Special Assistant for Gulf War Illnesses (OSAGWI) had taken pains to *rule out* hypothetical modes of illness, this equivocal conclusion was taken by many as an endorsement of the PB etiology. Source: "A Review of the Scientific Literature as It Pertains to Gulf War Illnesses, volume 2, Pyridostigmine Bromide," Beatrice Alexandra Golomb, prepared for the Office of the Secretary of Defense by RAND's National Defense Research Institute, Washington, D.C., October, 1999.

Six months later, however, scientific opinion began to swing in the other direction because the Israeli findings on PB's penetration of the brain were not duplicated by others. See, for one report, "Stress Does Not Enable Pyridostigmine to Inhibit Brain Cholinesterase after Parenteral Administration," E. Grauer et al., *Toxicology and Applied Pharmacology*, vol. 164, no. 3, May 2000, pp. 301–304. In the spring of 2000 John Feussner, the VA's chief of research, told the Special Oversight Board, the successor to the PAC: "We have learned a lot more about this agent [PB] than we had in the past, but at least at the moment there doesn't seem to be anything to impugn this as a cause of sustained illness." In the overall research program, a half dozen studies of the mechanisms of PB interactions were still ongoing. Source, for Feussner: Hearing of the Presidential Special Oversight Board for Department of Defense Investigations of Gulf War Chemical and Biological Incidents, Washington, D.C., April 4, 2000. Available at: www.oversight.ncr.gov/ xcript_hearing_4apr00.html. For a biomedical overview of the nerve agents and PB, see "Pretreatment for Nerve Agent Exposure," chapter 6, Michael A. Dunn et al., in *Medical Aspects of Chemical and Biological Warfare*, ed. F. R. Sidell et al., TMM Series, Part I, Office of the Surgeon General, Borden Institute, Walter Reed Army Medical Center, Washington, D.C., 1997.

Page 149 Senator Riegle twice used the line about the Pentagon's "mental problem" during the May 25, 1994, Banking Committee hearing, op. cit.

Page 150 My source for Blanck's statement that CFS and gulf war illnesses were the same is *Osler's Web: Inside the Labyrinth of the Chronic Fatigue Syndrome Epidemic*, Hillary Johnson, Crown Publishers, New York, 1996, p. 663.

Page 151 Blanck, after serving as its surgeon general for four years, retired from the army in 2000.

Pages 155–156 Sources for the 1995 developments: The Presidential Advisory Committee issued three reports: an interim report in February 1996; a final report in December 1996, which I have cited several times; and a special report in October 1997. All available through the U.S. Government Printing Office, Washington, D.C., or at www.gwvi.ncr.gov.

The *60 Minutes* program was "Gulf War Syndrome," *60 Minutes*, CBS News, March 12, 1995. Tuite's March 1995 report was "Persian Gulf Syndrome and the Delayed Toxic Effects of Chemical Agent Exposure." I got it from www.chronicillnet.org/PGWS/tuite/science4.html. The Duke toxicologist was Mohammed Abou-Donia, whose study was formally published the following year. I described this work on p. 385. The reported surge in CCEP enrollments is from "Gulf War Veterans' Health Registries: Who Is Most Likely to Seek Evaluation?," Gregory C. Gray et al., *American Journal of Epidemiology*, vol. 48, no. 4, 1998, p. 348. The news item about Timothy McVeigh is from " 'Gulf War Syndrome' a New Bombing Angle," Reuters, *Washington Times*, April 29, 1995.

Pages 156–157 The published report of the Medical/Scientific Panel of the Persian Gulf War National Unity Conference was "Progress on Persian Gulf War Illnesses—Reality and Hypotheses," Garth L. Nicolson, Edward Hyman, Andreás Korényi-Both, Damacio A. Lopez, Nancy Nicolson, William Rea, and Howard Urnovitz, *International Journal of Occupational Medicine and Toxicology*, vol. 4, no. 3, 1995, pp. 365–370.

All the theories that were put forward at the conference assumed that toxic agents, whether biological or chemical, had a determinative role in the veterans' illnesses. Earlier in these notes I discussed the possible role of vaccines (pp. 372–374) and pyridostigmine bromide (pp. 384–386). Also see two good reviews of the diverse toxic agents and their possible mechanisms of morbidity: "Gulf War Veterans' Illnesses: VA, DOD Continue to Resist Strong Evidence Linking Toxic Causes to Chronic Health Effects," Second Report by the Committee on Government Reform and Oversight, U.S. House of Representatives, Report 105-388, November 1997, and "Gulf War Syndrome—a Model for the Complexity of Biological and Environmental Interaction with Human Health," Goran A. Jamal, *Adverse Drug Reactions and Toxicological Reviews*, vol. 17, no. 1, 1998, pp. 1–17.

Here I limit myself to sketches of two agents that became popular in the veterans' community. One is biological and the other chemical.

Garth Nicolson, the organizer of the Medical/Scientific Panel at the Texas conference, and his wife, Nancy, promoted a mycoplasma, specifically *Mycoplasma fermentans.* These cryptic bacteria are tinier than other bacteria, lack a cell wall, and resist culturing in the laboratory, all of which makes detection difficult. Prior to the gulf war, mycoplasmas were known for causing respiratory infections and achy, flulike conditions; they were especially dangerous to AIDS patients. Nicolson, a scientist with good credentials in cancer research, claimed to find mycoplasmas in almost half the blood samples of ill veterans that he analyzed.

Nicolson never published a scientifically controlled study of his work. Moreover, the methods he used to test for mycoplasma were unique to his laboratory, he said. Thus when the army screened veterans' blood and found negligible mycoplasma infections, Nicolson countered that the army tests were not sensitive enough. He said that since this particular strain of mycoplasma could live "deep within the nucleus" of the infected cell, it was resistant to most antibiotics and tended not to elicit an antibody response in blood screening. The dispute may have remained academic, except that Nicolson had also devised a treatment for the mycoplasma. One antibiotic, doxycycline, was said to be able to knock out the germ. Not an M.D., Nicolson did not treat the sick vets directly, but he reported that three-quarters of those who adopted his heavy regimen of doxycycline were being cured of the gulf war syndrome.

Nicolson gathered a following. In December 1996 researchers at the Walter Reed Army Institute of Research reluctantly agreed that they ought to learn Nicolson's DNA-based methods of testing for mycoplasma, and so began negotiations with him on how to collaborate. Eventually his laboratory got a Pentagon contract, as did two other labs that were brought in to verify his test methods. Still, progress was very slow because of various objections by Nicolson to the collaboration as it went along. As for results, at this writing it appears that his test methods were nothing special.

I agreed with Nicolson on one thing: He looked beyond the gulf war illnesses and linked them to chronic fatigue syndrome and fibromyalgia. "There's no such thing as gulf war syndrome—there's no distinct syndrome," he has stated. "We have millions of civilians with similar symptoms." But Nicolson believed that "a majority of patients with chronic illnesses suffer from stealth infections that can be identified and successfully treated." He said this type of chronic illness started with flulike symptoms and worsened through discrete stages. It was moderately contagious but had a long latency before the signs and symptoms showed themselves.

Of all those ill, he said, the gulf war vets were a special case because of the way they contracted their mycoplasmas. Nicolson believed that the organism may have been used as a biological weapon by the Iraqis and may also have contaminated the vaccines given to U.S. troops, through either carelessness or irresponsible experimentation on the part of the Pentagon. He claimed to have evidence that the HIV virus was mixed up somehow with the veterans' mycoplasma.

Because of such ideas, darker and more daring than his basic theory of infection, Nicolson and his wife felt themselves under political attack. They charged that their phones had been tapped by the CIA, that assassins tried to poison them and run them off the road, that they were forced to leave Texas for California. When I interviewed him in the spring of 1997—a rumpled man with a thick, pageboy haircut and pale, deep-set eyes—Nicolson tossed out many accusations, which I won't repeat except for the strangest: that a high VA medical official, an important figure in the health controversy, had emigrated from an Eastern bloc (Communist) nation not very long ago, her Irish name notwithstanding.

For all that, the embattled scientist was feeling hopeful about the prospects of validating his ideas. "You get hammered from every direction," he said, "but now the tide is beginning to turn." His research company, the Institute for Molecular Medicine, was testing the blood of people with chronic illness, and he continued to recommend doxycycline widely.

In 1999, concerned because gulf war veterans were adopting Nicolson's regimen on word-of-mouth evidence, the government started a scientific trial to see whether doxycycline really worked. In a blind study, some five hundred symptomatic veterans were given either the antibiotic or a placebo, which they agreed to take for a year. In order to enroll, the subjects had to test positive for mycoplasma on a DNA-based assay (PCR) that was equivalent to Nicolson's. The experiment cost twelve million dollars. Results are pending. For Nicolson it was triumph enough that hundreds of mycoplasma-positive vets were produced for the trial—it appears they existed to the extent that he claimed.

For further information on Nicolson's research, the Institute for Molecular Medicine, in Huntington Beach, Calif., can be accessed at www.immed.org. In the popular press, see: "Finally, the Military Is Focusing on a Likely Cause of Gulf War Syndrome," Susan Duerksen, *San Diego Union-Tribune*, April 14, 1999, and "Gulf War Illness: Finally, an Answer," Gunjan Sinha, *Popular Science*, April 1999. For professional doubts, see: "No Serologic Evidence of an Association Found between Gulf War Service and *Mycoplasma Fermentans* Infection," Gregory C. Gray et al., *American Journal of Tropical Medicine and Hygiene*, vol. 60, no. 5, 1999, pp. 752–757.

Depleted uranium, DU, consists almost entirely of uranium-238. It is the material left over after uranium-235, the fissile isotope, is extracted from uranium ore for use in nuclear power plants and weapons. DU is weakly radioactive, but the energy emitted is less than that from raw uranium; it is and some two hundred thousand times weaker than that from plutonium, another nuclear material.

Because of its great density—translating into a capacity to deliver and take a heavy punch—DU was made into munitions and tank armor by the Pentagon in the 1970s. Its efficacy during the Persian Gulf War, the first time it was used, was stunning. No American tank with DU armor was disabled by Iraqi tank fire, and the DU rounds fired by the American M-1 tanks and A-10 tank-killing aircraft were devastating to the enemy equipment. The DU both penetrated and ignited on contact.

Friendly-fire incidents exposed American tank crews to their own side's DU. Thirty-three men came home with DU shrapnel in their bodies. Dozens more breathed DU dust when working on blasted tanks following the conflict. In addition, a large group of unknown size had what the Defense Department called fleeting contacts with DU. These people were in and around disabled Iraqi equipment or were downwind from fires, including a large munitions fire at a supply depot in which DU burned.

The Pentagon admitted that its warnings about the possible health risks of DU had been inadequate. As the gulf war illnesses mounted, depleted uranium joined the list of risk factors because it had been widespread on the battlefield. Veterans' advocates claimed that up to four hundred thousand may have been exposed, a figure that the Pentagon disputed strongly. No central figure, like Garth Nicolson, articulated a DU theory of illness for the veterans' community, but there were enough DU advocates with technical and medical backgrounds to make the case plausible in the news media.

The DU connection was dismissed by scientific panels that looked at the issue, such as the Presidential Advisory Committee. Maybe there would be an increased risk of lung cancer in the future, allowed the PAC, citing studies of uranium miners. The uranium miners of the fifties and sixties, most of whom smoked cigarettes and worked for years in unventilated spaces, were exposed not just to uranium dust but to the much more hazardous radon gas. These men had elevated rates of lung cancer. But the more the researchers looked into it, the less plausible was the connection to the current symptoms of the gulf war veterans.

Unlike the other substances on the battlefield, uranium had been extensively studied in industrial settings. Its health risks, radiological and chemical, were to the lung and to the kidney respectively. Still, outside the mines, the incidence of lung and kidney illness in the workplace was not remarkable, according to the studies. The Persian Gulf vets had been exposed to a less toxic form of uranium in lesser amounts over a much shorter period. Their exposures were closer to the background levels of uranium than to the industrial cases, for traces of uranium were in the soil, in drinking water, in all human bodies as a "natural" contaminant.

The few vets with DU demonstrably coursing through their systems had no kidney problems. According to the VA research, there was nothing remarkable about the health of this most exposed group except that, on a computerized test of problem solving, the men with higher levels of uranium in their urine did not perform quite as well as those with normal levels of uranium. On pencil and paper tests they all tested the same, however. The significance of the finding was murky. It may well have been due to inherent differences between the two small samples.

The VA and Defense Department attempted to respond to the fears in the veterans' community. In July 1998 the agencies announced a new medical program to evaluate those who were potentially exposed to DU. Urine would be tested, questionnaires administered. The fears, at this writing, have not been calmed.

My DU sources: On the failure to warn troops: "Operation Desert Storm: Army Not Adequately Prepared to Deal with Depleted Uranium Contamination," U.S. General Accounting Office, GAO/NSIAD-93-90, Washington, D.C., January 1993, pp. 4–5. On exposures in the field: "The Pentagon's Radioactive Bullet," Bill Mesler, *Nation*, October 21, 1996; "Pentagon Poison: The Great Radioactive Ammo Cover-Up," Bill Mesler, *Nation*, May 13, 1997; "Environmental Exposure Report: Depleted Uranium in the Gulf," Office of Special Assistant for Gulf War Illnesses, Department of Defense, Washington, D.C., August, 1998.

On the general health hazards of uranium and DU: Testimony of George Voelz before the Presidential Advisory Committee, Denver, Colo., August 6, 1996, www.gwvi.ncr.gov/0806gulf.html; Presidential Advisory Committee, Final Report loc. cit., 1996, pp. 119–120; "Depleted Uranium," vol. 7, "A Review of the Scientific Literature as It Pertains to Gulf War Illnesses," prepared by RAND's National Defense Research Institute for the Office of the Secretary of Defense, Washington, D.C., 1999; "Toxicological Profile for Uranium (Update)," prepared by Research Triangle Institute for Agency for Toxic Substances and Disease Registry, U.S. Department of Health and Human Services, Public Health Service, Atlanta, September 1999; "Special Oversight Board Analysis (Ver. 2) of OSAGWI's DU Report," Presidential Special Oversight Board for Department of Defense Investigations of Gulf War Chemical and Biological Incidents, Arlington, Va., February 19, 1999; "Gulf War Illnesses: Understanding of Health Effects from Depleted Uranium Evolving but Safety Training Needed," U.S. General Accounting Office, GAO/NSIAD-00-70, Washington, D.C., March 2000; "Health Effects of Depleted Uranium on Exposed Gulf War Veterans," M. A. McDiarmid et al., *Environmental Research*, Section A, vol. 82, no. 2, 2000, pp. 168–180.

Except for the articles in the *Nation*, the above constitute the mainstream scientific views of DU. For the most reasoned and well researched of the dissenting opinions, see: "Don't Look, Don't Find: Gulf War Veterans, the U.S. Government and Depleted Uranium,1990–2000," Dan Fahey, Military Toxics Project, Lewiston, Maine, March 2000. Available at: www.ngwrc.org/Dulink/DLDFReport.pdf.

Finally, for a historical account of the perceived hazards of exposure to nuclear materials, especially plutonium, see: "Atomic Overreaction," Jeff Wheelwright, *Atlantic Monthly*, April 1995, pp. 26–38. The DU controversy is but another example.

Page 158 The Pentagon analysis of its registry cases was "Comprehensive Clinical Evaluation Program (CCEP) for Gulf War Veterans—Report on 10,020 Participants," Department of Defense, Washington, D.C., August 1995. An account of the report is "Study Finds No Evidence of Gulf War Illness," Associated Press, *New York Times*, August 2, 1995. For criticism of the way that the report related the vets' symptoms to those of different medical populations, see: *Evaluation of the U.S. Department of Defense Persian Gulf Comprehensive Clinical Evaluation Program*, Institute of Medicine, National Academy Press, Washington, D.C., January 1996, pp. 13–14, and "Older Patients Used in Government Study of Gulf War Veterans," Thomas D. Williams, *Hartford Courant*, October 22, 1995, p. A10.

Pages 158–159 Two large epidemiology studies examined veterans' deaths and veterans' inpatient admissions. The first was "Mortality among U.S. Veterans of the Persian Gulf War," Han K. Kang and Tim A. Bullman, *New England Journal of Medicine*, vol. 335, no. 20, November 14, 1996, pp. 1498–1504. An update to this study by the same authors, subtitled "First Update through December, 1995," was issued in 1997 by the Environmental Epidemiology Service, Department of Veterans Affairs, Washington, D.C. The mortality figures contained one striking feature: Gulf war vets had more fatal accidents than their peers, and as a result, their death rate from external causes was higher. See p. 381 for details.

The second study was "The Postwar Hospitalization Experience of U.S. Veterans of the Persian Gulf War," Gregory C. Gray et al., *New England Journal of Medicine*, vol. 335, no. 20, November 14, 1996, pp. 1505–1513. An update to this study, by James D. Knoke and Gregory C. Gray, was published in *Emerging Infectious Diseases*, vol. 4, no. 2, April–June, 1998, pp.

211–219. This work didn't cover retired personnel. In 1999 Gray and colleagues published a paper attempting to extend their findings to veterans who had left active duty. They compared the diagnoses of those being treated in Pentagon hospitals with diagnoses of vets in VA and civilian hospitals. Using hospital admissions in California as a subsample, the researchers found there was not enough information on the *rates* of illness to make conclusions. But the *range* of the diagnoses was similar among the active duty and retired gulf war vets, and was similar in turn to the range of diagnoses among hospitalized military personnel who had not gone to war. Source: Gregory C. Gray et al., "Are Gulf War Veterans Suffering War-Related Illnesses? Federal and Civilian Hospitalizations Examined, June 1991 to December 1994," *American Journal of Epidemiology*, vol. 151, no. 1, 2000, pp. 63–71.

Page 159 Here are the studies of symptom prevalence (the relative rates of gulf war illness), in the order that I named them:

1. "Physical Health Symptomatology of Gulf War–Era Service Personnel from the States of Pennsylvania and Hawaii," Robert H. Stretch et al., *Military Medicine*, vol. 160, March 1995, pp. 131–136.

2. "Unexplained Illness among Persian Gulf War Veterans in an Air National Guard Unit: Preliminary Report—August 1990–March 1995," *Morbidity and Mortality Weekly Report*, U.S. Centers for Disease Control and Prevention, Washington, D.C., June 16, 1995, pp. 443–447. Three years later there came an in-depth report of Pennsylvania veterans by the same team: "Chronic Multisymptom Illness Affecting Air Force Veterans of the Gulf War," Keiji Fukuda et al., *Journal of the American Medical Association*, vol. 280, no. 20, September 16, 1998, pp. 981–988.

3. "Self-Reported Illness and Health Status among Gulf War Veterans: A Population-Based Study," The Iowa Persian Gulf Study Group," *Journal of the American Medical Association*, vol. 277, no. 3, January 15, 1997, pp. 238–245.

4. "Increased Postwar Symptoms and Psychological Morbidity among U.S. Navy Gulf War Veterans," Gregory C. Gray et al., abstract, American College of Epidemiology Annual Sessions, September 21–23, 1997. This work was published formally in the *American Journal of Tropical Medicine and Hygiene*, vol. 60, no. 5, 1999, pp. 758–766.

5. "Musculoskeletal Syndromes of Deployed Persian Gulf Veterans," André Barkhuizen et al., Portland Environmental Hazards Research Center, *Arthritis and Rheumatism*, vol. 41, no. 9, 1998, Supplement S133, Abstract #601. This study covered veterans in the Pacific Northwest.

6. "Health Status of Persian Gulf War Veterans: Self-Reported Symptoms, Environmental Exposures and the Effect of Stress," S. Proctor et al., *International Journal of Epidemiology*, vol. 27, no. 6, 1998, pp. 1000–1010. The study subjects were from New England.

7. "Illnesses among United States Veterans of the Gulf War: A Population-Based Survey of 30,000 Veterans," Han K. Kang et al., *Journal of Occupational and Environmental Medicine*," vol. 42, May 2000, pp. 491–501. In this, the VA's national survey, some 10,000 vets who were contacted did not respond, while twenty thousand did. Hence the difference between the title of the report and the numbers it analyzed.

As for the missing case definition of the gulf war illnesses, by 1999 a consensus appeared to be developing, within government circles at least, around the criteria devised by Fukuda et al. for the CDC survey of air force reservists in Pennsylvania. See above, op. cit. (2), 1998. This definition came to be known as the CDC multisymptom criteria for GW illness. A case of this illness was said to be a gulf war veteran who attested to at least one symptom in at least two of three possible categories. The three categories comprised chronic symptoms of fatigue; of mood and/or cognition; and of musculoskeletal pain.

Page 160 Examples of the failure to correlate symptoms with chemical exposures: "Symptoms in 18,495 Persian Gulf War Veterans: Latency of Onset and Lack of Association with Self-Reported Exposures," Kurt Kroenke, Patricia Koslowe and Michael Roy, *Journal of Occupational and Environmental Medicine*, vol. 40, no. 6, June 1998, pp. 520–528; "Increased Postwar Symptoms and Psychological Morbidity among U.S. Navy Gulf War Veterans," Gregory C. Gray et al., *American Journal of Tropical Medicine and Hygiene*, vol. 60, no. 5, 1999, pp. 758–766; "U.S. Gulf War Veterans: Service Periods in Theater, Differential Exposures, and Persistent Unexplained Illness," Peter S. Spencer et al., *Toxicology Letters, 102–103*, 1998, pp. 515–521. By contrast, limited correlations between exposures and symptoms were reported in "Health Status of Persian Gulf Veterans: Self-Reported Symptoms, Environmental Exposures and the Effect of Stress," S. P. Proctor et al., *International Journal of Epidemiology*, vol. 27, 1998, pp. 1000–1010. The poor reliability of accounts of exposure is explored in "Strategies to Assess Validity of Self-Reported Exposures during the Persian Gulf War," Linda A. McCauley et al., *Environmental Research Section A*, vol. 81, 1999, pp. 195–205.

Pages 160–162 Haley's three papers in *Journal of the American Medical Association* (*JAMA*), vol. 277, no. 3, were: "Is There a Gulf War Syndrome? Searching for Syndromes by Factor Analysis of Symptoms," Robert W. Haley et al., pp. 215–222; "Evaluation of Neurologic Function in Gulf War Veterans: A Blinded Case-Control Study," Robert W. Haley et al., pp. 223–230; "Self-Reported Exposure to Neurotoxic Chemical Combinations in the Gulf War," Robert W. Haley et al., pp. 231–237.

Dr. Philip Landrigan, a member of the Presidential Advisory Committee, wrote an editorial in the same issue of *JAMA* that was critical of the Haley studies. Landrigan summarized his criticism in an interview with the PBS program *Frontline*. The program, "Last Battle of the Gulf War," was broadcast on January 20, 1998. Landrigan's interview, only parts of which were aired, is posted at: www.pbs.org/wgbh/pages/frontline/shows/syndrome/interviews/landrigan.html.

Pages 165–171 Details of Khamisiyah: The *Times*'s initial report of the incident was "Gulf War Illness May Be Linked to Gas Exposure, Pentagon Says," Philip Shenon, *New York Times*, June 22, 1996, p. 1. See also "U.S. Troops Were Near Toxic Gas Blast in Gulf," Bradley Graham and David Brown, *Washington Post*, June 22, 1996, p. 1.

Of the volumes of information about Khamisiyah, I recommend the evenhanded account by the Senate Veterans' Affairs Committee, the last federal panel to weigh in on the affair: "Report of the Special Investigation Unit on Gulf War Illnesses," Committee on Veterans' Affairs, U.S. Senate, Report 105-39, Part I, Washington, D.C., September 1998. The summary statement that I quoted is on p. 21. As to whether there was a cover-up of Khamisiyah, the committee stated: "These denials [of chemical exposures by U.S. officials] appear to be the result of a negligent failure to investigate the facts fully and promptly, but there is no evidence to date that they resulted from a concerted conspiracy of silence" (p. 3).

In the months following the Khamisiyah revelation, the criticism of DoD officials was much sharper. The Presidential Advisory Committee, for instance, said that the Pentagon's handling of this and other chemical warfare incidents had sowed distrust and lacked credibility. For an independent and accusatory account of the government's handling of the chemical warfare allegations, including Khamisiyah, see *Gassed in the Gulf: The Inside Story of the Pentagon-CIA Cover-up of Gulf War Syndrome*, Patrick G. Eddington, Insignia Publishing Co., Washington, D.C., 1997.

Because of the failure to investigate Khamisiyah properly, Bernard Rostker, who had been serving as an assistant secretary of the navy, was named special assistant to the deputy secretary of defense for gulf war illnesses in November 1996. Rostker's office, known by the acronym OSAGWI, greatly expanded the investigation. It chased down all the publicized claims and reports of chemical exposures, starting with the oil fires and ending with Khamisiyah itself. Compared with the hares active in the veterans' community, OSAGWI was a tortoise with inexhaustible resources. As of this writing, it was still issuing what it called case narratives about suspicious events on the battlefield. OSAGWI for the most part minimized the significance of these events. The reports are posted, along with unclassified documents from the war and much other useful information, on a labyrinthine Website called GulfLINK, /www.gulflink.osd.mil.

The VA's preliminary look at health conditions associated with Khamisiyah was: "A Review of the VA Persian Gulf Health Registry and Patient Treatment File for the 21,799 U.S. Gulf War Veterans Stationed within 50km Radius of Khamisiyah, Iraq," Environmental Epidemiology Service, Department of Veterans Affairs, Washington, D.C., December 1996. The *Times*'s account of this work was "U.S. Links Chemicals in Iraq to One of Soliders' Symptoms," Clifford Krauss, *New York Times*, January 22, 1997.

As for the reconstruction of the Khamisiyah explosions and exposures, an effort that engaged both OSAGWI and the CIA during 1997, officials made a distinction between the March 4 and March 10 incidents. In the so-called Bunker 73 blast on March 4, the release of sarin was largely contained, according to the government analysts. The plume of gas, if any, was much smaller than the plume that was released on March 10. Thus the calculations of exposure were based solely on the latter incident.

The July 24, 1997, news release from the Pentagon, "Troops Not Exposed to Dangerous Levels or Chemical Agent," estimated the doses of sarin (agent) in the following terms: "Officials calculate the dose of agent was greater than the general population level of 0.01296 milligram-minutes of sarin per cubic meter, but well below the noticeable health effect level of 1 milligram-minute per cubic meter. The general population level, established by the Centers for Disease Control in 1988, is a level which 'long term exposure to these concentrations would not create any adverse health effects.' It takes an exposure of 35 milligram-minutes of sarin per cubic meter to incapacitate an individual and 100 milligram-minutes per cubic meter to produce fatalities."

To explain: A milligram-minute can accommodate many different exposure scenarios. For example, an exposure to one milligram of sarin (per meter of air) that lasts for one minute is rendered as 1 milligram-minute. So too is an exposure of a half milligram of sarin that lasts for two minutes. Or two milligrams lasting thirty seconds. If one milligram-minute is delivered to a soldier in a short time—within a very few minutes, say—he or she might feel uncomfortable. The pupils might narrow, the nose might run. But if one milligram-minute of sarin is delivered over twenty-four hours, as was likely after Khamisiyah, it would not be noticeable because the concentration of sarin vapor in the air at any one moment would be extremely low.

The *Times*'s story about the calculation of exposures was "New Study Raises Estimate of Troops Exposed to Gas," Philip Shenon, *New York Times*, July 24, 1997. (Shenon got a copy of the study a day early, so that his article appeared on the day of the Pentagon briefing.)

According to later reviews of Khamisiyah, the Pentagon went too far in estimating the health risks. The Senate Veterans' Affairs Committee judged that the exposure numbers were flawed on the high side and that "the government may have ended up doing more to confuse and alarm Gulf War veterans, both those healthy and ill, than to help them" (1998, op. cit., p. 36). The CIA, after acquiring new information and tinkering with the plume model, revised downward the number of people who could have been exposed.

The formal epidemiological study of the troops in the Khamisiyah area was delayed in part because no researcher responded when the Pentagon asked for bids on a study proposal in 1997. The next year the work was tasked to the Institute of Medicine, an arm of the National Academy of Sciences. Complicating the task was that officials realized that some of the warnings mailed to soldiers in 1996 and 1997 had been mistaken. Because the warnings could have tainted vets' accounts of their symptoms, the study planners were compelled to compare the health pictures of four groups of veterans instead of two: those who were potentially exposed and notified about it correctly; those who were not exposed but who were told, incorrectly, that they may have been; those exposed but not notified initially; and those not exposed and not notified.

The *Times's* early health assessment of Khamisiyah was "Legacy of Illness for Troops in Battalion That Destroyed Iraqi Bunkers," Philip Shenon, *New York Times*, August 11, 1996, p. 8.

Finally, regarding the veteran Brian Martin and the depiction of his "effusive symptoms" by the news media, see: "Gulf Lore Syndrome," Michael Fumento, *Reason* magazine, March 1997. The article is posted at www.reason.com/9703/fe.fumento.html/. Fumento is skeptical of the gulf war illnesses—too much so, in my view—and scathing about the press coverage of them.

Pages 175–176 Information about the EPA's Toxic Release Inventory and right-to-know is available at www.epa.gov/opptintr/tri.

Page 176 The public health was clearly wronged by the secret Hanford releases, but it may not have been harmed. After the details of the emissions were bared in the mid-1980s, scientists estimated the doses of iodine-131 delivered downwind of the plant. (Their model had more information in it than that for the Khamisiyah releases because amounts of radioactive iodine in the air and on the ground had been measured, sporadically, by the Atomic Energy Commission.) The exposures estimated were low, not threatening, said researchers. In addition, some thirty-four thousand people from the Hanford area were brought in for health exams. The number of thyroid abnormalities—this gland is the prime target of I-131—was low. Less than 1 percent had thyroid cancer, in accord with the background rate. Sources: Hanford Thyroid Disease Study, a project of Fred Hutchinson Cancer Research Center and the U.S. Centers for Disease Control and Prevention, Draft Final Report, January 1999. Available at the study website, www.fhcrc.org/science/phs/htds. See also, on the AEC's measurement of I-131: "Nuclear Health and Safety: Examples of Post World War II Radiation Releases at U.S. Nuclear Sites," U.S. General Accounting Office, GAO/RCED-94-51FS, Washington, D.C., November 1993.

Page 177 Regarding Rachel Carson and nuclear fallout, Paul Brooks, her editor and literary biographer, wrote: "With the coming of the atomic age, Rachel felt that certain deep convictions she had cherished since childhood were being threatened." Source: *The House of Life: Rachel Carson at Work*, Paul Brooks, Houghton Mifflin Co., Boston, 1972, p. 9. Before the publication of *Silent Spring*, Brooks wrote to Carson, "[T]he parallel between the effects of chemicals and effects of radiation is so dramatic that people can't help getting the idea. In a sense, all this publicity about fallout gives you a head start in awakening people to the dangers of chemicals." From: *Rachel Carson: Witness for Nature*, Linda Lear, Henry Holt, New York, 1997, pp. 373–375 and associated footnotes. The published allusions to fallout are taken from pages 39 and 6 of the reissued edition of her book (*Silent Spring*, Rachel Carson, Houghton Mifflin Co., Boston, 1962, 1994).

The estimate that up to 90 percent of cancers were environmental in origin was first postulated in a World Health Organization report, "Prevention of Cancer: Report of a WHO Expert Committee," Technical Reports Series No. 276, Geneva, 1964. See also: "Environmental Determinants of Human Cancer," Samuel Epstein, *Cancer Research*, vol. 43, 1974, pp. 2425–2435, and "Cancer: The Price of Technological Advancement?," Natural Resources Defense Council, *NRDC Newsletter*, vol. 5, no. 2, Summer 1976.

The change in scientific opinion was triggered by an influential review by epidemiologists Richard Doll and Richard Peto: "The Causes of Cancer: Quantitative Estimates of Avoidable Risks of Cancer in the United States Today," R. Doll and R. Peto, *Journal of the National Cancer Institute*, vol. 66, June 1981, pp. 1191–1308. For the current view that less than 5 percent of cancers are due to pollution, see: "Unfinished Business: A Comparative Assessment of Environmental Problems, Appendix I to Report of the Cancer Risk Work Group," Environmental Protection Agency, Washington, D.C., February 1987; "Actual Causes of Death in the United States," J. M. McGinnis and W. H. Foege, *Journal of the American Medical Association*, vol. 270, no.18, November 10, 1993, pp. 2207–2212; "What Causes Cancer?," D. Trichopoulos, F. P. Li and D. J. Hunter, *Scientific American*, vol. 275, September 1996, pp. 80–84.

Page 178 Gibbs's quote about the health effects of Love Canal is taken from the Preface of *Dying from Dioxin: A Citizen's Guide to Reclaiming our Health and Rebuilding Democracy*, Lois Marie Gibbs and the Citizens Clearinghouse for Hazardous Waste, South End Press, Boston, 1996.

A good introduction to the mind-body aspects of toxic exposures is: "Psychological effects of toxic contamination," Bonnie L. Green et al., in: *Individual and Community Responses to Trauma and Disaster: The Structure of Human Chaos*, ed. R. J. Ursano, B. G. McCaughey, and C. S. Fullerton. Cambridge University, Cambridge, England, 1993. See also "Modifiers of Non-Specific Symptoms in Occupational and Environmental Syndromes," A. Spurgeon, D. Gompertz and J. M. Harringon, *Occupational and Environmental Health*, vol. 53, 1996, pp. 361–366. From the abstract of the paper: "Many occupational and environmental health hazards present as an increased reporting of non-specific symptoms such as headache, backache, eye and respiratory irritation, tiredness, memory problems, and poor concentration. The pattern and number of such symptoms is suprisingly constant from hazard to hazard, suggesting that common psychological and social factors not directly related to the exposure may be involved."

Another specialist in this area is Evelyn Bromet of the State University of New York (Stony Brook). An expert on the sociological consequences of the Three Mile Island incident, Bromet was invited to an Institute of Medicine symposium, "Workshop on Preventing Unexplained Symptoms in Deployed Populations," sponsored by the Defense Department in July 1998, in connection with the investigation of the gulf war illnesses. Here is an excerpt from Bromet's presentation:

". . . [A]fter these kinds of events, like nuclear power plant accidents or toxic waste site exposure, a sizable percentage of people respond with somatic [bodily] complaints, or they tell you that they perceive their health as being compromised and is bad.

"Unfortunately, I can't put a number on that because it depends on how the question was asked about health and what the population was that was studied and whether they were part of litigation or not—many of these populations are part of litigation—and when the data were collected. . . .

"Number two, they report health complaints across their entire body. It doesn't matter whether you are talking about headaches and cognitive problems like memory problems, joint pain, backaches, gastrointestinal symptoms, cardiovascular type symptoms, or just simply asking people how do you rate your health, excellent, good, moderate, fair, or poor. People report symptoms; they report a variety of nonspecific symptoms.

"These kinds of problems seem to go on for years. They don't seem to arise and go away in many of these populations. Once they are there, they are very persistent. . . .

"In terms of risk factors, there is very little literature that helps us there. Some studies show that women report more of these symptoms than men, but women in general report more of these symptoms whether they are in a disaster situation or not. So that is not terribly helpful.

"Our study on Three Mile Island showed that people with prior mental health problems tended to report more health and mental health problems and somatization after the accident. On the other hand, people's retrospective accounts . . . about how they were before is very colored by how they are now. So I don't think that is a terribly exciting finding either.

"In natural disasters the severity of exposure has been shown to be a very powerful correlate of perceived health, but in technological disasters that's not necessarily the case. So it isn't necessarily the objective severity of the exposure that is at issue; it's how you perceive yourself to have been exposed and whether or not you perceive it to have been severe, which may have nothing to do with actually happened.

"Finally, what is very interesting about all of this and especially about the persistence of all of this is what accounts for it. A variety of issues have been talked about in the literature. For example, the media has been blamed as a source for all of these health problems and for their persistence, probably somewhat unfairly but maybe in some cases it's not so unfair."

Page 179 The JFK quote is from a presidential address to the nation in July 1963. I found it in *Secret Fallout: Low-level Radiation from Hiroshima to Three Mile Island*, Ernest Sternglass, McGraw-Hill, New York, 1972, 1981, p. 27.

Page 180 The Efron quote is from the Preface of *The Apocalyptics: Cancer and the Big Lie*, Edith Efron, Simon & Schuster, New York, 1984.

Page 183 The correlation between early life abuse and adult health problems is an important and emerging topic in the social science and medical literature. On the connection between abuse and MCS symptomatology, see: "Adult Sequelae of Childhood Abuse Presenting as Environmental Illness," Herman Staudenmeyer, Mary E. Selner and John C. Selner, *Annals of Allergy*, vol. 71, no. 6, December 1993, pp. 538–546; "Sensitization to Early Life Stress and Response to Chemical Odors in Older Adults," I. R. Bell et al., *Biological Psychiatry*, vol. 35, 1994, pp. 857–863; J.W. Pennebaker et al., "Psychological Bases of Symptom Reporting: Perceptual and Emotional Aspects of Chemical Sensitivity," *Toxicology and Industrial Health*, vol. 10, 1994, pp. 497–511.

On the connection between traumatic incidents and the development of fibromyalgia: "The Presence of Sexual Abuse in Women with Fibromyalgia," M. L. Taylor et al., *Arthritis and Rheumatism*, vol. 38, 1995, pp. 229–234; "Sexual and Physical Abuse in Women with Fibromyalgia Syndrome," M. H. Boisset-Pioro et al., *Arthritis and Rheumatism*, vol. 38, 1995, pp. 235–241; "Relationship Between Traumatic Events in Childhood and Chronic Pain," Richard T. Goldberg et al., *Disability and Rehabilitation*, vol. 21, no. 1, 1999, pp. 23–30; "Abuse History and Chronic Pain in Women," M. K. Walling et al., *Obstetrics and Gynecology*, vol. 84, 1994, pp. 193–206.

Finally, the following papers discuss the link between physical violence, experienced or witnessed when young, and the adult's development of physical complaints: "Somatoform Disorders in Victims of Incest and Child Abuse," R. J. Lowenstein, in *Incest Related Syndromes and Adult Psychopathology*, ed. R. P. Kluft, American Psychiatric Press, Washington, D.C., 1991; "Adult Physical Illness and Childhood Sexual Abuse," R. Fry, *Journal of Psychosomatic Research*, vol. 37, 1993, pp. 89–103; "Briquet's Syndrome, Dissociation, and Abuse," E. F. Pribor et al., *American Journal of Psychiatry* vol. 150, 1993, pp. 1507–1511; "Histories of Childhood Trauma in Adult

Hypochondriacal Patients," A. J. Barsky, C. Wool, M. C. Barnett, P. D. Clearly, *American Journal of Psychiatry*, vol. 151, no. 3, March 1994, pp. 397–401; "Sexual and Physical Abuse and Gastrointestinal Illness," D. A. Drossman et al., *Annals of Internal Medicine*, vol. 123, 1995, pp. 782–794; "Long-Term Correlates of Child Sexual Abuse: Theory and Review of the Empirical Literature," M. A. Polusny and V. M. Follette, *Applied and Preventive Psychology*, vol. 4, 1995, pp. 143–66; "The Relationship of Childhood Physical and Sexual Abuse to Adult Illness Behavior," P. Salmon and S. Calderbank, *Journal of Psychosomatic Research*, vol. 40, March 1996, pp. 329–36; "Dissociation, Affect Dysregulation and Somatization: The Complex Nature of Adaptation to Trauma," Bessel A. van der Kolk et al., *American Journal of Psychiatry*, vol. 153, no. 7, Supplement, 1996, pp. 83–93; "Gender Differences in the Reporting of Physical and Somatoform Symptoms," K. Kroenke and R. L. Spitzer, *Psychosomatic Medicine*, vol. 60, 1998, pp. 150–155; "Health-Related Quality of Life and Symptom Profiles of Female Survivors of Sexual Abuse," L. Miriam Dickinson, F. V. deGruy, W. P. Dickinson and L. M. Candib, *Archives of Family Medicine*," vol. 8, pp. 35–43, January–February 1999; "Physiological Correlates of Childhood Abuse: Chronic Hyperarousal in PTSD, Depression, and Irritable Bowel Syndrome," K. A. Kendall-Tackett, *Child Abuse & Neglect*, vol. 24, 2000, pp. 799–810.

Page 186 Research showing an overlap between the gulf war conditions and CFS, FM, and MCS includes: "Self-Reported Chemical Sensitivity and Wartime Chemical Exposures in Gulf War Veterans with and without Decreased Global Health Ratings," I. R. Bell et al., *Military Medicine*, vol. 163, 1998, pp. 725–32; "Chronic Multisymptom Illness Affecting Air Force Veterans of the Gulf War," K. Fukuda et al., *Journal of the American Medical Association*, vol. 280, no. 11, 1998, pp. 981–988; "Rheumatic Findings in Gulf War Veterans," E. P. Grady et al., *Archives of Internal Medicine*, vol. 158, 1998, pp. 367–371; "Medical Evaluation of Persian Gulf Veterans with Fatigue and/or Chemical Sensitivity," C. Pollet, B. Natelson, et al., *Journal of Medicine*, vol. 20, nos. 3 and 4, 1998, pp. 101–113; "Fibromyalgia and Chronic Fatigue Syndrome among Deployed Gulf War Veterans," André Barkhuizen et al., abstract, Conference on Federally Sponsored Gulf War Veterans' Illnesses Research, Persian Gulf Coordinating Board, Washington, D.C., June 1999; "Fibromyalgia in Gulf Veterans at a Phase I Comprehensive Evaluation Program Site," Thomas R. Roesel, abstract of a presentation, Conference on Federally Sponsored Gulf War Veterans' Illnesses Research, Persian Gulf Coordinating Board, Washington, D.C., June 1999, p. 103; "Prevalence of Chronic Fatigue and Chemical Sensitivities in Gulf Registry Veterans," H. Kipen et al., *Archives of Environmental Health*, vol. 54, no. 5, September–October 1999, pp. 313–318; "Multiple Chemical Sensitivity Syndrome: Symptom Prevalence and Risk Factors in a Military Population." Donald W. Black et al., *Archives of Internal Medicine*, vol. 160, 2000, pp. 1169–1176.

The "same elephant" quote by Dr. Buchwald was taken from the transcript of the Institute of Medicine workshop, "Difficult-to-Diagnose and Ill-Defined Conditions," Washington, D.C., March 1997.

Page 187 The CDC study of Pennsylvania reservists, which found gulf war symptoms in non–gulf war personnel, was by K. Fukuda et al., op. cit., 1998. Similar statistics can be found in the other prevalence studies cited on p. 391. For instance, Proctor et al., op. cit., 1998, comparing Persian Gulf veterans with military personnel who had been deployed to Germany during the war, observed: "It is interesting that the most prevalent symptoms are the same in the Gulf- and Germany-deployed groups, with the Gulf-deployed veterans simply reporting higher prevalence rates than the Germany-deployed veterans." The same finding is made in a more recent paper,

"Factor Analysis of Self-Reported Symptoms: Does It Identify a Gulf War Syndrome?," James Knoke et al., *American Journal of Epidemiology*, vol. 152, no. 4, 2000, pp. 379–388.

The VA trial of antibiotic therapy for gulf war vets was in response to Garth Nicolson's theory of mycoplasma infection. See p. 388. For the CBT trial see p. 401.

Extending his findings of a neurological disorder (*JAMA*, op. cit., 1997), Robert Haley presented and/or published work on putative organic signs of the gulf war illnesses. As before, his study subjects were drawn from the 24th Navy Seabee reservists. At a conference of the Radiological Society of North America in 1999, he and a colleague, James Fleckenstein, presented brain scans that they said indicated a loss of cells, possibly from a toxic injury. The work was later published as "Brain Abnormalities in Gulf War Syndrome: Evaluation with 1H [Proton] MR Spectroscopy," R. W. Haley et al., *Radiology*, vol. 215, no. 3, 2000, pp. 807–817. Also there was a publication on enzymatic differences between the sick vets and others: "Association of Low PON1 Type Q (Type A) Arylesterase Activity with Neurologic Symptom Complexes in Gulf War Veterans," R. W. Haley, et al., *Toxicology and Applied Pharmacology*, vol. 157, 1999, pp. 227–233. Third, the Haley team measured dizzy spells in vets that provided "subjective evidence" of brain damage: "Vestibular dysfunction in Gulf War syndrome," Peter S. Roland, Robert W. Haley et al., *Otolaryngology—Head and Neck Surgery*, vol. 122, no. 3, March 2000, pp. 319–329. And Haley made a spirited case that the "healthy-warrior effect" disguised the true extent of the gulf war syndrome in the veterans' population. See: "Point: Bias from the 'Healthy-Warrior Effect' and Unequal Follow-up in Three Government Studies of Health Effects of the Gulf War," Robert W. Haley, *American Journal of Epidemiology*, vol. 148, no. 4, 1998, pp. 315–323.

Chapter Four

Page 191 For my sources on irritable bowel syndrome, see: "Epidemiology of Irritable Bowel Syndrome in the United States," Robert S. Sandler, *Gastroenterology*, vol. 99, 1990, pp. 409–415; "Psychologic Considerations in the Irritable Bowel Syndrome," William E. Whitehead and Michael D. Crowell, Gastroenterology Clinics of North America, vol. 20, no. 2, 1991, pp. 249–267; "Irritable Bowel Syndrome," Richard B. Lynn and Lawrence S. Friedman, *New England Journal of Medicine*, vol. 329, no. 26, 1993, pp. 1940–1945; "Functional Somatic Syndromes," Arthur J. Barsky and Jonathan F. Borus, *Annals of Internal Medicine*, vol. 130, no. 11, June 1999, pp. 910–921.

In the last article Barsky and Borus note: "Patients with the irritable bowel syndrome have more psychiatric diagnoses, personality disorders, and psychiatric symptoms than patients with inflammatory bowel disease" (p. 913). In other words, the "organic" bowel condition, ostensibly more serious and psychologically worrisome than IBS, is not as likely to be accompanied by emotional distress as IBS.

For a small study comparing IBS patients with gulf war vets, see: "Is the Diarrhea in Persian Gulf War Veterans Caused by an Underlying Visceral Hypersensitivity?" J. M. Gordon et al., *Biomedicine*, vol. 44, no. 3, March 1996, p. 299A.

Chapter Five

Page 201 Regarding the number of health exams conducted through the VA and Defense Department registries: As of early 2000, some 78,000 exams had been administered through the

Persian Gulf Health Registry (VA) and 37,000 through the Comprehensive Clinical Evaluation Program (DoD). The total on the registry rolls was greater than 115,000 because some men and women declined health exams or, in fewer cases, were still waiting to take them.

Page 201 Two fine texts that comment on disease and illness are *The Nature of Suffering and the Goals of Medicine*, Eric J. Cassell, Oxford University Press, New York, 1991, and *The Birth of the Clinic: An Archaeology of Medical Perception*, Michel Foucault, Vintage Books edition, New York, 1994.

Page 204 I have supplemented Pete's account of his wartime duty with information from the military's official chronology, which was put together by the battalion historian. The document is "Battalion Landing Team 3/5, Command Chronology, 1 Jan–17 Mar 91," Marine Corps Historical Center, Washington, D.C.

Pages 205–207 The professional observations on the prebattle emotional state of the troops are from "Operation Desert Shield/Desert Storm: A Summary Report," Kathleen Wright, David Marlowe et al., Walter Reed Army Institute of Research, WRAIR/TR-95-0019, Washington, D.C., 1995. The quoted passage is on p. 35. McDuff's report on stress reactions during the war is "Classification and Characteristics of Army Stress Casualties during Operation Desert Storm," D. R. McDuff and J. L. Johnson, *Hospital and Community Psychiatry*, vol. 43, no. 8, August 1992, pp. 812–815. McDuff's personal concern about an allergic reaction to the sand of the region may not have been unfounded if the theory of a doctor named Andreás Korényi-Both has merit. See: "Al Eskan Disease: Persian Gulf syndrome," A. Korényi-Both et al., *Military Medicine*, vol. 162, no. 1, 1997, pp. 1–13. This doctor made a presentation at the Persian Gulf War National Unity Conference in 1995 (p. 156).

Page 210–211 Kurt Kroenke has written a treatise on the problem of nonspecific illness, from which I quote several times hereafter. It is "Unexplained Physical Symptoms and Somatoform Disorders," K. Kroenke, in F. V. deGruy, ed., *Twenty Common Behavioral Problems in Primary Care*, McGraw-Hill, New York (in press, 2001). For the *Washington Post* story that drew upon Kroenke's work, see: "Army Takes New Tack in Fighting the Unseen Enemy," David Brown, The Washington Post, November 23, 1998, p. A1. Kroenke worked for the army as a professor at the Uniformed Services University of the Health Sciences, in Bethesda, Md., until 1997.

Page 211–212 My discussion of the overlapping symptoms of functional somatic syndromes (functional illnesses) benefited from the following: "Functional Somatic Syndromes," Arthur J. Barsky and Jonathan F. Borus, *Annals of Internal Medicine*, vol. 130, no. 11, June 1999, pp. 910–921; "Functional Somatic Syndromes: One or Many?" S. Wessely, C. Nimnuan and M. Sharpe, *Lancet*, vol. 354, 1999, pp. 936–39; "Developing Case Definitions for Symptom-based Conditions: The Problem of Specificity," Kenneth C. Hyams, *Epidemiologic Reviews*, vol. 20, no. 2, 1998, pp. 148–156.

The Wessely paper pairs functional somatic syndromes with the medical specialties that have adopted them. As Hyams notes of such conditions, "The similarities are more consequential than the differences." Adapted from Wessely:

Gastroenterology	Irritable bowel syndrome
Gynecology	Premenstrual syndrome, chronic pelvic pain
Rheumatology	Fibromyalgia
Cardiology	Atypical or noncardiac chest pain
Respiratory medicine	Hyperventilation syndrome

Infectious diseases	Chronic fatigue syndrome
Neurology	Tension headache
Dentistry	Temporomandibular joint dysfunction, atypical facial pain
Ear, nose and throat	Globus syndrome [globus hystericus]
Allergy	Multiple chemical sensitivity

Page 213–214 For information on hepatitis C, I consulted Dr. Gary Roselle, an infectious disease specialist for the Department of Veterans Affairs, and the following articles: "The Unmet Challenges of Hepatitis C," A. Di Bisceglie and B. Bacon, *Scientific American*, October 1999, pp. 80–85; "The Shadow Epidemic," Jerome Groopman, *The New Yorker*, May 11, 1998, pp. 48–60; "Hepatitis C: How Widespread a Threat?," Denise Grady, "Science Times," *New York Times*, December 15, 1998, p. 1; "Old Blood Samples Offer New Clues to a Medical Mystery," Gina Kolata, *New York Times*, April 11, 2000, p. D1. The reader may also find information on the condition at www.hepcfoundation.org.

Page 216 Psychological diagnoses were issued by doctors for the Gulf War health registries in roughly one-third of the cases. See: "The Health Status of Gulf War Veterans: Lessons Learned from the Department of Veterans Affairs Health Registry," Frances M. Murphy et al., *Military Medicine*, vol. 164, May 1999, pp. 327–331, and "Adequacy of the Comprehensive Clinical Evaluation Program: A Focused Assessment," Institute of Medicine, National Academy Press, Washington, D.C., 1997.

A Pentagon researcher and clinician, Michael Roy, and his colleagues reported that in cases where the diagnostic scrutiny was increased, the finding of psychological and psychiatric conditions increased accordingly. See: "Signs, Symptoms, and Ill-Defined Conditions in Persian Gulf War Veterans: Findings from the Comprehensive Clinical Evaluation Program," Michael J. Roy et al., *Psychosomatic Medicine*, vol. 60, 1998, pp. 663–668. In another analysis of CCEP case files, Roy found that a mental disorder (depression, anxiety, somatoform, etc.) was "predicted" if the veteran had a high number of physical complaints (ten or greater) and/or was concerned about disability and serious illness. In other words, the people who were sickest by their own accounts were the most likely to be tagged with a psychiatric diagnosis. Source: "Clinical Predictors of Mental Disorders in a Group of Gulf War Veterans," M. J. Roy et al., abstract of a presentation to the Conference on Federally Sponsored Gulf War Veterans' Illnesses Research, Department of Veterans Affairs, Washington, D.C., June 1999.

Page 219 Kroenke's text is referenced on p. 399.

Page 221 Scarry's book, which ranges far beyond the pain of chronic illness, is *The Body in Pain: The Making and Unmaking of the World*, Elaine Scarry, Oxford University Press, New York, 1985.

Page 222 Engel's quote about somatization is taken from "Army Takes New Tack in Fighting the Unseen Enemy," David Brown, *Washington Post*, November 23, 1998, p. A1.

Pages 222–226 Publications by Daniel Clauw are available through the Georgetown Chronic Pain and Fatigue Research Center, Georgetown University Medical School, Washington, D.C.

Pages 223–224 For statistics on back pain and compensation claims, see: "Back Pain Prevalence in US Industry and Estimates of Lost Workdays," H. R. Guo et al., *American Journal of Public Health*, vol. 89, no. 7, July 1999, pp. 1029–1035, and "The Pain Perplex," Atul Gawande, *The New Yorker*, September 21, 1998, pp. 86–94.

Pages 227–228 For reports and commentary on the entanglement of injury, compensation and chronic pain, see: "Carpal Tunnel Surgery Outcomes in Workers: Effect of Workers' Compensation Status," P. E. Higgs et al., *Journal of Hand Surgery* (American), vol. 20, no. 3, 1995, pp. 554–560; "Repetition Strain Injury: The Australian Experience—1992 Update," D. C. Ireland, *Journal of Hand Surgery* (American), vol. 20, 1995 (3 Pt 2), pp. S53–56; "If You Have to Prove You Are Ill, You Can't Get Well," N. Hadler, *Spine*, vol. 21, 1996, pp. 2397–2400; "Compensation and a Psychiatric Model of Chronic Pain," R. Ferrari, *American Journal of Physical Medicine and Rehabilitation*, vol. 79, no. 3, 2000, pp. 310–311; "Effect of Eliminating Compensation for Pain and Suffering on the Outcome of Insurance Claims for Whiplash Injury," J. D. Cassidy et al., *New England Journal of Medicine*, vol. 342, no. 16, 2000, pp. 1179–1186.

Testifying on the compensation paid by VA for disabling injuries and illness after the Persian Gulf War, Joseph Thompson, undersecretary for benefits, told Congress that as of 1999 there had been 11,407 claims to VA for undiagnosed illness, of which 3,077 (27 percent) had been accepted and the remainder denied. The total claims filed under this category (the most germane to gulf war syndrome) represented less than 6 percent of the 202,000 decisions entered, said Thompson, which indicated that other service-connected disabilities were more important. In fact the most frequently compensated condition was knee injury. Thompson added that this war had produced the highest percentage of veterans in receipt of disability compensation, 16 percent, almost twice as much as for the Vietnam War or World War II. Source: Statement of Joseph Thompson before the Subcommittee on Benefits, House Committee on Veterans' Affairs, Washington, D.C., October 26, 1999.

Page 229 Cassell's book is referenced on p. 399.

Pages 232–233 For an overview of the worth of cognitive-behavioral therapy, see: "Cognitive-Behavioral Therapy for Somatization and Symptom Syndromes: A Critical Review of Controlled Clinical Trials," K. Kroenke and R. Swindle, *Psychotherapy and Psychosomatics*, 2000 (in press). According to the abstract: "A systematic review of the literature revealed 29 controlled trials . . . of the efficacy of cognitive-behavioral therapy (CBT) for symptoms and symptom syndromes. Physical symptoms, functional status, and psychological distress benefited in 71%, 47%, and 33% of the trials, respectively." See also the discussion of CBT in "Gulf War Illnesses: Causation and Treatment," M. Hodgson and H. Kipen, *Journal of Occupational and Environmental Medicine*, vol. 41, no. 6, 1999, p. 449.

As for the VA/Pentagon trial of the treatment, it was designed to test both exercise and cognitive-behavioral therapy. I don't have any results to report, but here was the shape of the project as planned in 1999: A total of 1,356 veterans with pain, fatigue, or memory problems were to be enrolled at twenty VA medical centers around the country. The subjects would be placed in one of four treatment groups: They would get either CBT; aerobic exercise; CBT and exercise together; or "usual and customary care." The last group was the controls, those receiving only what the VA provided them already. The hoped-for outcome was that the subjects participating in the exercise and the CBT wings of the trial would show more improvement than the subjects in usual care and that the vets getting *both* CBT and exercise would show the most improvement of all.

Enrollments lagged and the program was still seeking recruits as of the spring of 2000. Daniel Clauw told me that some veterans were being excluded from the trial because "their baseline function is pretty good, and we didn't think these interventions would make it any better, and/or they are already doing a fair amount of exercise (thus they wouldn't be likely to benefit from the exercise if they got randomized to that arm)." Overall, this trial was proving less popular than the antibiotic trial for mcyoplasma-positive veterans (p. 388).

Page 235 The Cunning Man, Robertson Davies, Viking, New York, 1995. The doctor/narrator of this novel also says, "I see diseases as disguises in which people present me with their wretchedness."

Pages 239–240 The Kroenke study of endoscopy seekers is "The Value of Screening for Psychiatric Disorders Prior to Upper Endoscopy," P. G. O'Malley, P. W. K. Wong, K. Kroenke et al., *Journal of Psychosomatic Research*, vol. 44, 1998, pp. 279–287.

Pages 241–242 The role of hiatal hernia (a.k.a. sliding hiatal hernia, hiatus hernia) and the treatment of gastroesophageal reflux disease (GERD) are discussed in any number of gastroenterological overviews. I was guided by the posting at www.postgradmed.com/issues/1999/06_99/szarka.htm. In addition, entering "hiatal hernia" as a search term in the Medline database of the National Library of Medicine (www.ncbi.nlm.nih.gov/PubMed), I gathered the following statements from the abstracts of recent journal articles: "Hiatus hernia is a common finding in healthy subjects, and it predisposes to gastroesophageal acid reflux." "Hiatus hernia is a not uncommon finding but often does not require treatment unless symptomatic." "Most hiatal hernias occurring in young adults are idiopathic."

According to "What Causes Gastroesophageal Reflux Disease," on www.WebMD.Lycos.com: "Although hiatal hernia may impair LES [lower esophageal sphincter] function, studies have failed to find a close causal association between gastroesophageal reflux and hiatal hernia. Some studies indicate that people with both GERD and hiatal hernia do have more severe gastroesophageal reflux."

On the correlation between GERD symptoms and the use of nonsteroidal anti-inflammatory drugs (NSAIDs, including aspirin and ibuprofen), see: "NSAID Consumption and Gastroesophageal Reflux Disease in a Medicaid Population," Jeffrey Kotzan et al., abstract of presentation to the American Association of Pharmaceutical Scientists, New Orleans, November 1999, and "Gerd Gymptoms, Medication Use and Endoscopic Findings in Elderly Patients with Peptic Strictures," J. P. Waring et al., presentation to the 62d Annual Meeting of the American College of Gastroenterology, October 31–November 5, 1997.

Chapter Six

Page 245 Source information on the two epigraphs: The full title of the first document is: *A Comparative Study of Warfare Gases, Their History—Description and Medical Aspects*, prepared by H. L. Gilchrist, colonel, Medical Corps, U.S. Army, and Chief, Medical Division, Chemical Warfare Service, Washington, D.C. The monograph was published by the army's Medical Field Service School, Carlisle Barracks, Pa., on September 19, 1925. Thanks to Jim Tuite for providing it. The paper by Kerr et al. was published in the *Annals of Internal Medicine*, vol. 11, 1937, pp. 961–992.

Page 249 In mallet toes, the joints cannot straighten and the toes curl under. The condition can be caused by athletic pounding or by being on one's feet too much, and it is aggravated by improper footware. Darren's problem began in bootcamp when he was issued boots that were too small, he said. In surgery he had two toes on the right foot straightened and pinned.

Page 250 The Rosenberg book is *Explaining Epidemics and Other Studies in the History of Medicine*, Charles E. Rosenbeg, Cambridge University Press, Cambridge, 1992.

Page 255 The Shorter book is *From Paralysis to Fatigue: A History of Psychosomatic Illness in the Modern Era*, Edward Shorter, Free Press, New York, 1992.

Pages 256–258 On the history of hysteria and neurasthenia, in addition to the Shorter work, loc. cit, see: For Briquet's study, "Briquet's Treatise on Hysteria: A Historical Perspective," François Mai and Harold Merskey, *Canadian Journal of Psychiatry*, vol. 26, 1981, pp. 57–63. According to a review by Harvard psychiatrist Bessel van der Kolk, Freud, when publishing his observations of eighteen hysterical patients in 1896, attributed the origins of the hysterical symptoms to childhood sexual trauma. Sources: "Dissociation, Somatization, and Affect Dysregulation: The Complexity of Adaptation to Trauma," B. A. van der Kolk et al., *American Journal of Psychiatry*, vol. 153, no. 7, Supplement, 1996, pp. 83–93, and "The Etiology of Hysteria," S. Freud, in *The Standard Edition of the Complete Psychological Works of Sigmund Freud*, vol. 3, ed. J. Strachy, Hogarth Press, London, 1896, pp. 189–221.

My references on neurasthenia include *American Nervousness: Its Causes and Consequences*, George M. Beard, G. P. Putnam's Sons, New York, 1881; "Old Wine in New Bottles: Neurasthenia and 'ME' [myalgic encephalomyelitis]," Simon Wessely, *Psychological Medicine*, vol. 20, 1990, pp. 35–53; "Neurasthenia in the 1980s: Chronic Fatigue Syndrome, and Anxiety and Depressive Disorders," Donna B. Greenberg, *Psychosomatics*, vol. 31, no. 2, 1990, pp. 129–137.

Page 260–261 Regarding William Baumzweiger: The TV documentary that brought him to the attention of Jackie and Darren was *Gulf War Disease: The Hidden Enemy*, produced by Tom Grant for KREM-TV, Spokane, Washington. It aired on December 1 and again on December 17, 1996.

Baumzweiger first explained his theory of the illnesses to a scientific panel of the Institute of Medicine in Irvine, Calif., in January 1996. The title of his presentation was "Brainstem Dysregulation Syndrome: A Neuropsychiatric Symptom Complex Caused by Multiple Sequential Insults to Immune-Attentional Brainstem Function as Seen in Case Studies of Gulf War Veterans and Environmentally Compromised Disability Applicants in Los Angeles, Calif." The IOM committee, on issuing its report, said about this theory: "The hypothesis suggests that two 'insults' to the brainstem, one early in life and one later (e.g., while in the Gulf region), could produce polysymptomatic illness. . . . No testable specification of this hypothesis has been presented and no study protocol has been reviewed by the committee." Source: *Health Consequences of Service During the Persian Gulf War: Recommendations for Research and Information Systems*, Institute of Medicine, National Academy Press, Washington, D.C., 1996, pp. 123–124.

Also that year Baumzweiger made a detailed submission to Congress. It was called "The Gulf War Disorders: A Family of Acquired Central Nervous System/Neuroimmune Disease Arising Subsequent to Exposure to Organophosphate Neurotoxin, in Conjuction with Other Environmental Risk Factors Present During the Persian Gulf War." See his prepared statement, Hearing of the Committee on Government Reform and Oversight, Subcommittee on Human Resources, U.S. House of Representatives, Washington, D.C., September 19, 1996.

The doctor's testimony before the Presidential Advisory Committee, in 1996, is available at www.gwvi.ncr.gov/0501gulf.html. His testimony before the Special Oversight Board for Department of Defense Investigations of Gulf War Chemical and Biological Incidents, in 1998, can be found at www.oversight.ncr.gov/thur.htm.

For press notices of Baumzweiger's work, see: "Congressman Accuses VA of Muzzling Its Critics," *Arizona Daily Star*, December 8, 1996; "Stricken Gulf Vets Feel Lost in Labyrinth of Bureaucracy," Norm Brewer and John Hanchette, Gannett News Service, March 11, 1997; "Illness from the Gulf: Seven Years Later, a Veteran and His Family Appear to be Infected with the Same Illness," Brewer and Hanchette, GNS, *Army Times*, May 4, 1998.

Page 261–262 The conditions known as POTS (acceleration of heart rate on standing) and neurocardiogenic syncope (fainting after a deceleration of heart rate and/or a drop in blood pressure) are poorly understood manifestations of a more general condition called dysautonomia. A good introduction to the subject can be found at the website of the National Dysautonomia Research Foundation, www.ndrf.org. See also: "Clinical and Laboratory Indices That Enhance the Diagnosis of Postural Tachycardia Syndrome," Vera Novak, Peter Novak et al., *Mayo Clinic Proceedings*, vol. 73, December, 1998, pp. 1141–1150; "Putting It Together: A New Treatment Algorithm for Vasovagal Syncope and Related Disorders," D. M. Bloomfield et al., *American Journal of Cardiology*, vol. 84, October 1999, pp. 33Q–39Q; "Postural Tachycardia Syndrome: Clinical Features and Follow-Up Study," P. Sandroni et al., *Mayo Clinic Proceedings*, vol. 74, November 1999, pp.1106–1110; "Neurocardiogenic Syncope," editorial, F. M. Abboud, *New England Journal of Medicine*, vol. 328, no. 15, 1993, pp. 1117–1119.

In 2000 researchers at Johns Hopkins University enrolled gulf war veterans in a study of POTS symptoms. See: www.med.jhu.edu/gws.

Page 268 Dr. Baumzweiger prescribed for Darren the following medications: sulfasalazine (the sulfa drug), 500 milligrams, three times daily; felodipine (calcium-channel blocker), 10 mg per day; Wellbutrin (antidepressant), 75 mg, three times daily; Ativan (sedative), 1.5 mg before bed; Motrin, 400 mg, three times daily; Tylenol #3 (with codeine), one before bed; Metamucil.

Pages 271–275 On the neurological effects of organophosphate insecticides: The pesticides used during the war and their possible role in the illnesses were topics addressed by the Presidential Advisory Committee on Gulf War Veterans' Illnesses. See the PAC's Final Report, 1996, loc. cit., pp. 96, 103–107. The report is available at: www.gwvi.ncr.gov.

For specifics on peripheral neuropathy, including the severe condition known as organophosphate-induced delayed neuropathy, see: "Human Toxic Neuropathy Due To Industrial Agents," H. Schaumburg and A. Berger, in *Peripheral Neuropathy*, P. J. Dyck et al., eds., 3d edition, W. B. Saunders Co., Philadelphia, 1993, pp. 1533–1547.

Dr. Robert Haley's probes of subtle nerve damage in gulf war vets are described in chapter 3. See also the notes on pp. 392 and 398. The measurements of eyeball reflexes were among the tests reported in "Vestibular Dysfunction in Gulf War Syndrome," Peter S. Roland, Robert W. Haley et al., *Otolayrngology—Head and Neck Surgery*, 2000, loc. cit. For a congruent assessment of neurotoxic injury, see: "The 'Gulf War Syndrome': Is There Evidence of Neurological Dysfunction in the Nervous System?," G. Jamal, *Journal of Neurology, Neurosurgery, and Psychiatry*, vol. 60, 1996, pp. 441–449. For a contrary view: "Evaluation of Neuromuscular Symptoms in Veterans of the Persian Gulf War," A. A. Amato et al., *Neurology*, vol. 48, 1997, pp. 4–12.

Regarding the precedents, the congressional witness whom I quoted on organophosphate health effects was Stephanie Padilla, an EPA neurotoxicologist. See her prepared statement to the Subcommittee on Human Resources and Intergovernmental Relations, Committee on Government Reform and Oversight, U.S. House of Representatives, Washington, D.C., September 19, 1996. Padilla provided an extensive bibliography, including results of toxicological experiments on animals.

Regarding the precedents, the most frequently cited studies of neuropsychological defects in agricultural workers were: "Chronic Neurological Sequelae of Acute Organophosphate Pesticide Poisoning," Eldon P. Savage et al., *Archives of Environmental Health*, vol. 43, no. 1, 1988, pp. 38–45; "Chronic Central Nervous System Effects of Acute Organophosphate Pesticide Intoxication," Linda Rosenstock et al., *Lancet*, vol. 338, 1991, pp. 223–227; "Chronic Neurological Effects of Organophosphaste Pesticides," Kyle Steenland et al., *American Journal of Public Health*, vol. 84, no. 5, 1994, pp. 731–736; "Abnormalities on Neurological Examination among Sheep Farmers

Exposed to Organophosphorus Pesticides," J. R. Beach et al., *Occupational and Environmental Medicine*, vol. 53, 1996, pp. 520–525. Also a textbook was often cited: *Pesticides and Neurological Diseases*, Donald J. Ecobichon and Robert M. Joy, second edition, CRC Press, Boca Raton, Fla., 1994.

As I indicated, conflicting reports were issued on the neuropsychological function of gulf war veterans. For the point of view that brain damage may have resulted from neurotoxic exposures, see: "Neuropsychological Correlates of Gulf War Syndrome," Jim Hom, Robert W. Haley and Thomas L. Kurt, *Archives of Clinical Neuropsychology*, vol. 12, no. 6, 1997, pp. 531–544. For the view that other factors, such as emotional distress, could explain the differences in test results, see: "Neuropsychological Deficits in Persian Gulf War Veterans: A Preliminary Report," S. Kotler-Cope et al., presentation to the International Neuropsychogical Society, Chicago, 1996, and "Gulf War Veterans: A Neuropsychological Examination," Monica C. Sillanpaa et al., *Journal of Clinical and Experimental Neuropsychology*, vol. 19, no. 2, 1997, pp. 211–219. For middle-of-the-road results and opinions, see: "Neuropsychological Findings in a Sample of Operation Desert Storm Veterans," Bradley N. Axelrod and I. Boaz Miller, *Journal of Neuropsychiatry*, vol. 9, no. 1, 1997, pp. 23–28; "Health Status of Persian Gulf War Veterans: Self-Reported Symptoms, Environmental Exposures and the Effect of Stress," S. Proctor, T. Heeren, R. F. White et al., *International Journal of Epidemiology*, vol. 27, no. 6, 1998, pp. 1000–1010; "Neurobehavioral Deficits in Persian Gulf Veterans: Evidence from a Population-Based Study," W. Kent Anger et al., *Journal of the International Neuropsyhological Society*, vol. 5, 1999, pp. 203–212.

Page 279 The seminal overview of wartime maladies is "War Syndromes and Their Evaluation," Kenneth C. Hyams, F. Stephen Wignall and Robert Roswell, *Annals of Internal Medicine*, vol. 125, no. 5, 1996, pp. 398–405.

Page 280 The original monograph about irritable heart is "On Irritable Heart: A Clinical Study of a Form of Functional Cardiac Disorder and its Consequences," J. M. Da Costa, *American Journal of Medical Sciences*, vol. 61, January 1871, pp. 17–52. For recent references to the condition during the Civil War, in addition to Hyams, op. cit., see: "Union Vets Lead Nation into Next Century," David M. Gosoroski, *VFW Magazine*, Kansas City, Mo., May 1997; *No More Heroes: Madness & Psychiatry in War*, Richard A. Gabriel, Hill and Wang, New York, 1987; and "Psychological and Psychosocial Consequences of Combat and Deployment with Special Emphasis on the Gulf War," David H. Marlowe, Prepared for the Office of the Secretary of Defense by RAND's National Defense Research Institute, Washington, D.C., 2000.

Marlowe gives the following account of the irritable heart: "The soldiers who presented themselves with this 'cardiac' disorder were capable of almost no sustained physical effort. Their heart rates were quite high, palpitations were common, and heart rate increased rapidly upon exertion. Overall weakness and fatigue were also characteristic. Few of the diagnostic techniques of the period could detect any known organic heart ailment that might account for these symptoms, and was extraordinarily puzzling to the military surgeons of the time."

In 1915, after irritable heart had cropped up in the next generation of soldiers, Thomas Lewis and two colleagues observed of their (British) patients: "They are men in whom the following prominent symptoms have arisen either gradually or suddenly, in some during the period of training, in other while serving actively in the trenches: Aching or sharp pain over the region of the heart, sometimes radiating but rarely severe, and breathlessness and palpitation on the slightest exertion, are the rule. So also is a sense of fatigue or exhaustion with effort: and sometimes giddiness, occasionally proceeding to actual fainting, may be present. . . . The pulse-rate is increased, often notably, and is peculiarly susceptible to posture and exercise. The blood pressure may show a noticeable fall as the patient passes from the lying to the upright posture. In many subjects there are other evidences of vasomotor instability. . . ." Source: "A Note on the 'Irritable Heart' of Soldiers," Thomas Cotton, Thomas Lewis, and F. H. Thiele, *British Medical Journal*, vol. 1, 1915, p. 722. Compare this description of the ailment to that of the modern autonomic disorder POTS on pp. 403–404.

Lewis's subsequent treatise was titled "The Soldier's Heart and the Effort Syndrome." The first edition was completed just before the end of World War I, and the second edition, from which I have quoted, appeared in 1940 (Shaw & Sons, London). The analyses by Paul Wood undercutting the organic basis of irritable heart were published sequentially in the *British Medical Journal*, vol. 1, 1941: "Da Costa's syndrome (or effort syndrome)," pp. 767–772; "Da Costa's Syndrome (or Effort Syndrome): The Mechanism of the Somatic Manifestations," pp. 805–811; and "Aetiology of Da Costa's Syndrome," pp. 845–851. The 1947 reference to irritable heart is from *The Principles and Practice of Medicine*, 16th edition, ed. Henry A. Christian, D. Appleton-Century Co., New York, 1947, pp. 994–995. The first edition of this text was written by the famous diagnostician William Osler.

Page 280 For understanding of shell shock I have relied on Hyams et al. and Marlowe, op. cit., and on two earlier texts: *Shell-Shock and other Neuropsychiatric Problems, Presented in Five Hundred and Eighty-Nine Cases Histories from the War Literature, 1914-1918*, E. E. Southard, W. M. Leonard, Publisher, Boston, 1918, and "Military Psychiatry: World War I," Edward A. Stecker, in "One Hundred Years of American Psychiatry," American Psychiatric Association, Columbia University Press, New York, 1944. On the broad application of the shell-shock label, the following comment is made by Southard, op. cit., p. 832: "The term Shell-shock appears to be a perfect term for the ordinary man, as it means much and little, connotes enormously and denotes a minimum and casts the lay hearer back upon the expert."

Page 281 The passage about "gas neurosis" and veterans' disability claims is based upon Lewis, 1940, and Marlowe, op. cit., and on *A Comparative Study of Warfare Gases*, H. L. Gilchrist, op. cit.

Page 283 The World War II text I quoted is "Men under Stress," Roy R. Grinker and John P. Spiegel, Blakiston, Philadelphia, 1945. In introducing the reprint edition (McGraw-Hill, 1963), the authors apologize for the rigorously Freudian interpretations of the original volume.

As for the Vietnam War, quite apart from its traumatic wounds, physical and mental, Vietnam service produced long-term health complaints. See "Health Status of Vietnam Veterans: II. Physical Health," Centers for Disease Control, *Journal of the American Medical Association*, vol. 259, 1988, pp. 2708–2714.

Page 285 For the evolving interpretations of hyperventilation, including the connection to irritable heart, see: "Some Physical Phenomena Associated with the Anxiety States and their Relation to Hyperventilation," Kerr et al., *Annals of Internal Medicine*, 1936, op. cit., "Hyperventilation and Hysteria, The Physiology and Psychology of Overbreathing and Its Relationship to the Mind-body Problem," ed., Thomas P. Lowry, Charles C. Thomas, Publisher, Springfield, Ill., 1967; and "The Grey Area of Effort Syndrome and Hyperventilation: From Thomas Lewis to Today," Peter G. F. Nixon, *Journal of the Royal College of Physicians of London*, vol. 27, no. 4, 1993, pp. 377–383. Recent overviews of hyperventilation are posted at www.emedicine.com/EMERG/topic270.htm and www.chestnet.org/education/pccu/vol13/lesson09.html.

For a valuable article on panic disorder, which can trigger hyperventilation, see: "Panic Disorder: Relationship to High Medical Utilization, Unexplained Physical Symptoms, and Medical Costs," Wayne Katon, *Journal of Clinical Psychiatry*, vol. 57 (supplement 10), 1996, pp. 11–18. For POTS and neurocardiogenic syncope, see the note on pp. 403–404.

Page 287 Dr. Short's source on toxic optic atrophy was "Chronic Intoxication of Organophosphorus Pesticide and Its Treatment," S. Ishikawa et al., *Folia Medica Cracoviensia*, vol. 34 (1–4), 1993, pp. 139–151.

Page 288 Hypochondriasis is officially defined in *Diagnostic and Statistical Manual of Mental Disorders, 4th edition: Primary Care Version (DSM-IV-PC)*, American Psychiatric Association, Washington, D.C., 1995. See also these references to the condition: "Somatization in Primary Care," C. C. Engel, Jr., and W. J. Katon, in *Primary Care & General Medicine*, J. Noble et al., eds., Mosby, St. Louis, 1996, pp. 1747–1756; "Unexplained Physical Symptoms and Somatoform Disorders," K. Kroenke, in: *Twenty Common Behavioral Problems in Primary Care*, ed. F. V. deGruy, McGraw-Hill, New York (in press, 2001); "Overview: Hypochondriasis, Bodily Complaints, and Somatic Styles," A. J. Barsky and G. L. Klerman, *American Journal of Psychiatry*, vol. 140, no. 3, 1983, pp. 273–83.

Page 290 Regarding the lack of follow-up on sick veterans, in June 1997, the General Accounting Office charged that "although efforts have been made to diagnose veterans' problems and care has been provided to many eligible veterans, neither DoD nor VA has systematically attempted to determine whether ill Gulf War veterans are any better or worse today than when they were first examined." Source: "Gulf War Illnesses: Improved Monitoring of Clinical Progress and Reexamination of Research Emphasis Are Needed," U.S. General Accounting Office, GAO/NSIAD-97-163, Washington, D.C., June 1997, p. 2.

In a report issued a year later, the Senate Veterans' Affairs Committee stated: "Perhaps even more critical is the VA's chronic and pervasive inability to generate valid and reliable data about the Gulf War veterans it serves. Repeatedly, this investigation found that the statistics generated by VA databases were inaccurate and inconsistent, and that too many times the VA simply could not answer questions about Gulf War veterans such as how many have undiagnosed illnesses, how many of those veterans also are receiving compensation benefits for that condition, how many are receiving health care, and whether those who have received care at VA facilities in the past are getting better or worse." Source: "Report of the Special Investigation Unit on Gulf War Illnesses," Committee on Veterans' Affairs, U.S. Senate, S. Prt 1-5-39, U.S. Government Printing Office, Washington, D.C., August 1998, p. 7.

Page 297 The quotation by B. A. van der Kolk on the extension of PTSD diagnoses from military to nonmilitary populations is from "Dissociation, Somatization, and Affect Dysregulation: The Complexity of Adaptation to Trauma," loc. cit. (Van der Kolk has since moved from Harvard to Boston University Medical School.) See also the citation by B. Green on p. 367.

On the association between PTSD diagnoses and increased health complaints in gulf war veterans, see: "Relationship between Posttraumatic Stress Disorder and Self-Reported Physical Symptoms in Persian Gulf War Veterans," Dewleen G. Baker et al., *Archives of Internal Medicine*, vol. 157, 1997, pp. 2076–2078; "Health Symptoms Reported by Persian Gulf War Veterans Two Years after Return," Jessica Wolfe et al., *American Journal of Industrial Medicine*," vol. 33, 1998, pp. 104–113; "Health Status of Persian Gulf War Veterans: Self-Reported Symptoms, Environmental Exposures and the Effect of Etress," S. Proctor et al., loc. cit.; "Can PTSD Cause Physical Symptoms? A Hypothesis Screen Using Registry Data," C. C. Engel et al., *Psychosomatic Medicine* (in press).

Patricia Sutker of the New Orleans VAMC and other mental health specialists found that graves registration duty, which involved picking up, analyzing, and storing bodily remains, was especially associated with high levels of psychiatric and physical distress. Sources: "Psychological

Symptoms and Psychiatric Diagnoses in Operation Desert Storm Troops Serving Graves Resgis-tration Duty," P. Sutker et al., *Journal of Traumatic Stress*, vol. 7, no. 2, 1994, pp. 159-171; "Symptoms of PTSD Following Recovery of War Dead: 13-15-Month Follow-Up," J. E. McCar-roll et al., *American Journal of Psychiatry*, vol. 152, no. 6, 1995, pp. 939-941; "Psychiatric Syn-dromes in Persian Gulf War Veterans: An Association of Handling Dead Bodies with Somatoform Disorders," L. A. Labbate et al., *Psychotherapy and Psychosomatics*, vol. 67, nos. 4-5,1998, pp. 275-279.

As stated on p. 368, Robert Haley challenged the PTSD surveys that were conducted by Pen-tagon and VA researchers. See: "Is Gulf War Syndrome Due to Stress? The Evidence Reexam-ined," *American Journal of Epidemiology*, 1997, loc. cit. As his title suggests, Haley conflated stress and PTSD, rejecting them both as sources of the gulf war illnesses.

Pages 298-299 On the correlation of childhood abuse and physical symptoms in adults, see the citations I offered on pp. 396-397. Here are additional commentaries:

Kroenke (2001, op. cit.) writes: "Abuse (sexual or physical), particularly during childhood, has increasingly been shown to have a strong relationship with somatization as an adult. This not only includes complaints like chronic abdominal. Moreover, there is a dose-response relationship between symptom counts and likelihood of abuse."

Barsky, in his 1994 paper, "Histories of Childhood Trauma in Adult Hypochondriacal Patients," loc. cit., concludes: "Hypochondriacal adults recall more childhood trauma than do nonhypochondriacal patients, even after sociodemographic differences are controlled for."

Kendall-Tackett, in her 2000 paper "Correlates of Childhood Abuse: Chronic Hyperarousal in PTSD, Depression, and Irritable Bowel Syndrome," loc. cit., observes that the severity of abuse is the main predictor of the severity of the physical symptoms. "From a biological perspective," she adds, " it appears to make little difference whether the abuse is physical or sexual."

Chapter Seven

Page 306 Thanks of a Grateful Nation was written by John Sacret Young. The executive pro-ducers of the movie were Young, Andy Adelson, and Tracey Alexander. The movie was broadcast on Showtime (pay cable TV) in 1998 and on NBC TV in 1999. The screenplay was provided to me with the permission of Tracey Alexander.

Page 307 Tuite's 1995 essay "When Science and Politics Collide" is available at www.chronicillnet.org/PGWS/tuite/collide.html.

Page 310 The army's experiments with OP nerve agents were summarized in three volumes published by the National Academy of Sciences, National Academy Press, Washington, D.C., under the main title *Possible Long-Term Health Effects of Short-Term Exposure to Chemical Agents*. The volumes are: *Anticholinesterases and Anticholinergics (Volume I)*, 1982; *Cholinesterase Reactiva-tors, Psychochemicals, and Irritants and Vesicants (Volume 2)*, 1984; *Final Report: Current Health Status of Test Subjects (Volume 3)*, 1985. Later in 1997 the VA and DoD asked the academy's Insti-tute of Medicine to undertake a follow-up study of the health status of the army test subjects. Results are pending. This was one of nineteen federal research projects—either in the works or completed—having to do with low-dose chemical weapons exposure.

A second OP precedent, also discussed at the Cincinnati conference, was the medical experi-ence of Japanese survivors of a terrorist gassing in the Tokyo subway in 1995. Twelve people were killed outright by sarin, and hundreds of others hospitalized. Both symptoms of PTSD and problems with balance, a neurological effect, were reported by some of the victims several years later. However, those people had been severely injured in the incident, so that their chronic effects could be connected to the acute effect of a specific exposure, unlike the cases of the gulf war vets. See: "A Preliminary Study on Delayed Vestibulo-Cerebellar Effects of Tokyo Subway Sarin Poisoning in Relation to Gender Difference: Frequency Analysis of Postural Sway," K. Yokoyama et al., *Journal of Occupational and Environmental Medicine*, vol. 40, no. 1, 1998, pp. 17–21, and "Chronic Neurobehavioral Effects of Tokyo Sarin Subway Poisoning in Relation to Posttraumatic Stress Disorder," K. Yokoyama et al., *Archives of Environmental Health*, vol. 53, no. 4, 1998, pp. 249–256.

Page 311 Tuite's first report for Riegle was "Gulf War Syndrome: The Case for Multiple Origin Mixed Chemical/Biotoxin Warfare Related Disorders," staff report to U.S. Senator Donald W. Riegle Jr., U.S. Senate, Washington, D.C., September 9, 1993.

Page 312 Regarding Abou-Donia's work and the possibility of adverse interactions among PB and other chemicals, see p. 385.

Page 313 For more information on Howard Urnovitz's biomedical work, consult his two Web-sites, www.calypte.com and www.chronicillnet.org. Calypte Biomedical is the name of his research company. ChronicIllnet, the site of his Chronic Illness Research Foundation, explores commonalities among AIDS, CFS, gulf war syndrome, and other illnesses. Recently Calypte and a corporate partner launched a subsidiary venture, Chronix Biomedical, whose focus, according to a Calypte announcement, was "novel ways to detect aberrant genes in individuals with chronic diseases."

Page 314 The reference to the Gulf War Research Foundation as a "group" is from "New Report Cited on Chemical Arms Used in Gulf War," Philip Shenon, *New York Times*, August 22, 1996, p. 1.

Page 315 Those wanting more of the point-counterpoint between Tuite and the CIA on the alleged exposures to nerve gas resulting from the January 1991 bombing of Iraq should obtain two documents: "Report on the Fallout from the Destruction of Iraqi Chemical Warfare Agent Research, Production, and Storage Facilities into Areas Occupied by U.S. Military Personnel during the 1991 Persian Gulf War," James J. Tuite III, submitted to Committee on Government Reform and Oversight, U.S. House of Representatives, Washington, D.C., September 19, 1996, and "Analysis of Weather Satellite Imagery of Fires and Fogs, and an Assessment of the Tuite Report Analysis for January 19, 1991," J. E. Cockayne, Science Applications International Corporation, undated report. SAIC was a contractor to CIA on matters of meteorology and exposure assessment.

There were other means by which chemical warfare agents were said to be present on the battle-field. For a summary of the most plausible incidents (excluding Khamisiyah), see the document prepared by the Pentagon in 1996, "Coalition Chemical Detections and Health of Coalition Troops in Detection Area," which is available at: www.gulflink.osd.mil/czech_french/czfr_refs/n08en011/coalitn.html. Much more detail on these and other incidents can be found elsewhere on the GulfLINK website. For an analysis that disputes the Pentagon accounts, see: *Gassed in the Gulf: The Inside Story of the Pentagon-CIA Cover-up of Gulf War Syndrome*, Patrick G. Eddington, Insignia Publishing Co., Washington, D.C., 1997.

Page 316 Tuite's comments about fallout to the Presidential Advisory Committee, which were delivered on April 16, 1996, can be accessed at www.gwvi.ncr.gov/0416gulf.html.

Page 322 *The Structure of Scientific Revolutions*, Thomas S. Kuhn, University of Chicago Press, Chicago, 1962, 1970, 1996.

Page 325 The Kizer letter, dated November 27, was published on the editorial page of the *New York Times* on December 4, 1996, under the headline "Gulf War Illness Findings Aren't Unexpected."

Page 327 As for the seven front-page stories of the *New York Times* in late 1996 in which Tuite was mentioned, all were written by Philip Shenon: "New Report Cited on Chemical Arms Used in Gulf War," August 22; "Report Shows U.S. Was Told in 1991 of Chemical Arms," August 28; "1991 Blast in Iraq May Have Exposed 5,000 G.I.'s to Gas," September 19; "U.S. Jets Pounded Iraqi Arms Depot Storing Nerve Gas," October 3; "Range is Expanded in Federal Search for Victims of Gas," October 23; "Ex-C.I.A. Analysts Assert Cover-up," October 30; "Pentagon Says Gulf War Data Seem to Be Lost," December 5.

Page 330 In September 2000 the Institute of Medicine produced a report on the agents of greatest concern to the veterans—sarin, pyridostigmine bromide, depleted uranium, and the vaccines to prevent anthrax and botulism. After reviewing the available medical literature the committee was unable to find evidence that would link exposures to these four agents to the chronic health problems of gulf war veterans. As of this writing the VA had not decided how it would act on the IOM findings—i.e., whether or not to pay compensation. See: *Gulf War and Health*, vol. 1, *Deplected Uranium, Sarin, Pyridostigmine Bromide, Vaccines*, Institute of Medicine, National Academy Press, Washington, D.C., 2000.

Chapter Eight

Pages 331–332 On the benefits (and losses) to health from war, see, from the World War II, Korea and Vietnam experiences: "Self-Concept Changes Related to War Captivity," W. H. Sledge et al., *Archives of General Psychiatry*, vol. 37, 1980, pp. 430–443; "Combat Experience and Emotional Health: Impairment and Resilience in Later Life," G. H. Elder and E. C. Clipp, *Journal of Personality*, vol. 57, 1989, pp. 311–341; "Vulnerability and Resilience to Combat Exposure: Can Stress Have Lifelong Effects?," Carolyn M. Aldwin et al., *Psychology and Aging*, vol. 9, no. 1, 1994, pp. 34–44; "Psychological Benefits and Liabilities of Traumatic Exposure in the War Zone," Alan Fontana and Robert Rosenheck, *Journal of Traumatic Stress*, vol. 11, No. 3, 1998, pp. 485–503. In the anecdotal mode, a recent best-seller dealt with the worth and gains of World War II veterans: *The Greatest Generation*, Tom Brokaw, Random House, New York, 1998.

As for the gulf war experience, Sutker's comment is from her pioneering study: "War-Zone Trauma and Stress-Related Symptoms in Operation Desert Shield/Storm (ODS) Returnees," Patricia B. Sutker et al., *Journal of Social Issues*, vol. 49, No. 4, 1993, pp. 33–49. The Pentagon-funded project in this area is titled "Measurement and Validation of Psychosocial Risk and Resilience Factors Accounting for Physical and Mental Health and Health-Related Quality of Life among Persian Gulf Veterans." The study, whose principal investigator is Daniel King of the Boston VAMC, is ongoing.

For the work of Richard Tedeschi, see: "Posttraumatic Growth: Positive Changes in the Aftermath of Crisis," ed. Richard Tedeschi, Crystal L. Park and Lawrence G. Calhoun, the Lea Series in Personality and Clinical Psychology, Lawrence Erlbaum Associates, March, 1998. Also: "The Posttraumatic Growth Inventory: Measuring the Positive Legacy of Trauma," R. Tedeschi and L. Calhoun, *Journal of Traumatic Stress*, vol. 9, 1996, pp. 455–471.

Page 350 The *C&EN* article was "Surviving Stress," Lois R. Ember, *Chemical & Engineering News*, May 25, 1998. Two other interesting reports on the physiology of stress that applied to gulf war vets were: "Acute Stress Facilitates Long-Lasting Changes in Cholinergic Gene Expression," Daniela Kaufer et al., letter, *Nature*, vol. 393, May 28, 1998, pp. 373–377, and the accompanying commentary, "The Stress of Gulf War Syndrome," Robert M. Sapolsky, ibid., pp. 308–309.

Page 356 The follow-up results of the Walter Reed SCP program are reported in "Rehabilitative Care of War-Related Health Concerns," Charles C. Engel et al., *Journal of Occupational and Environmental Medicine*, vol. 42, no. 4, 2000, pp. 385–390.

Index